Healthy Matters

Healthy Matters

Applying the Redox Lifestyle

RM

Dr. Lee Ostler

www.RedoxMatters.com

Copyright © 2022 Dr. G. Lee Ostler

All Rights Reserved. No part of this publication may be reproduced, distributed, or transmitted in any form or by any means, including photocopying, recording, or other electronic or mechanical methods, without the prior written permission of the publisher, or Dr. G. Lee Ostler, except in the case of brief quotations embodied in critical reviews, research articles, and certain other noncommercial uses permitted by copyright law, and with appropriate citation.

This is a profoundly important book for anyone interested in the science of cellular health and how cells communicate. It also provides a scientific basis for why many of our medications and supplements are not foundational enough to make as big of a difference in our health as we had originally anticipated.

Our bodies, our organs, and each and every one of our 70 trillion cells, is part of a cellular information superhighway. Cell to cell and intracellular communication is based on the constant flow of information, largely governed by the energy field of REDOX science. Over the past 10-20 years, we have realized that cellular health requires a complex surveillance system compromised of signaling molecules, which allows each cell to identify stressors and act in the defense of the cell and its micro-environment. This level of communication happens thousands of times each second and in each cell of our body. This regulatory surveillance system is at the core of how we age.

In the United States, more than 85% of adults suffer from metabolic syndrome (this includes hypertension, diabetes mellitus, atherosclerosis, and coronary artery disease), which makes Americans undoubtedly the least healthy people in the world. Dr. Ostler, in Healthy Matters, details how the effects of diet and lifestyle play a key role in this epidemic, but also gives the molecular basis for how healthy cells living in balance repair themselves on a second-to-second basis. Medications typically deal only with our symptoms, while inside each cell, our mitochondria and what Dr. Ostler calls the Redoxome, govern cell-to-cell communication and cellular repair. This is why REDOX medicine is synonymous with Cellular Medicine, and in my opinion, represents a core aspect of the future of medicine.

Our bodies cannot deal with the source of our cellular stressors, caused by continuous exposure to inflammatory foods, chemicals and toxins, stress, lack of sleep, and lack of exercise… Our cellular repair systems get overwhelmed and alarms go off (symptoms of distress). We get so accustomed to our symptoms that we fail to recognize they always reflect a weakness in our cellular repair capabilities.

If you want a deep-dive into the future of medicine where foundations of cellular health are emphasized, this is a great read that will empower you and guide you on your personal journey to achieve optimal health. We are moving into Longevity Medicine or Healthspan Medicine. Get on Dr. Ostler's train!

> *- Ahvie Herskowitz, MD, Clinical Professor of Medicine, UC San Francisco (2014), President, American College for Advancement in Medicine (ACAM)*

Dr. Lee Ostler's second book "Healthy Matters" so profoundly echoes again his heartfelt care and compassion for humanity. Well written and "easy to apply", this essay obviously springs from the same vein that inspired and generated his much acclaimed first book "Redox Matters," as it cleverly harmonizes and translates the fundamentals into actions and processes, providing the necessary situational awareness and the relevant guidance anyone may need to effectively identify and resolve a particular issue or situation.

In his first book, Dr. Ostler ensured to pleasantly navigate readers from all walks of life throughout the amazingly complex, yet enchanting open world of Redox Phenomenology. With great care, he left no stone unturned throughout a lengthy, thorough, and brilliantly precise demonstration enabling everyone to capture the real nature of what we are about... an intricacy of foundational multi-dimensional mosaics of various complex functionalities remarkably arranged to underlie and very effectively enable our natural resilience and health Balancing Acts, as well as the unbounded ever-changing connectivity and intricacies of our countless potentials for vulnerability to internal and external stressors and assaults.

In his second book, Dr. Ostler equally provides a thorough exploratory review of many extensive navigational references to enable everyone to identify, understand, and emphasize the need to "get easily into very significant long-term action" towards enhancing one's quality of Life with integrating the Redox Phenomenon into daily Lifestyle.

I wholeheartedly salute with a profound gratitude Dr. Ostler's educational contribution as I see it as a very timely distinctive literary achievement. He gallantly brings into global societal awareness about a considerable paradigm shift in Life Sciences that is part of the mounting global emergence of a novel understanding of the "mystery" of Life as per cellular performance, resilience, and survival mechanisms.

- Philippe A. Souvestre, MD, PhD, CES, FAsMA

Dr Lee Ostler, 'strikes again'! Not only has he clearly explained in, 'Redox Matters' the very foundations to all health, and how to regain what has been lost, with the first time ever human supplement of Redox signaling molecules. He now clearly places it in full context. "Healthy Matters: Applying the Redox Lifestyle" leaves no stone unturned to this end. Read this and you will be perfectly clear on exactly what you need to do to retain your optimum health or resurrect what you have long lost! This is clearly the journey of a doctor who has pursued what it takes to totally optimize one's health potential. I know because I have traversed the same journey. It matters not what provided the motivation, ill-health or simply 'What Matters' in the pursuance of the Holy Grail of optimum health, Dr Lee has eloquently extrapolated and explained here the quest of my life. What an extraordinary accomplishment and to follow so shortly after his monumental work on 'Redox Matters'! I said there, 'strap yourself in' for the ride of your life, now again I say strap yourself in for the story in full context, as there is more to add. Congratulations Dr Lee on such an amazing feat! Dr Ray

- Dr Ray Dixon DC, Naturopath

My friend, Dr. Lee Ostler, is a man of integrity. It is an honor to endorse his new book, "Healthy Matters: Applying the Redox Lifestyle." My 50-year Veterinary career in biomedical research, at the largest national and international laboratories, was dedicated to finding answers to important health questions for humans and non-human animals. Today, I am shocked to see science being turned upside down by deceptive leaders. I am 100% sure that Dr. Lee has researched and poured his exceptional knowledge into this book. We can be assured Dr. Lee put all of his effort into communicating the truth to his readers. Post exposure, please send him a note about your new vision of wellness. God bless.

- Martin Morin, DVM

Many of us have known for at least the past ten years or so that the breakthrough discovery that has resulted in the world's first and (so far) only redox based cell signaling supplement, is a transformational game-changer of the highest order and the deepest significance. Dr. Lee Ostler's second book (in a series) Healthy Matters: Applying the Redox Lifestyle represents another such game-changing moment in the evolution of our collective understanding of Redox Biology and precisely HOW the practical everyday application of this knowledge will help to establish this Redox Lifestyle into the mainstream. This Redox Lifestyle is destined to become the sturdiest foundation upon which to build the cellular wellness paradigm. This is a 'must read now' book!

- Russell Mariani, Health Educator, Digestive Wellness Expert, Author; Principle Eating: The No Diet Way to Complete Health

Once again Dr. Ostler has hit it out of the park! For those of us whose eyes start to glaze over when trying to follow biochemical molecular pathways, a book that gets right to the bottom line - the "what should I do" - of a Redox Lifestyle is wonderful indeed. As an integrative dentist and lifestyle practitioner, I am well aware of the huge impact an evidence based healthy lifestyle can have on both the prevention and reversal of oral and systemic diseases. But understanding the Redoxome and its role at the very foundation of health makes it possible to optimize the benefits of healthy living in a way never before possible. I highly recommend this groundbreaking book to everyone serious about maximizing health and longevity.

- Lon Peckham DMD, FAAOSH, Dip ACLM

Beyond excited for the rest of the book. Speaking to all the things that we influence; all the components involved in health, beyond the magic bullet mentality. As a naturopath, you are speaking my language. We look at how water, oxygen, rest, exercise, sleep, sunlight, and nutrition are the keys to health. Those are our tools of choice. Lifestyle!

- Carolyn Hoffman, ND, CNHP, LDHS

Dr. Ostler's groundbreaking book, Redox Matters, took an esoteric subject and made it relevant for everyone. In his new book, Healthy Matters, Dr. Ostler transforms the science of redox from analytical to practical. Knowledge is power, but the application of knowledge is transformational.

- Maureen Hayes, MD

Most people who have studied and practiced a healthy lifestyle know that life begins and ends at the cellular level. The foundation of optimal health is efficient cellular communication. Our cells must receive clear signals to repair damaged cells or kill cells off to be replaced if the damage is beyond repair. Clear cellular communication, good nutrition, sleep, exercise, and a healthy mindset all contribute to our optimal overall state of health and wellness. The foundation of efficient cellular communication is a proper supply of redox signaling molecules. Supplementing with redox molecules enables us to live a redox lifestyle of health, wellness, calmness, and happiness. In his new book, "Healthy Matters: Applying the Redox Lifestyle", Dr. Lee Ostler provides us the parameters to live the Redox Lifestyle with all its benefits. To get the most out of your lifetime here now, enjoy this read and put it into practice!

- Debbie Wetzler

Dr. Lee Ostler has done it again! In his latest book, Healthy Matters, Dr. Ostler takes the complex world of cellular technology out of the classroom and into the real world, opening our eyes to how a cell "thinks and acts." He boils down the science of redox signaling molecules into practical application and invites us to live our best life with what he calls the "Redox Lifestyle." As a nurse with 40 years of experience, I'm always looking for ways to help my patients make wise daily choices to boost their wellness and vitality. This exceptional book provides the tools to do just that!

- *Doria Stewart RN*

In his first book, "Redox Matters", Dr; Ostler skillfully lays out the recently discovered secret operating, energetic, communication, and adaptation systems for the cellular basis for nearly all life on this planet. It was amazing! Now with his new book "Healthy Matters" he gives us the owner's manual for living, and maximizing, a rich, fully loaded life in all its wondrous Redox Glory. This book shows us how to go beyond understanding the microscopic redox universe and teaches us to build a life that nurtures our "Redox Life Potential" on purpose. Be ready to change your health, fitness, nutrition, sleep, energy, life force, and effectiveness, with hope and power. You will be confidently different when your read this book.

- *Jerry White, PT*

Thank you for your time and expertise in writing this new book Healthy Matters. Redox Matters was a phenomenal book, and when people see what you have done to translate the foundational Redox biology science and how it fits into a lifestyle, they will be astonished. I have been involved in Redox supplementation for over five years. It has truly changed my life in a way I could not comprehend at first. Once I started using Redox with some high quality nutrition, it took it to another level. Your new book confirms what I have seen in my personal journey and with many others around the world. If people truly want to be healthy this book will help them understand how. It will be a guide for them for as they improve their lifestyle. The daily decisions and disciplines people make on what they eat and drink, their exercise and so much more is discussed in this book and will lead them to a healthier enjoyable lifestyle. Not everyone needs to know the deep science, but they need to understand the benefits and health longevity the science brings their way.

- *Leland Duyck- Orthopedic Surgical PA*

It is my honor to review this massive 'health game changer' from Dr. Lee Ostler, the sequel to Redox Matters – "HEALTHY MATTERS." Dr. Ostler and I have become good friends as we are helping people all over the world with the Friday global broadcasts of "The 5". When Dr Lee announced this new book, my response was OH MY GOLLY! Now to be able to review his latest book, what I will call a TOTAL HEALTHY MASTERPIECE, is my tremendous pleasure.

Healthy Matters changes the game of dealing with the confusion of different opinions of what to do for our health. Experiencing the changes in my body by having redox in my life for seven years, has been amazing. The medicines I have taken for 25 years for many lower back procedures, stopped when redox started. I am back to living a very active lifestyle. BUT my nutrition has never been the best. Now I have more peace in my life knowing that HEALTHY MATTERS is here, and I know Dr. Lee will simplify what most people struggle with - understanding nutrition - and best of all, grounding it on what he describes are "the rules of the cell." Dr. Ostler is a master at simplifying the complex. Just look at REDOX MATTERS - and now... learn the power of HEALTHY MATTERS from our teacher, Dr Lee Ostler.

- Jim Glenn

Dr. Ostler did an amazing job with his first book, Redox Matters, by making the science understandable. Now, this second book is so exciting! He has brought all the science into the practical application of everyday life. He teaches what I have taught for years, as a midwife, to my pregnant clients, with everything connected to redox. He links diet, exercise, and so much more, to the importance of redox signaling molecules and how they help our bodies function properly. I am thrilled to have this new resource that will help everyone understand what redox is and why we should live a redox lifestyle in order to be healthy, happy, and reach our full potential. You have knocked it out of the ballpark with this one Dr. Ostler! Thank you,

- Donnellyn Dominguez, LM, CPM

Not too long ago, the world of Redox was discovered and has slowly emerged into the world of healthcare and general wellness. As this foothold is being established and accepted and is picking up speed, along comes books like *Redox Matters* and now *Healthy Matters* which show us how to use these principles to change our lifestyles and change our life. Kudos to Dr Ostler for providing the world with a guide to teach us how to live the Redox Lifestyle - such an important topic in our modern world.

- Trish Schwenkler

The redox science that Dr Ostler laid out in Redox Matters flows beautifully into Healthy Matters, where it is applied into real life. The challenge and opportunity is to believe that this science and now the new redox lifestyle applies to you! It does! As Dr. Ostler says, these are the rules of how the cell functions, and therefore they are the rules which create health - because this is the essence of life itself. I said it about Redox Matters and repeat it here - the challenge is to believe that the science applies to you. Let your mind journey through the pages until your heart is grasped by the life-changing world of redox. Be brave. Live with no regrets.

- Carmen Keith, MD, IFMCP, Harvard-trained; triple board certified: Anesthesia, Pain Management, and Functional Medicine

Lee is most insightful and deep in his understanding of Redox physiology and biology. If Healthy Matters provides the expected application of Redox principles consistent with his last book, you are in for a treat. This will be a treasure for your bookshelf to be read and re-read along your journey to health.

- Stan Gardner, MD

Dr. Ostler has done it again! With Healthy Matters he has provided us a focused bookend to his Redox Matters published last year. With these two books he paints a clear focused picture of how to create a healthy "Redox Lifestyle" for ourselves that can spell longer, healthier life. I have been developing and teaching these principles in my integrative family medicine practice for 36 years. Dr. Ostler tells you how and why these recommendations work in this, his second *tour de force* self-improvement masterwork. Thank you, Dr. Ostler!

- Aaron Kaufman, DO

DISCLAIMER

The content in this book is not intended to be a substitute for professional, medical, dental, psychological, emotional, psychiatric, or other advice, nor to be used to diagnosis or treat ailments common or not common to the human experience. No medical claims are made or inferred. Always seek the advice of licensed and competent health providers familiar with this science and your specific health conditions, with any questions you may have regarding your health. While every effort has been taken to verify and provide accurate information contained in this publication, all content contained herein or made available through this book or it's related websites and online content, is for general information purposes only and cannot be relied on to replace professional health supervision and oversight. Note that nutritional supplements as a class, are not intended to diagnose, treat, or cure disease. All discussions related to redox biology in any of its forms or applications, whether mentioned herein or not, are not presented as cures or treatments for disease. The author and any company remotely connected or construed to be associated with this information disavows any liability related with the personal utilization or adoption of this information. The responsibility for the interpretation and use of the material lies with the reader. In no event shall the publishers, author, or potentially remotely connected interests, by liable for damages arising from its use.

Acknowledgements

I asked a prominent physician why it was so clear and easy for him to diagnose and solve a perplexing health condition which baffled many other physicians and related health professionals over many years. My comment and (almost) rhetorical question was meant as a compliment to him for his expert diagnostic prowess and wise treatment planning abilities. Graciously and with modest humility his response was instructive. He said, "It was easy! All the other doctors found out what it wasn't and narrowed the list down for us." Each had a role to play in a successful result. Gracious. Diplomatic. Self-effacing. And true!

In the same way, credit must go to many wise and ever intelligent colleagues and investigators who have gone before, upon whose shoulders this work stands. Collectively, their contributions to my understanding are immense. In writing this book, I stand on the shoulders of giants!

Because true science always leans forward, it bends to the discovery of new concepts that evolve and emerge with new understandings and technology, which seems obvious after their discovery. but was not so obvious in years gone by. The biggest discoveries and scientific breakthroughs are those that are closely associated with the development and understanding of Natural Law – rules and principles so grounded in their moorings that they affect everything! This certainly applies to the life sciences which are grounded foundationally with 'all-things-Redox!' Playing in the sandbox of notable experts, scientists, and the scientific architects who discover and explain foundational "natural law" is something to be cherished.

Sometimes your mentors know that they are your mentor, but often they do not. In this regard, the 'shoulders of giants' must include the critical thinkers and researchers and clinicians who pioneer these science concepts, too numerous to count or to credit individually, but without whom this book and all that goes with it would be impossible to research or write. I am humbled by their knowledge base and am thankful for their collective contribution in making any of this possible. They all had a role to play in my journey of discovery and helping me to better explain the science of health that is written into the redox code of life at the most foundational level. I cherish the experience of being so mentored!

Closer to home, this same thought applies to many in my "redox circle." I want to thank Dr. Richard (Dick) Walker who has brought such thoughtful insight and clear analysis and thinking into this discussion of what powers the human body to be healthy. Beyond his practice of medicine, his deep understanding of the workings of nutrition bless all of us who listen to and attend to his message. Likewise, thanks goes to those who serve on Medical Professionals Boards with me and are involved in deep redox-thinktanks.

I thank Dr. Ray Dixon, for his ever patient and wildly brilliant observations and assistance in proofreading the manuscript and providing amazing insights and suggestions, ever respectful and gracious in his outpourings.

Specifically, I thank Dr. Maureen Hayes, Terry Latham, Jerry White, Jim Glenn, Deni Robinson, Trish Schwenkler, and Alan Noble, who have each been a constant source of encouragement to me to get out of my shell and to boldly share my "stuff" with people far and wide. Their patience and inspiration and belief in me is highly prized. Special thanks to Deni Robinson for allowing me to utilize her artwork and memes which are so valuable and instructional in teaching redox principles.

I acknowledge the efforts of those within the business and redox-science arena, too numerous to mention here, who have contributed immensely to bringing the science of redox out of the shadows and onto the main-stage of modern society – and soon within the grasp of every health professional and common citizen. Tens of millions will be forever grateful, as am I, for their improved health because of your collective contribution.

I am also grateful for family, friends, and many colleagues who inspire and shout uplifting cheers from the sidelines, who are each like-minded in their collective beliefs and efforts to help as many other people as possible discover and apply these health principles in their lives. They, like me, believe that this is the answer to our larger problems of health and 'healthcare' and in having more healthy lives in our respective longevity.

I thank my wife Stephanie who has endured through my obsession with these 'Matters' – both Redox Matters and now Healthy Matters – and patiently allows me to investigate, research, experiment with new food choices, and at least tolerate my meager efforts to eat better and do more exercise and improve the health of our bodies and minds – and to make the

Redox Lifestyle something real. Home is always the best laboratory, and her encouragement is highly appreciated.

These are individually and collectively the giants upon whose shoulders I have had the privilege of standing, and who perform the always important role of 'making it real' and being a kind and wise sounding board.

I am grateful for their allowing me to see the Redox Landscape and the future from such a privileged viewpoint.

Dr. G. Lee Ostler

Table of Contents

Forward – Richard Walker MD ix

Preface xiii

Executive Summary – Healthy Matters xix

Part One – Introduction to Health, Diets, and the Redox Lifestyle 1

    The Deconstruction of The Redox Lifestyle 1

    Dietary Advice 17

    Dietary Philosophies: The Good. The Bad. The Ugly. 25

    Structured Diets 31

        7th Day Adventist Diet: 36

        The Word of Wisdom: 37

        Mediterranean Diet: 40

        Blue Zone Diet: 41

        Ketogenic diet: 41

        Paleo Diet: 43

        The Redox Lifestyle Diet: 44

Part Two – Metabolic Health and Disease 47

    What Does It Mean to Be Healthy? 47

        Liver Health 48

        Fructose, Sugar, and Health 54

        Gastrointestinal Health 61

    Metabolic Disease 69

        Insulin Resistance 73

        The Metabolic Healthcare Cliff 74

        The Modern Pill Mentality & Metabolic Disease 77

    The Metabolic Redox Machine 81

    Energy Metabolism, and Functional Ketosis 84

    Metabolic Flexibility, Krebs Cycle, and Energy Metabolism 91

Part Three – The Functional Redoxome 95

  Nutritional Ketosis 95

    Early Beginnings of Functional Ketosis 98

    Ketosis for Diabetes 100

    Redox Biology of Ketosis 101

    Intermittent Fasting 104

  Hormesis – The Dual Nature of Redox 111

    Nutrition and Hormesis 124

    Exercise and Hormesis 133

    Redox, Hormesis, and 'Anti-nutrition' 140

  Autophagy – Redox Driven Cellular Repair 149

    Fasting and Autophagy 155

    Carbohydrate Restriction and Autophagy 156

    Exercise and Autophagy 160

    Autophagy, Aging and The Redox Connection 164

    Cellular Death - Apoptosis 169

    Applied Autophagy and the Redox Lifestyle 171

    Autophagy and Diabetes 174

    Autophagy and the Brain 177

Part 4 – Redox Functional Nutrition 179

  Functional Nutrition in the Redox Lifestyle 179

    Applied Redox Nutrition 181

    Nutrition and Hormesis - Review 184

    Redox Micronutrients and Phytochemicals 187

  Functional Redox Nutrition - Supplementation 191

- Acetyl-L-Carnitine 191
- Alpinia Galanga 192
- Ashwagandha root extract 193
- B Vitamins 194
  - Vitamin B3 – Niacin 197
  - Vitamin B5 199
  - Vitamins B6 200
  - Vitamin B12 203
- GABA 204
- Garden Sage and Spanish Sage 206
- Guarana 209
- L-Theanine 210
- L-Tyrosine 213
- Nicotinamide Mononucleotide 213
- Panax Ginseng 215
- Phosphatidylserine 216
- Red Orange Complex® 217
- Rhodiola rosea 219
- Saffron extract 220
- Zinc Citrate 221
- Conclusion & Quick-Start Recommendations 223
- APPENDEX 229
  - Anti-Nutrients 229
  - Artificial Sugar 232
  - Biological Redox Switch 234
  - Brain Health and Function 236
  - Fats 237

Ketosis and Exercise 240

Metabolomics Study – The Supercharging of Krebs 242

Nutrition Philosophy and Science 251

Processed Food 260

Redox Detoxification 264

About the Author 270

End Notes 273

Forward – Richard Walker MD

When Dr. Lee Ostler asked me to write a foreword to this his second book pertaining to the impacts of redox on cellular health, I agreed immediately. Knowing Lee's sincere interest in exploring, understanding, and teaching the many wellness implications of redox I was very excited to read <u>Healthy Matters</u>. Little did I know how much I would learn that could be applied daily in order to live a fuller healthier life! This is truly a redox manual for a wellness lifestyle.

If you haven't read Lee's first book, <u>Redox Matters,</u> I would strongly urge you to do that. It isn't required to understand his new book, but it will give the reader a robust foundation for understanding the scientific principles of redox. There, he relates his journey of discovery and eventual understanding of redox biochemistry and physiology through the lens of it's surprising and unexplained impacts on his wife's severe health challenges. Having seen redox technology work it's wonders, Lee very much wanted to explore and explain why and how it worked. He explains this quite well in language all can understand.

In my long career as a physician, specialty-board certified in both Internal Medicine and Emergency Medicine, I have personally witnessed the amazing responses that many people have achieved when employing this technology. At first skeptical, I became convinced of this technology's effectiveness by validating the experiences had by many people. Of equal importance was my own, and later Dr. Ostler's, even more robust exploration of the documented scientific literature supporting this technology.

Together these two books provide an explanation of how redox functions to both enhance wellness as well as enable one's body to overcome illness and injury. To, as Lee points out, empower our "Inner Doctor." This new book is very timely as it references the veritable explosion of science related to the interface of redox with nutrition, lifestyle, and aging.

This is a book for anyone seeking a broader and deeper understanding of how redox biology impacts their health in profound ways. Having gained that knowledge it is also a book that teaches you how to engage with the natural laws of science and biology to dramatically enhance your health. We all live in a body made of trillions of cells all of which depend on a fully functional Redoxome to maintain health and longevity. We ignore that fact at our peril! For some this book contains knowledge not previously explored and for others it contains a robust extension of information known to be crucial for achieving an enhanced state of wellness. The interrelationship of the Redoxome to energy metabolism, metabolic flexibility, ketosis, fasting, insulin resistance, exercise, autophagy, longevity, and much more are explained in a way anyone can grasp.

I find it very interesting that many people, especially in the medical world, confine themselves to certain silos of knowledge that are defined by their educational expertise. Medical doctors, dentists, naturopaths, chiropractors, acupuncturists, massage therapists, athletic trainers, nutritionists, on and on, are often reluctant to look beyond their field of expertise to newly discovered scientific breakthroughs. Maybe it's education, maybe something else, that determines who will remain open to the vast world of information that exists outside these narrowly defined boundaries of information. What determines who will be resistant to new ideas and technologies that arise from elsewhere in the ever-expanding universe of information, I don't pretend to understand.

For anyone involved in healthcare who is interested in understanding this new field of redox science and redox medicine I strongly urge you to read this book. It will give you access to a potent new mechanism for adding value to your patients' lives.

For many reasons I have found myself to be an information seeker for as long as I can recall. I believe this thirst for knowledge is what brought Lee and I together and why I was asked to write this forward. I'll admit I didn't grow up wanting to be a doctor. In fact, I grew up on a farm, not in a family that was medically oriented and neither of my parents had a college degree. However, I unfortunately suffered a serious trauma as a teenager and saw up front how medical expertise could be life saving

So, I chose Medicine. I've never regretted that decision and several years later I was accepted and eventually graduated from the University of Iowa College of Medicine. But my career choice had a few twists and turns and didn't end there. As it turns out, I really didn't have a clear understanding of what a standard medical education would teach me. I soon realized there was scant attention being focused on prevention. "How do you keep people well?"

I grew up in a household with a mother that was very much oriented toward prevention and wellness before it became the 'thing' to know about. So, I decided to find a way to add those areas of knowledge, to fill that void in my medical education. I very much wanted to learn more about keeping people healthy! I was firmly convinced that drugs and surgery were important but by no means the only answers to health challenges. In this regard Dr Ostler and I were kindred spirits before we ever met. We both keep asking ourselves "How do we do a better job of keeping people well. What other 'tools' could we employ or recommend?"

Fortunately, I was able to address those shortcomings in medical education during a one-year sabbatical in the School of Public Health. There I achieved a master's degree in Preventive Medicine and Environmental Health with additional nutritional education. The knowledge gained there has established my career-long interest in new advances in health, wellness, and anti-aging technologies. Because of that interest when I first encountered references to a profound breakthrough in biology known as 'redox cellular communication' I was convinced this held the key to some very interesting breakthroughs in health and wellness.

Lee and I are both firmly grounded in the conventional worlds of dentistry and western medicine. In addition, we also share an openness to exploring new modalities that hold promise for positively impacting the health of those we encounter in our lives and practices. In other words, we are on the open-minded end of that continuum. If something works, we want to know about it. One very important step further, we want to understand how and why things works. I began that journey of discovery a few years before Lee, however Lee has far surpassed my search for knowledge and now has much to share with all of us who want to further understand the tremendous degree to which redox concepts impact our lives.

This is not simply a book about the chemistry of electrons moving from one molecule to another, back and forth, defining the process of reduction-oxidation. It is about life and how to live it in accordance with predetermined principles of redox. This book is about using the non-negotiable scientific principals embodied in the Redoxome. Doing so at the very least, to be as healthy as possible, to live as long as possible, and to avoid disease as long as possible.

When it comes to your health nothing could be more real or more important!

Dr. Dick Walker MD, FACP, FACEP, MpH

Preface

There is a great deal of confusion in modern society about what constitutes health. The very word itself - "healthcare" - is a bit of a misnomer, since too often it is anything but!

This is more than unfortunate since the business of "health-care" is enormous. The arena of "health" is so complex and bloated that it is simply out of control. US health care spending has grown at almost 10% per year, reaching $4.1 trillion ($12,530 per person) and accounts for 20% of the Gross Domestic Product in the United States. This is simply unconscionable.

Much or most of this would simply go away if health were really what the word meant – caring for health! It's almost surreal to consider, but what would happen if more people were well and didn't require medical intervention?

The real answer to the crisis we call healthcare is for each person to awaken their "Inner Doctor." This requires a will to be well, personal responsibility and action, and an awareness of how to make it happen.

The purpose of Healthy Matters is to take personal health out of the dark and present the topic of health and wellness in new light. New understandings about the ground rules of cellular health shine needed light and answers important concerns about the 'game of life.' Just as every game requires rules, it is difficult to win the game if the rules are unknown or cloaked in mystery – or are even concealed from the participants!

Healthy Matters will reveal these rules, now emerging from decades of scientific inquiry, but which have been in operation since time immemorial. Knowing the rules of how cells work grants new powers to individuals and families to activate the human body's "Inner Doctor" with its inherent ability to defend, heal, and repair. We will make the point that this goes beyond 'just' managing disease processes and controlling symptoms.

The answer is all about lifestyle! The Redox Lifestyle! It is about "redox" because these are the rules! These rules are bounded by laws that govern the control of everything in our body – right down to the tiniest sub-cellular parts of how atoms, molecules, and cells function in a bioenergetic world.

While that may sound complex, it isn't! Health is really quite simple. Create and give the body and its cells what they want and need to operate properly, and health results! Leverage that with a redox lifestyle and agents that activate healthy pathway genes, and it works even better! However, provide bad fuel, deficient building blocks, poor maintenance, and an unbalanced bio-electrical redox landscape, and disease results.

Cells always play by the rules! Sickness results because those rules were followed. Health happens when cells are playing by the rules of health. No exceptions! They are governed by laws of physics and the pluses-and-minuses of bio-electrical law. This is at a level below and more foundational to the DNA programming – in fact redox tells the DNA when and how to execute its programming. This is why it is important to know the rules! Especially of what health is and is not.

This takes us back to today's problems with health. In today's world, the working definition of health has morphed into being the absence of symptoms – by any means possible. This usually implies via medical intervention. If the symptoms or the lab values or the problems are kept well managed and under control, then one is said to be in good health. The focus is on management of disease and the evidence of "health" by this definition is the absence of symptoms and good laboratory values. Broadly speaking, in today's world good health equals good disease management!

A premise that is made in this book, and its predecessor "Redox Matters," is that health is more than the absence of, or even the good management of symptoms. Expert medical intervention does not create health. Or wellness. It keeps us alive and functioning through reactive measures, until our appointed date with destiny when longevity runs out.

The overall focus in our modern world has been on intervention and treatment. This is interwoven into our modern institutional and systemic healthcare system and mindset. Precious little attention has been given or 'paid' to prevention. In a wellness model, being healthy and resistant and strong means that cells are fully functional, robust, and able to deal with the insults and stresses they experience. That is the definition of real health - cellular health.

There is no escaping the stresses and assaults of the environment around us or inside us. That's a part of living. However, how the body responds to these insults and stresses is a function of the cell's ability to mobilize natural defenses and guard against changes in cellular oxidation. That is at its most "root" level the root cause of all disease! Any and all downstream inflammation and disease begins first with perturbations of this basic redox phenomenon. Being healthy is about having an awake and responsive defense.

The differences in opinions about what health means has created two main camps. Modern medicine has evolved around the concept of managing disease with after-the-fact intervention, while others focus on empowering the body to heal itself with a prevention mindset, using 'natural' means where possible.

The truth is that both are necessary!

In a world of 7+ billion people, and even in the life of one person living 78 years (average), it is not remotely practical or feasible to believe that medical intervention is not or would never be necessary. The odds are not in anyone's favor that they can escape a lifetime of insults and bad choices and remain in perfect health. And if that is true, then we want to have competent medical intervention to remedy the damage. However, it is also true that people individually and collectively can and should do more to prevent that necessity.

To illustrate this point let us consider "the health cliff."

Every day, a sizable number of people fall off the edge of the "health cliff" to crash-land at the bottom of the cliff. Maybe it is a heart attack, a tragic accident, diabetes, or any of a thousand reasons – but fall and crash they, and we, do. And when it happens, we all want a capable and immediate response from medical care teams to put the proverbial "Humpty Dumpty" back together again.

Up on top of the cliff, where all the action began, there are throngs of people pressing the edge, flirting with danger – some completely unaware of where the edge is or what the danger entails or what it feels like to fall. Some justify the risk because of the pleasures of living at the edge.

Wisely, there are people within and about that group who are warning of the edge, teaching, and trying to oppose the forward momentum and push toward the edge. Maybe they were one of the lucky ones who clawed their way back up on top after a nasty fall, or maybe they are just more awake and aware, but either way, these experts work to advise people to move back away from the edge. They put up warning signs and fences and guardrails to protect and keep people from falling. Their argument is that if you stay away from the edge, you can reduce if not eliminate the risk of falling and landing with the other broken bodies at the bottom where that wonderful medical intervention is waiting. This top-side activity is different from that which occurs at the bottom. It is prevention.

The truth is that both groups of experts are necessary. They have two different missions and drive in two different lanes. Those on top are not mending broken bones, and those mending the brokenness are not focused on prevention. There is little need for argument or overreach from either, toward the other. This is the 'real' world!

While we will never see the two sides resolve their differences and come together in harmony, we must accept they are both needed. There is an appropriate time for medical intervention. But there is also an appropriate time and place for primary prevention. And – if that has already failed, then for secondary and tertiary prevention. At some point the Inner Doctor must be awakened if real health is to be realized.

The good news is that we can individually act within our own lives to have this happen. And well-meaning folks on both sides will celebrate this as it happens.

While staying away from the edge and invoking prevention strategies is ideal, the first concern of a person floundering at the bottom of the cliff should not be about cellular health or prevention. It's too late! Rather, it should be about surviving! Once that is assured, then secondary and tertiary prevention measures can be initiated to climb back up the cliff and reassume life up on the plateau - but with renewed effort to not fall again (and to help others also not make the same plunge).

In the final analysis, the "wellness lightbulb" turns on differently for each person in both time and place. It is a function of education, societal and family exposures, access to care, how badly one is hurting, and many other factors and variables. However, at any point along the path – whether atop the cliff or while lying at the bottom or while climbing up its face – the mind can be educated and informed and brought to value and understand the proper role for medical intervention and prevention.

In the end, successful pre-vention always trumps intervention. And even "re-vention" can help to diminish the amount of inter-vention needed after-the-fact. That is the essence of understanding and mastering redox biology in personal living. Aside from trauma and a handful of other situations at the bottom of the cliff, the redox mindset is a prevention mindset – even when instituted after-the-fact.

Learning to prize the idea of prevention – by Awakening the Inner Doctor – is what the redox lifestyle is all about. It is the difference between medical management and health. It is the difference between intervention and prevention. It is the difference between longevity and healthspan. It is the difference between managing disease and being truly well. It is the difference between remaining ignorant and being informed.

In the end, it is all about choice! And wise action!

Executive Summary – Healthy Matters

The first book in this series, Redox Matters, introduced the foundational redox signaling biology that orchestrates everything related to life, energy, health, and disease. In this book, Healthy Matters, I will build upon this grounding to translate the principles of redox signaling into an empowering old, yet very new, Redox Lifestyle.

As you proceed, it will be helpful to keep in mind the basic ground rules of what "redox" is and how it works in the body. It is upon these principles that life exists! And the degree to which these principles are followed, is the degree to which health is enjoyed. These are principles. These are rules. This is *natural law*!

The designs of our universe from its broadest expanse to the tiniest parts of sub-cellular space, rely upon the creation and movement of energy, first in the form of photons and then through the movement of electrons and their influence along many metabolic and physiologic pathways. This system is uniquely designed to transfer power from the ultimate source of all energy to the end user. These laws govern everything and give life-force to everything. Although recently discovered, they have always existed!

As this translates to the human experience and the biological world we live in, the transduction or movement of electrons from one molecule to another, from one atom to another, is the essence of everything! They play by their rules, not the rules we make up for them or wish that they were. It is these rules that matter! When we bend or break ourselves against these rules, we bend and break! If we follow them, we heal and stay strong!

The objective in Redox Matters and here in this book Healthy Matters, will be to simplify and translate this vast and deep redox science to the extent possible into how following these laws support a healthy lifestyle – what we will call a "Redox Lifestyle." This really is 'the bottom line!'

Because this is grounded in redox biology, it will help to read or review Redox Matters and keep in mind at least a basic understanding of reduction and oxidation as it relates to redox biology. This will serve you well as you begin to apply these principles in making daily, if not hourly decisions about your health in the form of food, drink, shopping, exercise, activity level, supplementation, mental and emotional state, and much much more.

There is no shortage of information in the public space, and many voices and vested interests who would persuade and entice you to their ideology, products, and services. Some of this information is well grounded. However, much is also conspiringly deceptive. Knowing the difference between the two is helped by being informed and aware of the grounding rules of redox science - or in other words, knowing how the cell thinks. When you know the rules, you can make informed decisions about your meal planning (energy metabolism, polyphenol consumption, and nutritional ketosis, in 'science-speak'), your activity level (hormesis and exercise), managed cellular repair (autophagy) - and your medical care (how to prevent the need for).

As habitual lifestyles shift toward a more robust and responsive redox lifestyle, you will begin living by the rules the universe designed, and not as marketers, taste buds, or habits want them to be.

Reduction Oxidation and Metabolic Function

The very process of energy metabolism (Krebs cycle in mitochondria) relies integrally on the movement of electrons between molecules that are reduced and oxidized in a continuous chain of bioelectrical reactions. Food is the fuel that provides this energy source to the body – effectively transferring the sun's energy through the food chain into our bodies. We digest and process it and extract this biological energy in the form of ATP/ADP molecules which power life.

Along the way, a myriad of reactions occur that are dependent on, and can be manipulated by the type, amount, and quality of this fuel source, and the amount of glucose, fatty acids, and amino acids which are present in the blood stream and body - over time.

The type, amount, and quality of this food/energy source, along with the timing of its consumption, are all independent variables. They are the factors tightly linked and interwoven into the fabric of our health. Varying any of these variables has profound influence over how this energy metabolism functions and the degree of cellular function it supports. Or does not!

Factors related to where and how energy comes from and how its by-products regulate health and disease, are more important than any other consideration in a "lifestyle" discussion. Of everything a person can do to improve or re-establish their health, nutrition with all that involves is more influential than anything else! We are what our cells are, which is why "we are what we eat." And - this is also why "you can't outrun a bad diet." Nutrition trumps everything!

This is because chronic metabolic disease is a consequence of the fouled and mismanaged conversion of food into energy, along with the mishandling of the redox platform – all of which sabotages cellular function (a result of the Standard American Diet, SAD, which doesn't help with "Healthy Matters").

Through all of this, oxygen is the vital ingredient in the process. Oxygen acts integrally with redox-couples and the electron transport chain, to act as the ultimate electron acceptor within energy metabolism, and in creating many oxygen derivatives that are essential redox signaling messengers. This is what makes oxygen so vital to biological life. Without it, electrons do not flow, energy creation ceases, and cellular communication stops.

However, inside mitochondria the reduction of oxygen is not a complete process. This means 2-3% of the oxygen molecules remain in an oxidized state - meaning they are not fully reduced (as we will learn, this is an important design feature and should not be extinguished outright!). This incomplete reduction of oxygen creates a reactive oxygen molecule called "superoxide." This molecule is then converted to hydrogen peroxide (by the antioxidant superoxide dismutase), which is then converted to carbon dioxide and water by glutathione.

These molecules are used in the immune system to help degrade and kill bacteria (the "oxidative burst" of phagocytosis in white blood cells) as well as to help regulate cellular function for self-renewal and preservation.

However, within and alongside these processes, and because they are still 'reactive oxygen species,' these altered oxygen molecules also become a source of oxidation and damage within the cell – especially if left unchecked.

This produces damage to cell membranes and proteins, including DNA, and causes enzymes and proteins to fold and twist improperly, thereby altering their function. Taken together, all of this damage and the changed 'reduction-oxidation' (redox) state of the cell, affect cellular function.

Much of the damage these oxidants cause from this state of elevated oxidation results in inflammation. This elevated state of chronic oxidation and inflammation is compounded when because of aging and disease, the body is less able to respond in healthy ways to this oxidation.

Alterations in the way mitochondria burn fuel (energy metabolism) affect mitochondrial function, and this mitochondrial dysfunction affects the process of healthy energy metabolism. These cyclical effects are intensified from having too much energy (being overfed), having problems with cellular metabolic function (insulin resistance), and from impaired cell function due to poor redox signaling (aging, poor nutrition). Collectively they lead to higher amounts of oxidation from the mitochondrial dysfunction they create.

Problems with food quality (processed food), outward toxicity, undue radiation, poor sleep, untoward stress, hypoxia, and infection (to name a few) also contribute significantly to increase this state of cellular oxidation stress.

Compounded together – the internal oxidative stress from energy production, and the oxidation created by the external environment, profoundly impacts the cell.

The Sea-Change in Cellular Defense and Renewal

The prevailing belief has long been that the solution for these problems of oxidation and free radicals was to take antioxidant supplements. Vitamins and plant-based antioxidants have been used for decades to reduce highly reactive molecules generated in the creation of cellular energy. This practice is so well entrenched in our society and within wellness circles that it is viewed by many as "the Holy Grail" of prevention and health. And to a limited extent, they can 'work.'

In fact, a thriving supplement industry has grown up around this idea, which is expected to reach $9 billion by 2026 with an annual growth rate of 5.3%

per year (Antioxidants Market Size, GlobalNewswire.com). The prevailing belief of many is that 'normal' nutrition was not sufficient to provide the quality of plant-based polyphenols needed for cellular repair and antioxidant function. Considering the state of the agricultural and food production industries, a good case can be made for modest supplementation. This has resulted in much debate, an abundance of 'junk science,' and a great amount of commercial competition.

However, there has been a sea-change of late - a substantial change in understanding about the other role oxidation plays inside the body. It isn't all bad after all! The sea-change in thought isn't so much about the merits of antioxidant usage in controlling oxidation, as it is about the role of oxidation itself.

Rethinking and establishing new guidelines for nutrition and antioxidant usage based on this emerging redox-based science, is the sum and essence of the redox lifestyle – and is the only path to health, wellness and anything that resembles anti-aging. To be sure there is a proper place for supplementation, but it is often far different from what many suppose. As it turns out some oxidation is good, and it should not be overly suppressed! In fact, to some degree it should be encouraged – but only if done 'right.'

This is a paradigm shift of massive proportions because it affects everything in the "modern" world of 'enlightened' healthcare. It ties directly to the core rules of a cell's ability to detect stress and execute a responsive action which protects itself in the face of challenging conditions – be they self-imposed or otherwise. Ultimately, this is about the definition of health itself. It is what defines our "Inner Doctor" and is the science of using lifestyle to activate its power in our life.

To be sure, emerging science is showing us that oxidants are not wholly the villains they have been made out to be. In fact, they are important and essential in their role as the primary signaling molecules which activate pathway genes - which in turn drive healthy genetic expression. Because these energized molecules are created in the mitochondria in the reduction and oxidation reactions of energy metabolism, and because they are used 'downstream' in other redox reactions to modify and manage cellular functions, they are called redox molecules, or redox signaling molecules.

Redoxome

This has led to the development of a new science discipline called the "Redoxome." We have known about other science "-omes" for decades (namely the metabolome, proteome, transcriptome, and genome). Each one refers to a different level of the workings of the biological body ranging from the genotype outward to the phenotype – in other words from the hidden cellular genomic programming to how their work appears in real life. This new deeper Redoxome science is the 'granddaddy' of them all! In fact, it sits at the bottom and foundation of all the others.

Each of the established -omes has extensive science and practical medical application to healthcare and treatment. Each can be measured and diagnosed and "treated" with medications when they are not working well. This will continue to be so forever.

Treatment for problems seen within the higher-level -omes allows doctors to intervene and manage signs and symptoms, prolong life, and make life more enjoyable and functional. There is a place for that! However, because "treatments" rarely if ever reach the Redoxome level where the "root-cause" originates, true wellness cannot be assured or maintained.

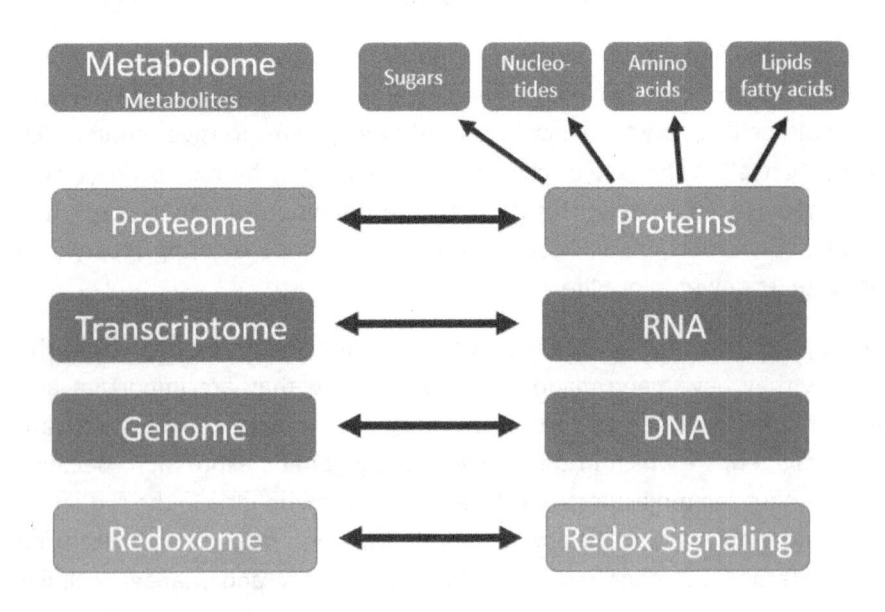

Metabolome (Metabolites)	Sugars	Nucleo-tides	Amino acids	Lipids fatty acids

Proteome	⟷	Proteins
Transcriptome	⟷	RNA
Genome	⟷	DNA
Redoxome	⟷	Redox Signaling

This is because problems in the higher more visible -ome levels occur due to problems upstream, or said differently, in the more foundational level of the Redoxome. Chronic lifestyle diseases will not resolve on their own or through "treatment" of symptoms, unless or until the foundational metabolic redox-level problems are addressed through corrections in lifestyle and energy metabolism and improved redox functioning.

Because this new category in health of the Redoxome is at a level below the genome, it is sometimes referred to as the "epigenome." This give it influence upon and overlays the DNA, controlling and modulating how genes express – good and bad.

Broadly speaking this is all referred to as the "redox landscape." How these principles of redox signaling function and operate within this landscape is referred to as the *redox species interactome*.

Ultimately, the answers to any questions about how cells work and the disease conditions which result when they are impaired, are found at this level. The Redoxome is wholly concerned about how the body senses stress and responds to it. This is a critical proposition for the survival of any and all living organisms with environmental stress, whether from internal or external sources. These collective stresses, and how the cells respond to them determine metabolic function, metabolic health, and metabolic disease.

Hormesis and the Redox Switch

At the heart of the Redoxome platform is the discovery that mild intermittent stress is protective to the body, not harmful. Mild intermittent oxidative stress provokes an adaptive cellular response governed by redox molecules. This awakens internal mechanisms which improves survivability, counters disease, and improves health.

The redox principle which governs this marvelous ability is the principle of hormesis. The discovery and application of this concept finally clarifies the reasons why bio-oxidative, mitochondrial-focused, and redox-based systems and supplements have positive effect on cellular health. It clearly explains the two-sided effect of oxidation within a cellular environment – good and bad.

The concept that every person has a hormetic zone, lives each day on "the hormetic curve," and utilizes everything in their lifestyle knowingly or unknowingly to impact this principle – can be life changing!

This speaks to the far-reaching effects of oxidative stress across the entire system as a whole, as well as the importance of following the innate "rules" of the cell and the maintenance of homeostasis and cellular repair. It also speaks to solutions that address the deficiencies and dysfunctions that occur at the cellular and sub-cellular level. It also explains why improved lifestyle measures are effective in promoting healthy outcomes, because they play on these same pathways to increase native redox signaling.

These pathways and mechanisms in the Redoxome contain many redox regulatory "switches" and systems which are responsive to changes in oxidative status. This is the 'grand secret' to health! The *modus operandi* and biological mechanism of action for how the body senses, detects, interprets, and responds to changes in oxidation (i.e., stress), is that redox-sensitive molecules stimulate pathway genes to activate and call for a defensive and reparative response. This is called *stress adaptation*. The degree of success in this adaptation ultimately determines the resulting degree of health or disease the organism experiences.

Again, this is the principle of hormesis in action. Small amounts of oxidation challenge the cell apparatus in a way that it responds with cellular defense and repair. Large amounts of the same agents of oxidation provoke inflammatory disease. However, mild levels of oxidative stress within the physiologic hormetic zone, constitute the basis of understanding for everything that results in health. Anything that promotes health does so because it enlivens the redox-sensitive pathways which is what activates cellular defenses and repair. Period!

Within this rule lives the explanation for how good nutrition, exercise, stress reduction, infection control, and good sleep produce and maintain health - and how their opposites lead to disease. This makes positive lifestyle measures a bio-oxidative stimulus to the cell. This means they respectively produce a mild or sub-toxic level of oxidative stress, which in the throughput of the redox interactome causes the sensing mechanisms to upregulate pathway genes, which then activate nature's very own "Inner Doctor."

Recall that redox molecules are not "standard" biomolecules. They are electrically charged reactive species. As such they have the ability to interact with each other, exchanging cellular 'information' by way of bio-electrical action up and down and across the landscape, possessing an extended web of intra- and inter-cellular interactions throughout the cellular space. Because of this they are predisposed to react with redox agents and redox-sensitive sensors. As such they can switch on and switch off pathway genes as dictated by the source and level of ambient oxidative stress in the cell. This defines the "Redox Landscape."

In science-speak, this describes the pleiotropic roles of redox molecules. This means that one molecule or process participates in many physiological processes in an amazingly complex array of biological reactions. These are set in motion to regulate an organism living in a constantly changing environment and continuously synchronized across the body at all times. This management of the many different biological processes in the body, often unrelated in purpose and function, is connected together by the same redox mechanisms, using redox-sensitive sensors to conduct the business of the cell. It is a "one-to-many" model that runs contrary to the reductionist "one-to-one drug model" of modern medicine.

This is in part what makes the two approaches to health so disparate and hard to reconcile at this level. It also explains why redox molecules cannot be considered in the same light as drugs (which operate on specific receptor sites with specific actions).

This new category of redox health demands that supplements and redox lifestyle measures be viewed with different expectations than traditional healthcare and medications. The objectives are to correct redox deficiency and target base-level cellular dysfunction - and not to suppress symptoms which occur as a result of that dysfunction.

This defines the difference between *inter-vention* and *pre-vention*. Correcting redox deficiencies is about prevention and about awakening the *Inner Doctor* so that cells can self-correct the health problems which originally came about from dysfunction. Intervention is generally about mitigating the effects of the dysfunction – and to intervene in life-extending ways (lifespan) - thus preventing morbidity from becoming premature mortality.

Different from mainstream and pharmacologically based medicine, the business of the Redoxome is to manage energy metabolism, bioenergetics, antioxidant defenses, the immune system, cellular 'repair and replace' mechanisms (cell cycle), and more. The vertical "redox spine" connections which interconnect all of the parts and processes through the interconnecting redox pathways depend on and use the same redox molecules that are created in the cell from the creation of energy in a saline salt-water environment within mitochondria. The same is true for the redox-related functions within the horizontal redox landscape, operating with synergy throughout the Redoxome.

Ironically, thinking that they were categorically bad, these redox molecules have been and still are maligned and targeted by well-meaning but (now) uninformed health professionals and health enthusiasts, who attempt to discount their importance or to eliminate them altogether through the use of antioxidants (the old paradigm that all oxidation is bad).

Redox Supplementation

Today, "the rest of the story" has come out and is changing everything. It is time for a new landscape and a new lifestyle. These are the (new) rules of the cell, where the truth is found in balance and in not suppressing nature's mechanism so carefully designed for its own protection and repair.

This is why the discovery and breakthrough of stabilized redox signaling molecules is so important and significant. Almost regardless of the degree of insult or stress, a supplemented mild oxidative stress operating within the hormetic curve can produce and enhance these nature-bound mechanisms. They "work" because they adhere to the rules laid down by nature itself. They provide a significant advantage in helping manipulate the redox landscape for good - by providing a bio-identical tool to activate redox-sensitive switches and healthy pathway genes.

This new chapter of stabilized redox in healthcare had its humble beginnings in a bioresearch laboratory. Understanding the various roles which reactive redox molecules play in the human body, researchers set out to duplicate this process by fractionalizing saline, or salt water, into its component parts (in real life called ROS / redox molecules). They discovered that while the mitochondria produce them during energy metabolism, they can also be created and stabilized in a laboratory setting from the same materials mitochondria use, saline - in a process of physics called electrolysis. Their original objective was to duplicate the body's ability to make these native molecules, and to create new solutions for very troubling diseases which hijack the body's immune system, and which create distressing amounts of inflammation by-products which can profoundly injure its victims.

This effort fell short not because they weren't successful, but because the researchers were too successful! Because they are native to the body and have no toxic effect at any dose, they were unable to qualify it for drug therapy, and accordingly developed it as a supplement. Now broadly available, this adjunctive solution fits perfectly with a redox lifestyle strategy to support all cells of the body. It does so through the principle of hormesis and redox-sensitive switches which help the body manage genetic expression. Rather than being a specific solution to a narrow base of specific diseases, it is now a redox-based solution for redox deficiency generally - which applies the mild hormetic-based oxidative stimulus needed to upregulate healthy pathway genes.

This discovery is one of the most important breakthroughs in health today because redox signaling molecules are the deepest cell-signaling messengers ever discovered. They work and live at the interface of energy and matter where cellular communication activates biological programming and modulates all cell processes – including the energy of life itself.

When combined with living a more complete Redox Lifestyle - which is the point of this Healthy Matters book - it becomes a powerful strategy for the proper management and support of the Redoxome. Ultimately, this is the key to antiaging medicine, wellness and in awakening the "Inner Doctor!"

The Redox Lifestyle

This is where the metabolic dynamics of energy metabolism and metabolic flexibility enter the picture. The slight nutritional stress from low carbohydrate consumption (low blood glucose and low insulin levels) produce a mild increase in oxidation (nutritional stress) within an individual's hormetic zone, which induces a redox state that upregulates cell-protective genes which protect health. They are responsible for inducing autophagy, and apoptosis when needed, and for activating cellular antioxidant defenses which powerfully affects metabolic health. All of these are at their base, redox processes borne of redox-sensitive mechanisms and transcription factors that drive gene expression and cellular response. In other words, mild oxidative stress produces a stress-adaption that has been conserved to help assure survival and health. Follow the rules! Natural law!

The science of the role of redox molecules and the redox switches which control gene expression is an exciting discovery. It explains the usefulness and role of ROS oxidants inside a cell and how they can be manipulated with nutrition, exercise, stress reduction, sleep, infection management, and supplementation to optimize our health.

While it is still true that too much oxidation is dangerous and creates inflammation and disease, it is refreshing and empowering to discover that a small mild amount of controlled oxidation plays such an important role in activating cellular health. This places immense control for better health directly in our own hands – and mouths! This forms the basis for how a person can create and manage a redox lifestyle for their own life.

This is what gives redox-based lifestyle factors such great power for hope and change to improve health. It is why lifestyle matters.

Regardless of whether it is about primary, or secondary prevention, making improvements across the Redoxome is always helpful. This strategy always works – whether it is "felt" or not!

Without this new knowledge and ability, we remain victims of our own ignorance and the persuasive marketing agendas, ideologies, and even guidelines that too often run counter to the rules cells operate with.

These rules rule! They were designed this way and have been conserved in nature throughout all time and are grounded in the foundations of life. They provide answers to some of the most important and basic biological concerns.

As you read this book and its companion Redox Matters, you will discover answers to these and many other questions that are directly affecting your life. More importantly, you will learn to ask better questions, so that you get better answers! For example:

- What is cellular biological stress?
- How is cellular stress created?
- How does a cell know when it is in trouble?
- How does the cell (and body) respond to this stress?
- Is the response to stress good or bad?
- Is oxidation always bad? Or can it be helpful?
- What is the relationship between oxidation and inflammation?
- How does a cell repair itself when damaged, and how does it restore balance and improve its function?
- What can I do to better follow metabolic and redox rules and improve my life?
- If I need to make changes to my lifestyle, which are the most important?
- What supplements are truly health-friendly?
- What supplements work the best with the Redox environment?
- How can I sort through the confusing and conflicted voices of health advice?

With a better understanding of the rules of how your personal Redoxome functions, you will better recognize and sort through the shortcomings, flaws, and half-truths in the world of nutrition and health advice around you. Knowing these rules will allow you to make better choices which will activate cellular renewal, and which will change the trajectory of your health and healthspan.

This is more than a philosophical construct. It is more than an ideological bias. It is about learning the natural laws which dictate how cells function, and then aligning and positioning your lifestyle to be in accord with those laws.

The redox-driven science and lifestyle is not an irrelevant philosophical or theoretical abstract! It is very real! In fact, it is the only true 'doctrine' for how healthy cells work. Redox-driven stress-adaptation is real science - based on biochemical, bio-electrical, and physiological truths.

Governed by these laws, they operate to impact hormesis, energy metabolism, nutritional ketosis, autophagy, redox-sensitive transcription, pathway gene activation, redox signaling, metabolic health, and so much more.

Discovering these rules and knowing how to apply them in your life, is what this book is about.

Being Healthy Matters!

> "There is no particular virtue in being uninformed. Certainly, no virtue in ignorance."
> — Richard L Evans

The Deconstruction of The Redox Lifestyle

Part One – Introduction to Health, Diets, and the Redox Lifestyle

The Deconstruction of The Redox Lifestyle

Any discussion of health should begin with a grounded discussion of what makes us healthy. This would include understanding the core principles of how cells function and survive. While staying uninformed may serve the interests of stakeholders who benefit from our ignorance, in matters of personal and national health it does not serve us well.

Richard L Evans notably said that "there is no particular virtue in being uninformed. Certainly, no virtue in ignorance." Being healthy matters - and knowing why and how to make that happen will be our focus in this book.

Chronic metabolic diseases are the most prevalent and costly health conditions in the world. They kill 41 million people and account for 71% of all deaths globally[1]. Presently, sixty percent of all Americans suffer from at least one persistent disease condition[2]. This list includes cancer, diabetes,

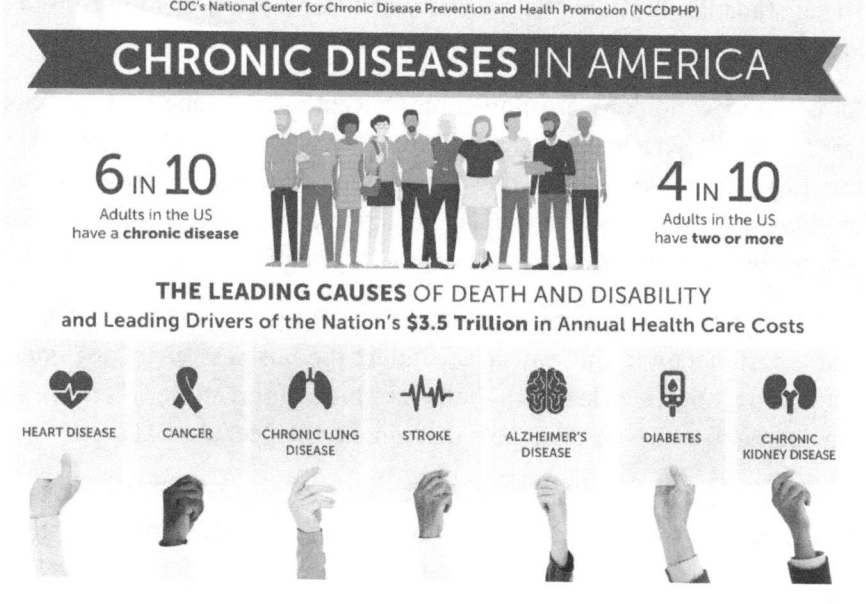

The Deconstruction of The Redox Lifestyle

hypertension, stroke, heart disease, respiratory disease, arthritis, obesity, and oral disease, to name a few. It is an easy assumption that these statistics hold true for the global population at large – especially those who participate to any degree in the modern way of life.

In the United States, $5,300 USD is spent per person annually on these conditions. This equals 75% of the aggregate healthcare spending in the US. In terms of public spending, fully 96 cents per dollar within the Medicare insurance program is devoted to the treatment of chronic persistent disease conditions[3]. Fully seven out of 10 deaths are attributed to or are caused by these conditions, which means these deaths are universally 'premature'. The national healthcare spending has risen steadily for the last four years[4]. These statistics illustrate the enormity of these health, or rather disease. Problems. They absolutely affect every family!

> **90% of the nation's $3.8 trillion in annual health care expenditures** are for people with chronic and mental health conditions.

All of these conditions are non-communicable – meaning they are non-transmittable, which begs the question, how does one acquire these diseases? The answer is that these conditions are consequences of energy metabolism gone awry – of cellular reduction / oxidation dysfunction. This is as we will discover, the root-cause of all metabolic disease!

This means that before any of these health problems set in, there is/was first a dysfunction in the way cells conduct the business extracting energy out of food, how cells deal with the by-products of this energy reaction, and the degree to which cells are able to maintain their cellular balance.

The factors that affect our cellular environment include nutrition, oxygen status, redox stability, cell communication, radiation, toxicity, stress, infection, and inflammation.

The Deconstruction of The Redox Lifestyle

Due to the nature of how these disease conditions come about, and how the medical establishment deals with them, there is a universal misunderstanding about the nature and course of chronic disease. The problem is not that they cannot be passed from one person to another, it is that these diseases are actually symptoms of underlying metabolic and cellular disorders. What are commonly referred to as "disease" are actually the symptoms of a precursor metabolic disorder. As far as wellness is concerned, this misdirection is a major distraction.

This does not minimize the enormous impact these conditions and symptoms have on individuals and families, nor is this an attempt to malign the well-meaning physicians and institutions that attempt to "treat" them. What it calls for, however, is the need to sharpen the focus on the true root-causes of disease, and to redirect serious attention to where these problems begin.

Notwithstanding the need to be focused on upstream health and risk factors, the "Bigs" (as we will refer to them) have been very successful in 'educating' us that symptoms are disease. Whether intentionally or through 'innocent' ignorance, the "Bigs" treat symptoms as the disease. This has shifted us away from core issues that should constitute true healthcare.

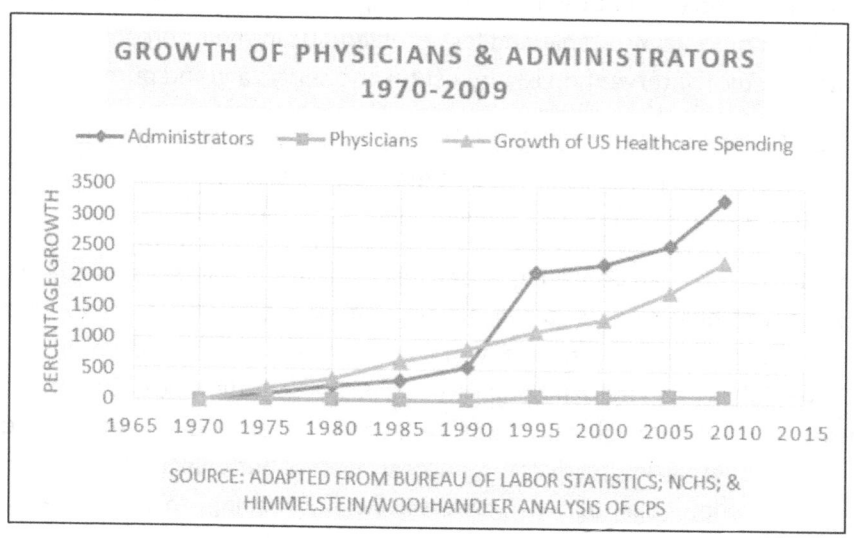

GROWTH OF PHYSICIANS & ADMINISTRATORS 1970-2009

SOURCE: ADAPTED FROM BUREAU OF LABOR STATISTICS; NCHS; & HIMMELSTEIN/WOOLHANDLER ANALYSIS OF CPS

The Deconstruction of The Redox Lifestyle

In addition to the institutional 'Bigs,' common people in the 'real' world also believe the symptoms are the disease. This is what they have been taught. All of this creates a massive re-direct away from important foundational and lifestyle matters that cause true disease.

A complicating factor is when stakeholders are financially benefited from these definitions and distractions which control and regulate the public mindset and professional guidelines. When this happens, it is akin to letting the fox guard the hen house!

The strong convergence of Big Agriculture, Big Food, Big Medicine, Big Pharma ad Big Media, has changed the world of nutrition and healthcare forever. While that may be judged a cynical worldview, it is nonetheless how the world turns on several levels.

The truth is that drugs seldom if ever treat the causes of chronic disease. The defining conditions and assumptions within this statement relate to the definition of the words "treat" and "cause and "disease." Understanding how these three words are used will be the defining thesis of this book and will ultimately determine your understanding of the Redox Lifestyle.

With some rare exceptions (often genetic based) drugs seldom resolve the upstream causes that underlie metabolic disease. However, to their credit they can and do prevent them from spiraling out of control and make living with them more comfortable and less problematic in their outcome. In this regard, medical intervention is very useful and serves a grand purpose.

The better solutions must include dealing with the foundational disorder. This however is difficult to teach and maintain in an era of modern social- and pleasure-eating, and in the enlightened "take-a-pill" culture.

Admittedly, this is a nuanced look at disease, at least by today's standards. Anyone with high blood sugar or elevated blood pressure expects to have good management to prevent worse outcomes. Using medications to achieve stability and to maintain normal levels, is considered treatment and does prevent undesirable outcomes. However, medications are very limited if not completely ineffective for addressing foundational and causative underlying metabolic disease process. Acknowledging this requires a

The Deconstruction of The Redox Lifestyle

significant paradigm shift and in understanding the rules that make cells work.

Our focus here is not on symptom management. It is on the ground-level metabolic disorders that underlie these health problems. These arise from dysfunctions in cellular metabolism related to the effects of how cells metabolize food for energy and cell signaling. The impact of why this matters is witnessed by the fact that chronic metabolic disease represents three-fourths of all diseases and roughly 75% of all disease and healthcare spending.

Accordingly, any discussion of metabolic health must involve how food is converted to energy. This is the definition of energy metabolism. How efficiently food is used as a fuel source determines cellular function, and health. The science of cellular energy metabolism and fuel sourcing is a central and pivotal part of cellular health and redox function.

The "Bigs" would have us believe that food is food! Whether it is processed in factories or comes straight from the garden or pasture, it does not matter. They preach that all food provides the necessary calories and nutrients that keep us powered and nutrified – even if it has to be added to the final food product via 'fortification' or enrichment.

A valid point can be made for such food production practices given the modern world we live in. That can be a debate for a different time. The discussion in this work is about the cellular and biology side of how cells use this food, and especially the effect of this biochemistry. In today's world this has turned into a very messy and convoluted landscape.

There are many points of view and belief systems which are based on differing views of the science, often co-mingled with philosophies that embrace the interests of conflicted stakeholders. Out of these varying ideologies and interpretations –guidelines arise that are meant at least on the surface, to support good health and wellness – but often do not! They too often fall short of what truly constitutes metabolic health.

A main objective of this book is to explore what the science really says about how the body works with regard to energy metabolism and the underlying

The Deconstruction of The Redox Lifestyle

powers of the Redoxome as it operates throughout the redox landscape[5]. Learning how to apply this information for personal benefit, and to create and live a redox lifestyle is a major objective here. As we will show, without this level of operational and functional redox wisdom, we remain trapped in a self-defeating cycle of redox roulette.

While there is abundant debate and public discussion about all-things food, there is little about its effects on the Redoxome. Even food labels that may indicate the packaged food's ingredients say precious little about what is done *to* food, and what happens *to* cells when it is consumed.

The latter point about what it done to food and its effect on us, is about food processing. This includes what is added to or taken away from food as it is prepared for the marketplace. Pointedly, what is missing in the guidelines is the effect processed food has on cells, and how it affects the liver, the gut, the brain, or the redox landscape altogether. (Those would certainly be annoying food labels to most people – probably only slightly more pleasant than tobacco warning labels).

For anyone who believes food is food, they do not understand the effect of processed foods on the body. Food processing matters because it changes food. It is true that food processing (added chemicals, removed fiber, etc.) increases shelf-life, storability, freeze-ability, and 'improves' color and texture and blend-ability and taste. These features take on important roles within the modern agricultural and food production machine. Processing leaves its mark by stripping nutrients and adding agents which are not friendly to liver cells or the gut, and with that it is unkind to our health.

With exceptions that arise from depleted soils, "real food" arrives in its original form as a complete package of nutrition. Plants contain enzymes, co-factors, phytonutrients, antioxidants, minerals, fats, carbohydrates, proteins, and fiber. These are vital for their growth and protection and are beneficial for the humans and animals which consume them.

Plants are the source of all nutrition on the planet. Through photosynthesis they capture the sun's energy and combine it with nutrients obtained from soil and air, and store these in a form that can be eaten and transferred to

The Deconstruction of The Redox Lifestyle

animals and humans. This provides an energy source and for phytochemical nutrition, along with the building blocks for cell repair and survival. Altering this time-honored formula is the root-cause of disease.

(At this point we are not taking sides about plant-based verses non-plant-based nutrition. The upstream origin of how the sun's energy is transferred into our bodies begins with photosynthesis and how vegetative organisms create fats, starches, cellulose, and proteins, and incorporate polyphenols as they grow. This is high in the food chain and all of it passes to those organisms which feed on them.)

Plant-based nutrition from 'real food' is readily available to humans. However, much of it is altered or removed with unkind processing and cooking methods which occur between planting and consumption.

As mentioned above, the reasons for this processing serve many purposes - some good, and some not so much! In addition to those reasons previously cited, are convenience, improved packaging, and shipping, making food for restaurant and 'fast-food' consumption, meeting global and seasonal demands, maintaining cosmetic stability, enhancing taste, and of course optimizing agricultural yields and maximizing commercial profits. The 'bottom-line' for this is that processing affects nutrient levels and adds chemicals to protect against bacteria and pests, and to avoid oxidation (rancidity), and to enhance flavor, aesthetics, palatability, and sweetness.

In today's world what is done to food is given scant consideration. It is rarely mentioned in nutritional guidelines, food channels, cooking shows, or in celebrity diets. The British Medical Journal reported that more than half of the food in Western diets is regrettably 'ultra-processed'[6].

Fast foods are consumed by 37% of adults on any given day[7], frozen and convenience foods are an everyday experience with a microwave used to even make it faster, backyard vegetable gardens are rare and are virtually non-existent in dense urban settings. Almost all meats and dairy are raised, or at least fattened and "finished," in CAFOs (Concentrated Animal Feeding Operations - even if they started off free-range). The New York Times reported that added sugar is used in 60% of the foods found in a typical

The Deconstruction of The Redox Lifestyle

American grocery store[8], and the University of California San Francisco reports it is hiding in 74% of packaged (processed) foods[9]. This holds true for a high number of proclaimed diet products, meal replacement and weight loss programs. While the latter may claim short-term success (in weight) they too often disobey important laws of metabolic cellular health.

If a food product has a food label, then it has been processed, handled, bagged, or boxed, and most often altered, somewhere along its journey from the farm to the home. Processing tampers with nature's antidotes, which are present in 'real' food and help prevent metabolic disease. Antioxidants are removed from foods to make them less bitter, and fructose is added to sweeten them. The removal of nature's remedies and the addition of metabolic poisons impact cell metabolism and redox physiology and perpetuates damage.

"Poisons" may sound like a harsh descriptor as it often implies willful mal intent. While the purposeful use of chemicals and processes are utilized in all the above, the term poison is used here to describe the effect of a process or food additive on specific cellular metabolic pathways. If the resulting effect of their use impairs or harms cell function, then it will be seen as toxic to the cell and organism and is therefore poisonous!

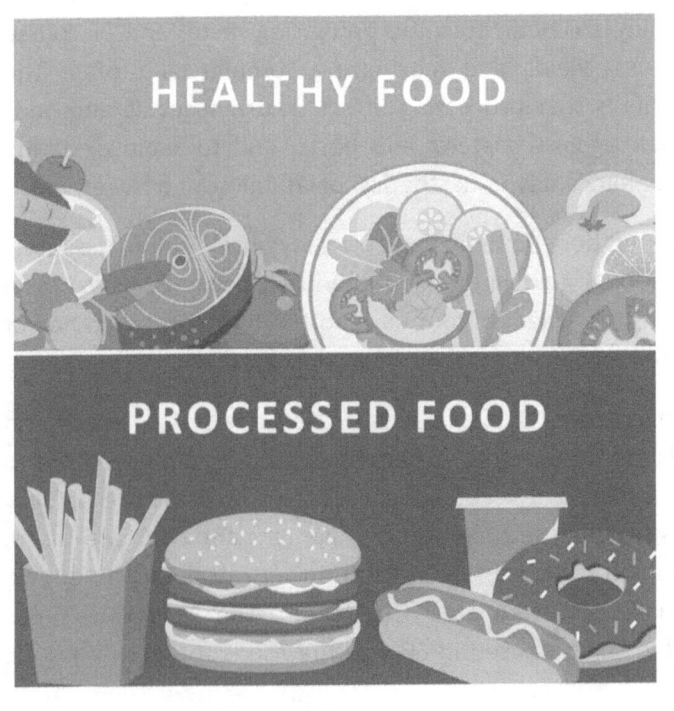

Fructose is a prime example and is one that is rightly receiving

The Deconstruction of The Redox Lifestyle

an increasing amount of attention. It acts in a very harmful manner within the liver cells to create disease and disfunction. There is simply no justification for its use other than to improve profit margins (fructose is sweeter and cheaper than other sugars) and attractiveness (sugar addiction). The most extreme offenders for sugar are the soft-drink industry, along with all processed food producers adding sugar (called "added sugar" on the label) to their packaged food products. [see the appendix for additional information on fructose.]

Removing fiber to increase shelf life and freeze-ability, adding chemicals that inhibit bacterial growth and spoilage, and adding sugars to sweeten food to make it more palatable may create consumer-friendly food, but overall, these processing practices are not cell-friendly, or healthy. Instead, they create problems for the gut and the liver that were largely unknown prior to this modern era of convenience-based food processing. One might argue that it is all part of the modern way of providing more food to an increasing global population, which may or may not be a valid argument, but at what cost?

While processing extends shelf-life and increases food availability, it also alters food which the body has relied on for eons, creating foods that work crossways with how the body is designed to work. And that is the point!

But it hasn't always been that way!

In looking at "yester-years" diet we must acknowledge that whatever those diets were, they existed without the benefit of refrigeration, fast transportation, and modern food science. These "primitive" conditions were the ones which the human body was designed to work with. Throughout history, societies were designed around the availability of food and water, whereas today food and water is designed around the needs, wants, and locations of their citizens - regardless of where or how they live. Through all this history what we can safely assume is that the programming and needs of cellular health and energy metabolism have not changed.

While our knowledge is limited about what life was like in past millennia, we can nonetheless make some general observations that should guide us

The Deconstruction of The Redox Lifestyle

today. The operating premise of this argument is that there is a design written into our cellular blueprint which dictate how cellular health occurs. Anyone and anything that operates outside these rules, is simply wrong – as far as the cell and our health are concerned!

Today we implicate grains as a big health concern, especially for those with GI disorders such as irritable bowel, celiac, and gluten sensitivities. We are concerned about added sugar, the presence or absence of omega-3 oils, and whether food is organic or not. Current culture obsesses over the best diets and exercise for fast fat reduction and new wardrobes, about which herbs work best, and which medications will finally cure and erase chronic disease.

But was it always that way? Think about what your cells know and how they function.

Consider that in past centuries cells were not exposed to herbicides and pesticides. People did not process their grain in a manner to bleach or remove the fiber, protein, bran, oils, and vitamins. Their ground wheat produced whole flour that was nutritionally complete, and the bread made was either non-leavened or prepared with gut-friendly fermentation (sourdough) which dramatically reduced or eliminated the threat of gluten proteins.

All crops were raised with 'real' organic fertilizer and in nutritionally rich soils that were not depleted of their nutrition or microorganisms. Arable farmland was routinely rested and allowed to remain fallow for one or more production cycles to recover and restore organic matter and collect minerals, and to disrupt the lifecycles of pathogens which would otherwise devour their host plants.

Historically, animals were raised on natural grass with high omega 3 containing grass and complete nutrition. They were not fattened for slaughter in grain-fed high-density farming practices. This was true of their dairy products and eggs as well. A chicken's diet was grubs and beetles and natural vegetation (instead of fortified feed pellets).

The Deconstruction of The Redox Lifestyle

All foods in these historical diets were consumed close to where they were farmed or raised because there was no refrigeration, transportation, and food preservation methods. While this may seem like a negative (compared to modern conveniences) it assured that food was nutritious, and whole. Preservation methods would have included healthy practices like fermentation with no added chemicals. Foods were not stripped of fiber, nutrition, or native enzymes. Oils were natural and high in omega 3. There was no "added" unnatural sugar to unduly tax the gut or the liver.

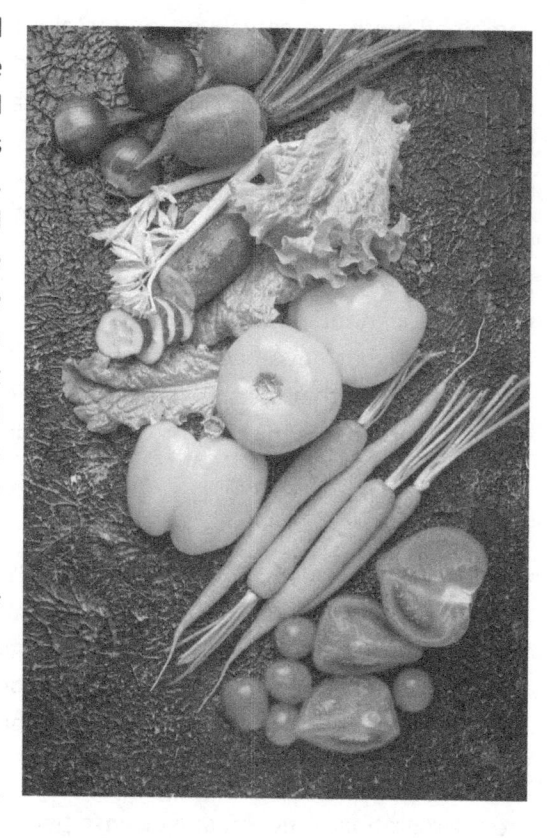

Fast-forward to the present. Today we push these limits in the name of production and outcome, suppressing pathogens and restoring soil nutrition with chemical herbicides and fertilizers. Regardless of the merits, the fact is that cells are not designed with these modifications and amendments in mind.

The grains we utilize today are not the 'same' grains used in previous eras or settings. Today grains are processed into flour and are then made into fiber-poor cereals, bread, flour, cake, crackers, and granola, many with a high glycemic index (boost blood sugar rapidly).

An honest inventory of most food products in modern grocery stores (and certainly any convenience store), finds these processed ingredients are

The Deconstruction of The Redox Lifestyle

combined with preservatives and stabilizers, enriched with synthetic vitamins, and made into a thousand-and-one different foods, mostly prepared for convenience, fast-food applications, portability, longer shelf life, and taste.

Even "cooking from scratch" today generally requires the use of these processed grains, quick-rise yeast, and a variety of other processed ingredients. However, even this is better than frozen waffles or breakfast cereals, doughnuts and pop-tarts, sugared fruit drinks, or any number of other foods that have been put into a package or box with an imprinted "nutrition" label that doesn't come close to informing what was done to the contents, or what is missing, or what is added to it with unpronounceable chemicals.

From the way the food is grown and harvested (pesticides/herbicides/fertilizers), to the way it is handled and recombined and processed for the food marketplace (addition/subtraction), and then finally to the way it is prepared for the end consumer (added chemicals, oil fryers, high heat) - the food we consume today is a far cry from what our bodies and its trillions of cells were designed to function. And therein lies the problem!

From a metabolic function and disease perspective, this is the point!

From a health point of view food that is unreasonably processed becomes adulterated and has a profound effect on how the gut and the liver process and metabolize it. This has profound implications for cellular and intestinal health – and for the family and national budget.

While we acknowledge the modern agricultural and food processing realities that exist today, we must lament and resist the changes (at least at a personal level) which have occurred over the decades resulting in the degradation of our food supply. In a practical sense we must concede that at the broad institutional and cultural level this battle has forever been lost. Without returning to a higher standard, and without top-level reform to change farming, agricultural, and food processing standards to align with cellular health principles (unlikely), and without improved education to

The Deconstruction of The Redox Lifestyle

inform the public about the dangers of food manipulation (also highly unlikely), and without incentives for nutritional health practices and policies (quickly vetoed) - it is a very long bet that anything will change anytime soon!

Therefore, the answer must rest squarely with the individual and the family. Personal responsibility must be taken to be educated and practiced in higher quality food production, shopping, preparation, and better dietary strategies and lifestyle habits. Otherwise, the collective societal drumbeat will remain overpowering and remain suspect – even if the guidelines and the Bigs were well intentioned.

While this viewpoint may appear overly sour, it is nonetheless true that modern society does in fact march to a new 'drummer'! Big Media is in it for the clickbait and ad revenue. Big Agriculture and Big Food are in it for their monopoly in food production. Big Pharma is in it to treat the metabolic disease that arises from poor lifestyles. And Big Government profits from taxation, control, and regulatory lobbying from all the above. Perhaps that is a jaundiced view. The reader may decide on their own. However, if denied, or even only partially true, there is a lot of explaining needed to dismiss these modern realities.

What is certain is that this new nutritional playing field creates opportunities for all sides, both good and bad. This creates a rich environment for, and leads to, the raging diet wars, 'fad' diets, and niche nutrition ideologies. It even sets conflicting (and conflicted) experts against each other, all lobbying for or presenting their highest authority to establish their cause. Unfortunately, much of it is based on hotly contested opinion and half-truth misinformation and is secured upon a grounding of commercial profit.

It is the profit motive aspect that especially benefits vested stakeholders in the marketplace - each championed by a nutritional or fitness guru, celebrity physician or 'Hollywood' endorsement, acclaimed science center, or whatever. Each one is driven by a different philosophical approach, ideological grounding, and varied scientific approach. Few of them are based on foundational principles of cellular redox biology and the full picture of nutritional biochemistry and energy metabolism.

The Deconstruction of The Redox Lifestyle

While our earlier ancestors and progenitors weren't as knowledgeable about cellular biology and nutritional redox biochemistry as we are today, there is no question that they were 'on to something' in how their bodies related to existing fuel and nutrition sources of the day. They obviously were missing many elements of sophisticated nutrition science and had variable access to food choices through each year, but those are the conditions for which their bodies and our bodies have been adapted to exist in – including the lean times when food wasn't as plentiful, or food sourcing had to change.

Their health and mortality problems revolved around public health, sanitation, clean water, infection, and accidents. Human longevity then was nowhere like today, and everyone can agree that modern medicines, public health, and better healthcare are to credit. However, it is hard to argue that from a cellular health standard, the refined, processed, chemically laden foods we "enjoy" today are superior to the foods they 'enjoyed.'

The existence of metabolic disease then was nothing compared to the rising rates modern humankind has experienced in the last half century. Historically, redox lifestyles were richly rewarded with quality nutrition, balanced energy metabolism, physical activity, sunshine, and lean times – features sadly missing with today's more 'enlightened' lifestyles which deny us of the ketosis, autophagy, and redox-sensitive properties of yesterday's redox-friendly lifestyle.

To be clear, this isn't to say that issues like diabetes, cancer, and heart disease were not present in past centuries. What we're calling out is the abrupt change in incidence of metabolic disease beginning in the mid-20th century along with the changes made in food processing which parallel the establishment of a processed food-science industry.

While this may sound negative, fatalistic, or even conspiratorialist in its approach and thinking, it is important to not overlook that the discussion here is on cellular function and how the body uses food for fuel and nutrition and redox signaling. This is a discussion about cellular and metabolic health in the real world of the Redoxome and how the foods we eat fuel and signal the body.

The Deconstruction of The Redox Lifestyle

The take-home message is that not all 'food' is food! Real food is food! Real food is the kind that plays by the rules of healthy cellular energy production, healthy redox gene expression, and the cellular "repair and replace" mechanisms – all of which are the subjects of this book. Any abuse of 'real food' and of the redox lifestyle landscape lays the groundwork for cellular dysfunction and disease. This is our focus.

The important paradigm shift is that the body needs to be fed and treated like the physiologic machine it is - and not with what makes brain-reward centers and food handlers happy, in the shortest time possible.

Knowing the rules of nutritional health and redox biology and how cells are programed to utilize food for energy, matters. This awareness enables better decisions and practices which support health. In this way the advantage can be gained against all the forces that rob our health, because how health can be reverse engineered back to what's best for the human cellular engine.

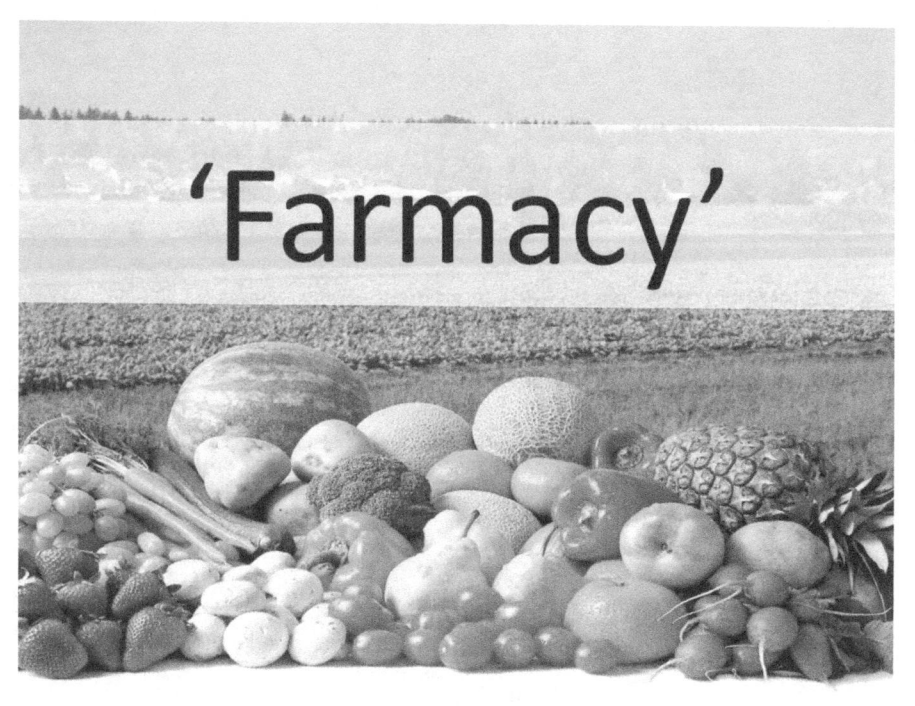

The Deconstruction of The Redox Lifestyle

Fortunately, we are now at a place where redox-based nutrition can even be discussed intelligently. The science is coming in!

A central organizing thesis of this book is that metabolic diseases, as a class, are not "drugable." However, they are "foodable!" That is because they are a part of the *redox interactome*. Translated, this means they are responsive to and can stress-adapt to redox-sensitive stimuli provided through nutritional strategy, improved lifestyle, and with supplementation. If you want to avoid sick, there is no other way.

This is about choice! And better choices require better information, and better information means sorting through the many voices of confusion and knowing what questions to ask.

We go there next.

Dietary Advice

Dietary Advice

Change Your Food. Change Your Life!

But how?

So far, we have discussed the immense challenges that work against anyone in the modern age wanting to redesign their life around redox-based nutrition principles. However, it is true that if we change our food and activity level, we can change our life! In a world filled with conflicting advice and full of processed food and convenience at every turn, how can this be accomplished? Whose advice should be followed, and at what cost?

Because of the uphill slope, converting to a redox-based lifestyle can be harder than it looks on the surface. That is why having a good working understanding of the principles that drive health are so empowering. Choices that support change are rooted in better information. Without knowing the operating rules for health, it is much easier to get taken in with false and misleading information, and to succumb to habits and hormone mis regulation that drive disease.

With even a modest grasp of the rules of the cell, the areas of food, exercise, gut and oral health, sleep, stress, and supplementation become much easier to navigate. It's like having a personal copy of the "owner's manual" as a reference guide in your back pocket.

Since metabolic health and a redox healthy life are so tightly tied together with diet and nutrition, it is reasonable and wise to address this issue head-on. However, what makes this problematic is the fact that there exists a multitude of different diets, nutrition facts, interest groups, regulatory bodies, and profit centers that have to be sorted through to come to the "truth" for any given person – let alone for what is true at the cellular health level.

A good basis for knowing what nutrition truth is, is to compare available recommendations and advice against nature's standard for how cells function in the body. There is as it turns out, a redox standard, and these rules are not bend-able! Even if you are a celebrity endorser, or a popular

Dietary Advice

physician spokesperson, or have a deliciously wonderful diet to sell or follow or think that your style of exercise is the best, it does not matter. If cellular health rules are not followed, health is shortchanged.

One of the reasons why there are so many diets, and exercise and health programs, is that most of them don't work. For a reason! They are sabotaged from the beginning because they are not founded and grounded on the cellular rules of energy metabolism, nutritional ketosis, hormesis, autophagy, redox signaling, and appropriate supplementation.

This is why we will give so much attention to the science that is the basis for energy metabolism in the Redoxome. A good dietary and lifestyle strategy should be based on how food affects cellular function. This is a different standard from whether it tastes good, or what hunger hormones are demanding, or what works in social and family budgets, or even what the health authorities of the day are saying.

With a better working knowledge of the "rules," it becomes easier to see the agenda of "the Bigs" and to counter those forces with informed decisions and actions. Health truth should not be based on a food processors or supplier's profit margin (Big Food), or upon what works for medical business concerns (Big Medicine and Big Pharma), or upon media voices paid to create and protect the marketplace (Big Media), nor upon regulatory controls which claim to protect the best interests of others (Big Gov and Big Insurance).

The real "Big" that ought to be considered first is "Big Metabolism" – yours!

Recognizing real nutrition truth requires learning to recognize what is not true. This includes half-truths, strawman arguments, obfuscated 'facts,' twisted or false logic, distractions and 'red herrings,' the vested interests of the "Bigs," and more. Knowing redox-based nutrition and health principles enables a person to better judge and sort through the confusing cacophony that is everywhere present.

To illustrate this point, consider the following list of readily available health advice that is sampled from an assortment of nutrition experts, physician councils, medical associations, and government agencies - and represent

Dietary Advice

nutritional and health "best practices." As you read through this list, evaluate what you presently judge to be good and bad advice. [Author commentary and questions are inside brackets.] Understand that this list of nutrition advice comes from our 'real-world' marketplace available from today's nutrition, medical, and government sources readily available online. This advice is conveyed through 'authoritative' websites, diet experts, and from numerous health and nutrition guideline.

- There is plenty of healthy nutrition in the normal average diet. [What is a 'normal' or 'average' diet? Why is there so much illness in people eating a normal and otherwise adequate diet?]
- There is no need to take vitamin supplements if you eat a good diet. [What is a 'good' diet? Who or what decides the right level of vitamins in a diet? Do vitamin levels that prevent deficiency (RDAs) also assure optimal health? Does 'good' food contain all necessary vitamins?]
- Eat breakfast [Inadequate information. What kind?]
- Cells don't know the difference between nutrition-based chemicals. (Synthetic vitamins) and those found in natural food sources [Vitamins and phytochemicals come packaged in nature for a reason.]
- Eat more protein if you want to grow strong bodies and stay healthy. [How much? What does 'grow strong' mean? How does protein, as opposed to other macronutrients, prevent disease?]
- Keto diet pills are just as effective as keto diets. [Can I eat anything I want as long as I take keto diet pills? Can I safely take diet pills 24/7/365 – ongoing as a way of life? Is this better than following a diet of keto-based real food?]
- Eat good snacks and bad snacks. [What is a good snack? How will this effect energy metabolism, blood sugar levels, fat burning, and metabolic health?]
- Cut down on processed foods. [That is good, but why not eliminate processed foods? If I only 'cut down,' what effect will those processed foods I do eat still have on cell metabolism and inflammation? How do any processed foods affect the liver and intestine?]

Dietary Advice

- Don't starve yourself. [Does this mean I should always be in a "fed" state?]
- Don't shop for groceries when you are hungry. [Why be hungry in the first place? Is there a diet that prevents hunger hormones? Can my nutrition awareness counter-balance hungry driven shopping?]
- Always count calories. [Why? Can I always do this as a rule 24/7/365? Will knowing my number improve my health? Does this assume caloric restriction, and if so, will I ever tire of feeling starved – especially if I don't limit carbs?]
- Limit sugar. [What kind? What does 'limit' mean? How much is too much?]
- Use sugar substitutes and artificial sweeteners. [Aren't there better ways to manage blood sugar levels and so-called 'empty calories? What effect does artificial sugars have on cell metabolism, inflammation, brain cells, liver health, and gut health?]
- Diet beverages are better. [Then what? And why? Are artificial sugars healthy?]
- Avoid added sugar. [Good advice on the surface. Does food with "no added sugar" automatically make it healthy? What if the food is still processed processed?]
- Eat low-fat. [What effect does a high-carb diet have on metabolic disease? If not eating fat, are processed carbs, okay?]
- Eat protein to decrease hunger pangs between meals. [How much is safe for kidney function? How does protein affect ghrelin hormone? Why not eat healthy fat which does this better?]
- Eat fats to decrease hunger pangs between meals. [Good, but what kind of fats? Can I eat carbs at the same time? Are bad fats, okay?]
- Don't cut out carbs – eat more vegetables. [It is misleading to assume that eating a low-carb diet means not eating vegetables and fruit. Fiber-rich carbs fit into low-carb diet.]
- Drink fat-free milk; eat low-fat dairy products. [Why? Do healthy fats help balance macronutrients and promote ketosis?]
- Don't skip meals. [Why not? Intermittent fasting improves metabolic health, and it can be done w/o hunger.]

Dietary Advice

- Drink plenty of water. [Good advice, but incomplete info. What kind? How much?]
- Fat burning diets do not work. [Incomplete info. Why not? What kind?]
- Enjoy all foods in moderation. There is no such thing as "bad" food, only expired food. (Really? What is 'moderation'? Literally - are 'all' foods good? And the definition of bad food is when it exceeds its 'use-by' date?]
- Maintain a ratio of 25:15:60 percent in fat:protein:carbs. [Is this grams? Calories? Since carbs are metabolized first if present, will dietary fat ever be metabolized or just stored? How does the body handle excess carbs?]
- Avoid anything that had a mother or a face. [A no-animal or vegan / vegetarian diet is okay metabolically as long as protein mix is sufficient and refined carbs are low or none, and oils/fats are healthy. Energy and redox metabolism cares about the relative ratio of fats, proteins, and carbs; less about their source.]
- Eat plant based. [Incomplete info. Oreo cookies and corn and potato chips, and all refined carbs and processed oils, are 'plant-based.' That doesn't make them metabolically healthy!]
- Eat a carnivore diet. [How much protein is too much for kidneys? Does this imply no vegetables? Is omnivore more descriptive? Effective if done right, this requires much discipline, education, and frequent testing to manage.]
- Clean your plate – people in China are starving. [Mom's advice! The supposed ethics of not wasting food ignores the impact on human health for over-consumption beyond metabolic needs.]
- Eat only until till you're full. [What does 'full' mean? Full of what types of food? Processed foods? How much is too much?]
- Only eat until you are satisfied. [Does this include the consumption of refined and processed foods? Is the primary concern about satiety?]
- Manage "Hangry" – tolerate hunger. [Good advice, but how? We've been 'educated' that candy bars solve being 'hangry.' Is it possible to not be in a "fasted" state and not feel hunger?]

Dietary Advice

- Fat-loss pills are a good way to lose weight. [Stimulants ramp up metabolism unnaturally. Cannot sustain this 24/7/365? And without lifestyle changes?]
- Understand the process of fat adaptation and carb addiction. [Good advice as being metabolically flexible leads to metabolic health.]

This sampling of dietary advice presents a few good principles, but most of it contains inaccurate and incomplete information made available by popular and well-known voices of authority. The fact that this advice is so quickly accepted demonstrates the power of these voices and perhaps how willing the public is to accept it without question.

The point is that what is prepared and presented by the "experts" is broadly accepted by consumers with little investigation or knowledge of how cells function or maintain health. One's ability to evaluate nutrition advice and judge it by the cell's standards is a function of how knowledgeable a person is in matters related to redox biology and their own metabolic health. Self-education is key.

Without further education it is impossible to know the mechanisms and effects on health, of: low-carb, low-fat, high-fat, high-carb, high-protein, plant-based, carnivore, vegan, fasting, exercise, processed food, organic, good fat vs bad fat, refined carb vs complex carb, high glycemic or low glycemic, caloric restriction diets, meal replacements, muscle building diets, smoothies, nutrition bars, juices and juicing, brain health nutrition, gut-friendly diets, added sugar, artificial sweeteners, soda pop, alcohol, agricultural herbicides, probiotics, prebiotics, shifting standards and guidelines, and on and one.

Which is best? Plant-based? Vegan? Vegetarian? Zone? Keto? Atkins? Fasting? Carnivore? Religious oriented? Low fat? High fat? DNA Personalized? Weight loss? Muscle building? Organic? Caloric restriction?

Without further education and public awareness, it becomes difficult to sort through the guidelines, commercial advertising, and the myriad of diets available in the marketplace – all of which promises to be our friend. In

Dietary Advice

today's day and age, if you expect to be metabolically healthy, it is very important to know your enemies!

[For further analysis of the good and bad advice common in the marketplace and especially given by "knowledgeable experts," see appendix "Nutrition Philosophy and Science"]

This begs the real question: Is it possible to have a diet that is kind to the liver and brain, friendly to the gut, improves digestion, provokes, and stimulates fat metabolism, reduces inflammation, enhances the immune system, creates metabolic flexibility, improves insulin sensitivity, manages satiety and hunger hormones, regulates blood sugar levels, keeps blood pressure and cholesterol under control, and is kind to the brain, and facilitates health - across the wide Redoxome landscape?

And if so, where does this health and nutrition information exist? If redox-based nutrition is so important, how is it that there isn't (yet) a mainstream swell with millions of voices pointing to these standards?

If anything has been learned so far, it should be that what we are doing isn't working! Admittedly, nutrition is not the most alluring or captivating subject. However, next to oxygen, it is by far the most essential aspect of our lives! If it is ignored or done contrary to the rules that govern cellular health, there are great penalties attached - often not experienced or suffered for years. This is why knowing the rules and following them is so critical.

In the process of knowing what works best, it is helpful to understand what nutrition philosophies do not work for health. And why!

Dietary Philosophies: The Good. The Bad. The Ugly.

Dietary Philosophies: The Good. The Bad. The Ugly.

Our level of nutrition awareness and our relationship with food greatly impacts how we choose a diet that is right. Should it be that hard?

Which diets are bad? Which diets are good? And does it really matter?

Beyond 'the diet,' the problem extends to food shopping, preparation, the timing of eating, the amount and type of snacking, soft- and hard-beverage consumption, what restaurants are frequented, and so much more. It even extends to a having an informed strategy for dealing with stress, emotional eating, food in social settings, and supplementation.

The competing philosophies surrounding food and nutrition spark intense debates that too often do disservice to the discussion of real health. Many points of advice and guidance are well intentioned but are not based in redox biology. At best they are confusing, and at worst they are simply wrong.

Much is based on now outdated science that occurred before the redox landscape was discovered, and/or uses study protocols that incorporate wrong assumptions into their control groups and conclusions. Unfortunately, there is much that is also influenced by the vested interests of the "Bigs"!

In almost every case, the "diet and nutrition wars" are fought over turf that is either not grounded in science, or so misrepresents the science that it makes the battles irrelevant - except for the mass casualties they produce. Many are simply ignorant of or are unwilling to acknowledge the effects of their advice on redox status and cellular function. This means they fail to address the most glaring violations and abuses of cellular health – which is the impacts they have on liver and gut health, energy metabolism and their effect, or lack thereof, on redox stability.

Examples of this come from both sides of the vegetarian debate with each side justifying and using processed foods. Notwithstanding the emphasis on whole vegetables, both vegetarian and omnivore diets can be, and often

Dietary Philosophies: The Good. The Bad. The Ugly.

are, filled with processed foods. The same is true for both organic and non-organic foods.

To stretch that point, cookies, potato chips, and junk food can now be green, sustainable, renewable, pesticide-free, dolphin-safe, whole-grain, free-range, certified, natural, and earth-friendly! Potato chips are now organic and baked – but they are nothing like the original food they started as! Despite their supposed social, environmental, and health-virtues, few if any are gut-healthy, nor do they protect the liver, or support or improve cellular metabolic health! And that's the point! All of the aforementioned dietary practices can and do include processed foods – and many do so without 'batting an eye' of concern for how their brand of 'virtuous food,' meal replacements, or flash-in-the pan diets affect the mitochondria and the Redoxome.

The predominant diet and nutrition advice in the popular media and professional circles has a fixation on losing weight. The vast majority of the popular advice written up in the alluring magazines next to the grocery store's checkout counter seldom if ever deal with metabolic health (despite their headlines). It is all about weight loss in one shape or another (pun intended). This is readily observed in nearly every weight-loss program, device, pill, herbal formula, and diet program available. And nearly all of the science they claim to be founded on is irrelevant, faulty, or misapplied. Why – because they do not understand or obey the rules of metabolic health and how a cell works at the redox level! This witnesses the industry's commitment for what sells, and their collective lack of focus on what matters (intentional or otherwise).

The 'weightier' considerations, the ones that have more gravity and health-related importance (regardless of the dietary persuasion one wishes to live in) have to do with how foods impact energy metabolism within the redox environment, and how they impact the liver and the gut. These concerns do not always align with what tastebuds, hunger hormones, and brain neurochemistry demand, nor what is socially fashionable, or that which fits the diet-of-the-month club.

Dietary Philosophies: The Good. The Bad. The Ugly.

True dietary health is about metabolic health. Therefore, the best diet is a metabolic diet. It is first and foremost concerned with the effect on mitochondrial and cellular function. This means it follows the rules of a healthy cellular blueprint. Good diets protect metabolic function, energy metabolism, and redox signaling, first and foremost - not obesity concerns.

From a metabolic perspective, placing weight loss, or satiety, or blood sugar, or blood lipids, or blood pressure as the dominant objective is the 'tail wagging the dog.' Obesity and the other metabolic 'symptoms,' as a rule, follow metabolic health.

Accordingly, from a metabolic diet perspective, what matters most is having the right metabolic diet and redox lifestyle. This is about having the right mixture of metabolic fuels (proteins, fats, and carbohydrates), supplied in proper amounts, and consumed with optimal timing. It includes phytochemicals and antioxidants, vitamins, enzymes, and fiber.

As importantly, a metabolic diet is also about what should not be consumed – which is processed, adulterated, changed, refined, enriched, highly heated, overly sugared, and fiber-poor "food."

A metabolically sound diet respects the liver, the gut, the energy metabolism systems, and the redox signaling properties of a cell.

What matters is consuming "Real Food!" That is what cells were designed to feed and fuel on.

The principles of metabolic health has been around for eons. Nature figured this out long ago. What is different now is the effect of the modern diet and modern food production methodologies on health. This has changed everything!

When considering the good, the bad, and the ugly as it relates to a nutrition and diets, the guiding philosophies should be aligned with the rules that are universally programmed into the genetic blueprints of our cells. This is true regardless of the name of the diet or which celebrity or 'authority' endorsement it has, or how they have 'worked' for a friend. If the favored

Dietary Philosophies: The Good. The Bad. The Ugly.

diet does not enhance cellular balance and healthy cellular renewal, it is not favoring metabolic health.

The intent of this book is to present these rules in a principled manner so that better decisions can be made. An educated and informed mind is free to choose because it knows the options and the reasons. Without this information, one is left at the mercy of outside influences, as well as the 'inside influencers' such as habit, tastebuds, and compulsive hunger.

The good news is that there are basic changes in one's redox lifestyle that can be made which follow cellular rules and provide better outcomes. Even amidst heavily promoted and even biased information, you can learn to discern and interpret and choose and not be fooled with misinformation.

As this health and nutrition paradigm shifts in your mind, you will discover that the all-important considerations are not about whether one is vegan or vegetarian, plant-based, carnivore, omnivore, low-fat, organic, or whatever. It is about whether cellular rules for metabolic health are being followed. The specific diet strategies that obey these rules, will become apparent.

To be healthy, the only "dogmatic" rules that should be followed are those set by nature itself; not from the ever-changing guidelines and mal-alignments of vested interests and regulators – or those guided by your tastebuds and hormones!

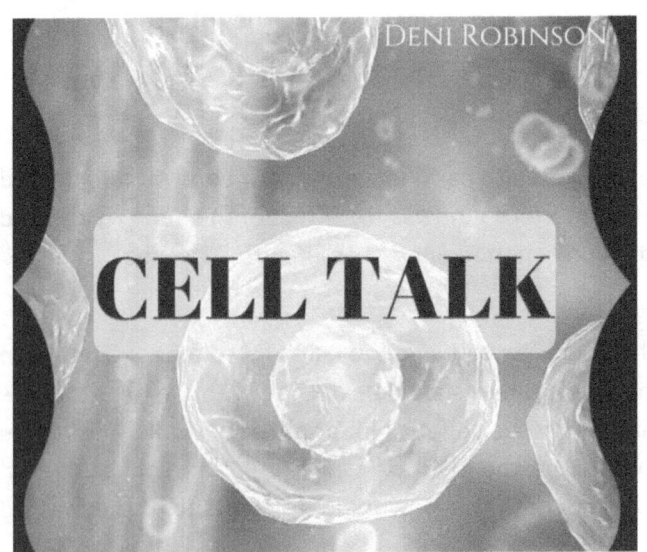

The truth is that our bodies benefit best with Real Food - whole food nutrition, untainted, nutritionally rich,

Dietary Philosophies: The Good. The Bad. The Ugly.

and which follow the rules of healthy energy metabolism and native redox signaling.

A quick way to begin seeing significant improvement in cellular health and function is to begin with redox supplementation. Jump start redox-based activation for all of your cellular health processes by quickly replenishing the mild oxidative state that characterizes all healthy lifestyle practices.

Eliminate processed foods and refined, fiber-poor grains. Cut out all sugared and carbonated beverages. (Do not drink your calories. Water is good!) A good place to start is to simply to eliminate fructose and "added sugars" in any and all packaged foods. Just stop! This is a "low-hanging-fruit" approach to begin making massive changes in metabolic health quickly.

Change the way you relate to food and think about it when you are grocery shopping. Become educated about what this means and how to shop and prepare food differently. Menu plan and restaurant plan a shift toward "real foods" which are packaged with nature's antidotes and redox stimulating properties. Increase vegetables and fruits which provide a hormetic stimulus that is nature's form of redox stimulation.

Then gradually layer other redox-sensitive health strategies such as fasting, ketosis and low-carb cycling, exercise, and other redox-based strategies (that will be discussed later) - as much as possible.

Avoid and don't be deceived by so-called 'healthy' diets that promise quick this or that - such as quick weight loss, flat abs, fat-burning, and the list goes on. Basically, anything that is headlined or featured on a magazine cover or inside the many health channels now available. It isn't that you can't quickly lose weight, but you want to do so in a metabolically healthy way.

If you want to change your life, change your lifestyle. Begin eating and exercising like your redox biology demands.

While the truth can be blunt, it is refreshingly liberating! And it will save your life!

This is the redox lifestyle way!

Dietary Philosophies: The Good. The Bad. The Ugly.

Before we launch into the principles of metabolic health directly, let's discuss diets in a more direct manner. We will begin to weave into this presentation certain metabolic rules that will be expanded upon in later sections.

Structured Diets

Structured Diets

Giving an overview of specific diets at this juncture and discussing their metabolic effect on metabolic health may be premature but will begin to set the stage relative to the overall strategies for developing a healthy redox lifestyle. Upon completion of this book, with a fuller grasp of metabolic health, it may be helpful to come back and review this section. This will be a good exercise as you combine and synthesize the rules of the cell together with dietary and lifestyle approaches that have as their primary result, improved metabolic health. This will be helpful, because it seems that all most people really want to know is what specific diet should they follow. "Tell me what to do and I'll do it!"

Before reviewing specific diets, it would be well to mention the prevailing reasons most people cite for "dieting," which would be to lose weight, look nicer, get into smaller clothes, etc. These 'outward' reasons are far distanced from the reality of the value of real dieting, being metabolic health.

Nonetheless, the prevailing model in the dieting and weight loss world is that energy expenditure must equal or exceed energy intake. These are the glaring headlines on every fitness and health-related magazine.

This model of "calories in – calories out' (CICO) emphasizes the importance of reduced caloric intake and increased caloric expenditure. This is achieved through portion control, meal replacement, eating a lot of salads and low-calorie food, frequent eating to minimize the effect of hunger hormones, and increased exercise and physical activity to "burn" calories.

This CICO model also emphasizes the importance of maintaining dietary carbohydrate intake due to the small storage capacity in the body for carbohydrates (glucose and glycogen). This accepted orthodoxy generally holds that carbohydrates are the primary and most important source for energy metabolism in the body, and therefore carbohydrate intake must be maintained at reasonable if not a high and steady levels to maintain energy and to avoid runaway hunger hormones that lead to more energy intake.

Many justify this carb-friendly posture in order to maximize vegetables and fruits with their associated fiber and phytochemicals, suggesting that if they

Structured Diets

eat less carbs, it will deprive the body from needed nutrition (an interesting half-truth that is often reflected in the base assumptions of 'leading' science studies biased against protein- and fat-leaning diets). [See Appendix for more analysis on "diet science."]

Caloric restriction by itself can and does often drive down available glucose levels to the point that fat and proteins must be metabolized to survive. In these states, protein is also utilized through gluconeogenesis to produce the necessary glucose fuel, with resulting weight loss not always coming from fat storage. The question almost categorically unanswered is – is it metabolically healthy? Also, more practically, can it be sustained?

This dietary and weight loss philosophy is very simplistic. It argues that since fat equals 3,500 kcal per pound, which tipping the balance to 3,500 less calories would equal one pound of fat (weight) loss. Thus, 500 less calories per day for a week equals roughly a pound of weigh lost per week. Do this for ten weeks and ten pounds and a dress size is reduced! It obviously assumes that everything else in life is equal and controlled. Simple!

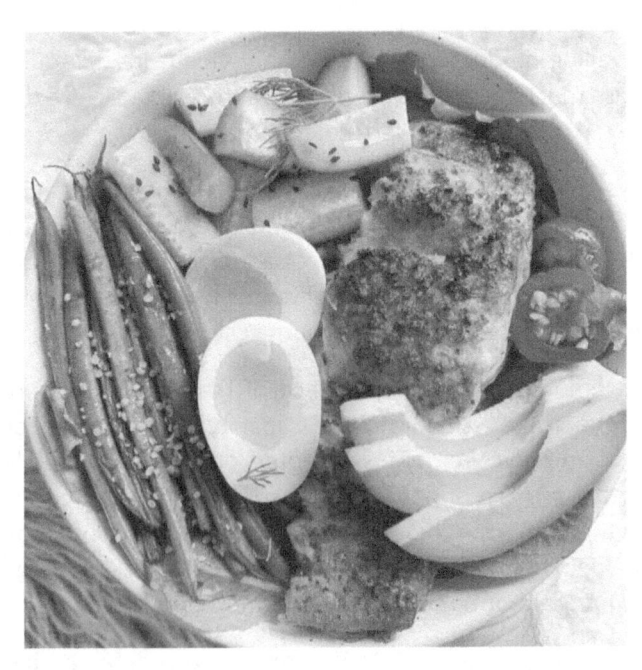

The problem with this, and the reason why it is so polarizing, is that the calories-in calories-out model overlooks many important variables in the metabolic energy equation. The human body is an energy system and rarely conforms to such simplistic energy equations. There are simply too many variables. It is very dynamic.

Structured Diets

If this simple model of CICO were correct, it begs many questions: Why people lose more weight with keto or low-carb diets? Why can some people eat "whatever they want" and never gain weight, while others restrict their eating and still gain weight over time? Why can't people with poor thyroid or pituitary function easily lose weight when eating very few calories? Why do we gain weight as we age, even when eating and exercising the same as always? How do we explain weight-loss plateaus? What effect does high-carb low calorie food have on insulin levels (or insulin supplementation if diabetic)? What is better, low carb or low calorie?

Multiple factors affect the "calories in – calories out" model and include:

- Carbohydrate: timing, frequency, quantity, refined, complex
- Exercise: ability, intensity, duration, frequency, type, etc.
- Sleep: autophagy ability, rest and recovery, systemic inflammation from apnea
- Sodium: intake and metabolism
- Metabolic disease: insulin resistance, polycystic ovary syndrome, fatty liver, etc.
- Medications: pharmacokinetics of drug metabolism and underlying metabolic disease
- Hormones: thyroid, catecholamines, steroids, cortisol
- Oils: dietary omega 3, processed
- Intestinal health: absorption, inflammation, leaky gut, calories absorbed
- Food: energy and nutrient density, social habits, calories absorbed
- Beverage: sweetened, fructose, etc.
- Appetite: hormone regulation
- Assessment: discrepancy of actual caloric intake

To the last point, a landmark study found a broad reaching discrepancy between actual calories consumed and expended, over what is counted or reported[10].

The "eat less move more" model is a significant oversimplification of what is really happening in the body at the metabolic and cellular level, and one which demands attention or metabolic consideration of the many moving variables in the equation.

Structured Diets

On the other hand, a cycling keto diet (see below) increases fats with modest amounts of protein and increases satiety with reduced appetite. It eliminates highly processed calories and foods that would be "legal" in a CICO diet. Drinking calories is greatly lessened with reduction of sugared, or artificially sweetened beverages, or fruit drinks with no fiber. Elevated ketone levels provide an energy-efficient fuel and help to suppress appetite. Autophagy and redox signaling are increased. These are all healthy metabolic features that will be analyzed in greater depth in the following sections.

To be sure, caloric restriction does reduce weight, just like outright starvation causes people in 3rd world conditions to be skinny. But it isn't healthy!

As you sort through these various diet strategies, or even those you are presently following or considering, do so with the thought in mind of whether or not they are supporting metabolic health within the redox landscape. It is a poor tradeoff to lose weight and not improve metabolic and redox health and be miserable in the process!

There are several diets that have gained particular attention and even notoriety over the decades because of their observed effect within their respective groups and/or locations. These deserve at least a passing mention. Understanding the principles of redox biology and energy metabolism as we do, it is easier to understand the good effects and outcomes of these stratified strategies and explain better why and how they work as well as that they do. (It should also inform us about other types of diets which do not follow these same principles and help us understand why they are not healthy or effective).

As a general rule, many of these diets are plant-based or focused, and as such would be expected to have higher levels of plant polyphenols, and come from fiber-rich sources – i.e., "real food." Being "plant-based" is not necessarily the same as a carbohydrate diet. Said differently, being carb-based does not necessarily mean that there are abundant vegetables and fruits (in that order of importance) in the diet. One can eat "plant-based" and still eat high amounts of processed grains with poor nutritional quality.

Structured Diets

Notwithstanding, many of the time-honored diet strategies and 'formulas' are on the whole successful for a reason, and most of these 'time-honored' eating practices are dated from decades and centuries ago. Processing and refinement and 'enrichment' was not a part of their food supply until recent times.

As such, the "strategies" were their normal everyday diet due to few other options. This means that their food was "real food," high in fiber, rich in phytochemicals, rich in omega 3, eaten close to points of food production (even the back yard or family farm), and meats and animal protein consumed were also benefited because of their free-range and pastured livestock methods.

"Back in the day" these population groups ate food native to their surroundings, and often did not have plentiful abundance of food, meaning they experienced stress-adaptation and hormesis effects that increased their metabolic health and cellular function. Metabolic disease did not enter the picture in any significant degree until food processing methods began to alter the food.

In a generic sense, the focus for good eating rules must be measured against the standards of metabolic health – how the cell 'thinks. Is the diet pro-inflammatory or anti-inflammatory? Does it create oxidation or suppress oxidation? Does it take advantage of hormesis and periodically create ketotic metabolic adaptability, or is it predominately otherwise?

The standard for healthy diets should be set within the cellular parameters of metabolic health, not whether it causes weight loss. Yet as pointed out earlier, the latter is the dominant focus of the media, food, and medical establishments. Any and nearly every magazine or diet and health book focuses on weight loss and available energy. They focus on exercise to burn calories, build body form, and give scant attention to the effects of high-carb and processed food's effect on cellular metabolism and redox signaling. Rarely will you find these words or concepts bundled together in leading health magazines, health guidelines, health cookbooks, etc.

Structured Diets

In the following review, be mindful that the pervasive threads and impacts of food processing has infiltrated and interwoven themselves into each one of these dietary strategies, which fundamentally changes them over time. Early vegetarian-based diets or those with emphasis on whole-foods and plant-based consumption, have been subverted and sabotaged from their original intent, and those now following them often find themselves in no better health than their contemporary neighbors. This is witnessed in the disease and health statistics that show a much narrower spread today than yester-year, in isolated or ideologically stratified population groups (easier to study) such as Seventh-day Adventists and members of the Church of Jesus Christ of Latter-day Saints – comparing their past and present population groups. This is due to the adoption of modern food processing and moving away from the original metabolic-rich standards of their earliest guidance.

These two religious-based groups make reasonably good study populations because there is reasonably good coherence and solidity through their respective church membership, to ascribe to and follow specific dietary rules they set forth. This would not be unlike other religious faith groups and their dietary proscriptions such as Jewish, Hindu, Muslim, and so forth.

Their faith orientation helps congeal together a higher level of compliance through their varied congregants. Notable universities sponsored by their respective churches, such as Loma Linda and Brigham Young University, each respectively produce research[11] that provides data which demonstrates the efficacy of their health guidelines.

What follows is a brief outline and overview of diets, notable population groups and their dietary standards and strategies, and other diet philosophies that have gained some acclaim, beginning with these two mentioned religious groups.

7th Day Adventist Diet:

The Seventh-day Adventist diet is a plant-based vegetarian diet, rich in whole foods and excludes most animal products, alcohol, and caffeinated beverages. Some within this group choose to expand those standards with

Structured Diets

low-fat dairy, eggs, and certain amounts of meats or fishes. These dietary guidelines to their members began at their inception in the mid-1800s and grew from the belief that mortal bodies are temples and should be fed the healthiest foods – as outlined in the biblical Book of Leviticus. This extends to physical exercise for the same reasons. Seventh-day Adventists have a lower risk than others of certain diseases, and researchers hypothesize that this is due to dietary guidance they follow.

The Adventist Mortality Study[12] was a large population size study and demonstrated an overall association of vegetarian dietary patterns with lower mortality compared with nonvegetarian patterns. This study showed that reduced meat consumption is associated with lower risk of death. Within the intricacies of the analysis, it is hard to separate the effect of a higher plant polyphenol diet on metabolic health, contrasted with the alleged negative effect of eating animal meats. Broad assumptions must be made with regard to the number of processed foods used, the amount of the carbohydrate portion comprised of high-fiber foods, etc. However, the main takeaway from the study was the positive effect of diets rich in plant-based foods.

The Word of Wisdom:

In the early 1800s, the Church of Jesus Christ of Latter-day Saints adopted a health code that became known as "The Word of Wisdom." It is most noted worldwide for its advice against tobacco, alcohol, and hot drinks (at that time tea and coffee). However, there was much more mentioned within it and the general "code" for healthy living which included "wise" recommendations for a healthy lifestyle - including nutrition, sleep, stress, and physical activity.

This health code emphasizes the use of grains, fruits, vegetables, seasonal eating, improved sleep, balanced work and rest, and managed stress. Each of these has now borne the scrutiny of time and scientific investigation.

Some wonder about the accuracy of these recommendations given the difficult time some people have with grains today – especially given that the original language identified it as the 'staff of life.'

Structured Diets

We have addressed the issue of grains, then and now, previously. Simply put, the grains and flours available today which are in common usage, are far different in their creation, and their effect on our metabolism, than the grains from decades and centuries past.

The recommendation then to use grains would today need to be bundled with the caveat that they are not refined or processed grains. The 'hot drinks' issue related to what was available as such in the early part of the 19th century. Recreational drugs were not specifically mentioned because they were not present or a concern in that era. Neither was the presence of processed foods. Wisdom and logic would update the remainder of the advice to reflect current realities and circumstances, relative to what is healthy and what is not. If it is not healthy, then it is not "wise"!

Regarding the sensitive issue of alcohol, which has been around since fermented grapes and grains were 'invented,' the truth is that there is no amount of alcohol that is healthy, metabolically. This is said with full knowledge of what the "science" and marketing behemoths have postured with regard to the heart-healthy effect of mild alcohol consumption.

Deeper and honest investigation would reveal that the health effect of "alcohol" is almost entirely due to the presence of proanthocyanidins in grape seed extract and skins (wine). These are polyphenols which exert their health benefit in wine due to the hormetic effect in cellular biology, by stimulating a stress-adapted response to improve antioxidant defenses and cellular renewal.

This effect in wine alcohol is color dependent, as grape seed proanthocyanidins are higher in the colored cultivars than in white grapes[13]. This would suggest that white wine cannot stand the same scrutiny as red wine – simply from the "heart-health" argument perspective. In other words, the heart healthy effect is far less to do with alcohol and much more (if not 100%) to do with plant polyphenols and their redox effect.

This information may not sit well with the vast population who love their wine and beer. Perhaps they believe that their health- or social-driven

Structured Diets

imbibing is good for their vascular health and the "social grease" justifies it, but from a metabolic perspective it defies the evidence.

The truth is that 90+% of alcohol is metabolized in the liver by the liver enzyme system using alcohol dehydrogenase and cytochrome P450, placing a metabolic tax on the liver to process and dispose of these alcohol molecules. Additionally, the break-down product acetaldehyde is also highly reactive, as is the increase in reactive oxygen species created[14].

Alcohol's dependency on liver metabolism is on par with the near 100% requirement for fructose to be metabolized in the liver, which is why both of these situations increase the risk for fatty liver disease (alcoholic and non-alcoholic).

The gradual and eventual liver damage, whether in the form of cirrhosis or 'fatty liver,' lowers the rate of alcohol oxidation and elimination from the body. Because there is no storage mechanism for alcohol (unlike glucose and fatty acids), alcohol remains in body water until eliminated and there is little if any hormonal regulation to pace the rate of its elimination[15].

Those who drink alcohol for its "health effects" are either unaware or in denial. While they may believe themselves untouched by its affects, they disregard the very real nutritional deficiencies associated with alcohol abuse due to alcohol and its metabolism preventing the body from properly absorbing, ingesting, and using nutrients. They also overlook the truth that any purported health effect comes from the polyphenols in their original packaging (grapes) and is equally present in non-alcoholic grape juice, which avoids the health risks assumed with alcohol consumption.

Additionally, these risks relate to the fact that from a cancer perspective (which is a metabolic disease) there is zero benefit from alcohol. This means there is no amount of alcohol that is safe from a 'zero-risk-for-cancer' analysis[16]. Lancet recently published a study that "finds unequivocally that alcohol use is a leading risk factor for the global disease burden and causes substantial health loss,"[17] and that risk is proportional with increasing levels of consumption.

Structured Diets

This says nothing about the undeniable impact alcohol has on societal problems related to DUIs and traffic accidents, impairment at work, family abuse, and alcohol abuse generally (attend family court at your local justice center, or a few Alcoholics Anonymous meetings if you are in doubt or want to challenge that point).

While adherents of many religious faiths similarly abstain from alcohol and may apply a spiritual faith focus to these practices, there is no doubt that avoiding dangerous drugs and chemicals found in these substances have proven to be a healthier way to live from a metabolic perspective, than not.

In a world where alcohol is a socially accepted and even a reverenced health practice and pastime, this seems like a hard line to take with something in such common use. It took many decades for tobacco to be finally recognized and accepted as the danger it is. To date this level of public opinion has not transferred to alcohol and remains an individual matter. Nonetheless, those who continue with it should understand the metabolic insult it represents to health.

Returning to our discussion of the Word of Wisdom specifically as it was originally given, in addition to the avoidance of harmful substances it is clear that it is intended as a focused strategy to consume whole foods, with an emphasis on seasonal fruits and vegetables which have high amounts of natural enzymes and phytochemicals, and high fiber content. It was decidedly not an anti-meat or strict vegetarian approach to nutrition, but one of balance and emphasis.

All of this, as we shall see, along with many other of these healthy diets, obeys the rules and principles of cellular health - and explains why they work when people 'work' them.

Mediterranean Diet:

This diet is inspired by the eating practices of people who live near the Mediterranean Sea. The diets of the people in this area included high amounts of olive oil, legumes, unrefined cereals, fruits, and vegetables. There was also moderate to high amounts of fish, moderate dairy, and wine consumption. This diet has received extensive attention in the science

Structured Diets

literature and is associated with lowering all-cause mortality and risks of chronic metabolic disease. The focus on fiber-rich fruits and vegetables and omega 3 rich proteins and fats is noteworthy.

Blue Zone Diet:

The "Blue Zones" are those parts of the world with the highest longevity in their populations. Five pockets of the world that exhibit this level of longevity include Okinawa, Japan; Sardinia, Italy' Nicoya, Costa Rica; Icaria, Greece, and Loma Linda, California.

The blue zone diet is mostly plant-based. The diets of people living in the Blue Zones are about 95% vegetables, fruits, grains, and legumes – in other words a whole food plant-based diet. These include whole grains such as corn, wheat, and rice; greens; tubers like sweet potatoes; and beans – often the cornerstone of the diet. When meat is eaten it is usually fish with milks and cheeses with little sugar – and almost zero processed food, including meats.

High fiber foods improve the feeling of satiety and helps manage weight and lowers risk for cancer generally.

Ketogenic diet:

A ketogenic diet is defined as a diet that forces the body into a process called ketosis. In this state, fats are selected as the energy fuel for metabolic catabolism in the mitochondria. These fats or fatty acids are generally sourced from fat depots (adipose) in the form of triglycerides. When carbs and glucose are unavailable through fasting or low-carb diets, cells shift to fat as the fuel source.

Variations of the "keto" diet incorporate diets that are focused on animals (carnivore), high fats, and said to be "primal." High protein diets, usually supervised with medical oversight, also fit this category, but due to the high protein effects on kidney health and overall metabolism, must be approached with caution and supervision generally.

Often these diets are said to be "fasting mimicking." That means that with very low carbohydrate consumption they create the same effect on energy

Structured Diets

metabolism and metabolic flexibility that shifts to fats for energy, as if fasting outright. These strategies are often combined and managed over time, since the main focus is to control the amount of glucose and insulin are available in the blood stream.

The ketosis that is produced with the micromanagement of fuel source and the timing of eating, is called *nutritional ketosis*. This is different from diabetic ketosis (ketoacidosis) which is an extreme metabolic crisis for Type One diabetics, and very brittle Type Two diabetics.

From a metabolic perspective, the objective is to trigger cellular defense and renewal (autophagy) without aggravating the cell's nutrient sensors and the hormone regulation of the body.

Keto or ketogenic diets are very mindful to manage the macronutrient ratio – meaning the relative amounts of fats, proteins, and carbohydrates. The objectives of this ratio management is to reduce carbohydrate ingestion to low levels of 5-10% of total calories consumed. Typical keto diet ratios are 75 / 20 / 5 % ratio, respectively for fats, proteins, and carbs. These numbers relate to the numbers of calories consumed in grams as a percentage of the whole.

The overarching objective of a keto diet is to train the body to run on fat more than carbohydrates. The word "train" is meaningful. The ability to reliably burn fat instead of glucose – and to enjoy the myriad of health benefits in so doing - is something that happens with time and acclimation. As the flexibility and metabolic efficiency is improved, and fat-burning becomes the norm being supported with a keto-friendly lifestyle, then even when carbs are consumed for a meal or two, the benefits of a fat-burning and metabolically healthy metabolism are less affected.

In this regard, this becomes the working definition of having a metabolically healthy lifestyle. Base levels of metabolic health and support will have shifted and transitioned to be more able to support healthy gene expression, cellular support, hormonal balance, and immune support – generally.

Structured Diets

While a keto-based diet is stricter in terms of managing macronutrient amounts, it isn't necessarily a vegetarian or carnivore-based diet. One can conduct a keto diet strategy and obtain fats and proteins from plant-based sourced foods while the carbs that are consumed maintain are high-fiber, or one can incorporate more meats in the diet and still be able to portion their foods according to a keto-ratio prescription. Many find that a keto diet is very satisfying due to the high fat content, and report that food cravings are reduced, and they find fat loss easy. There are solid scientific explanations as to why this is so, as a fat-based diet is able to metabolically deal with hunger hormones much better than a carb-based diet which requires more frequent eating to manage hunger due to "carb-addiction" or the inability to be metabolically adaptable.

Paleo Diet:

The Keto and Paleo diets are very similar in that they focus on whole foods and management of macronutrient ratios. While keto diets exclude rich sources of carbohydrates, paleo diets allow more fruits and some natural sweeteners.

Sometimes called "the caveman diet," paleo focuses on eating foods that were available to early humans during the 'hunter-gatherer' era. This diet is oriented around eating healthy within a hunter-gatherer framework (meat, fish, eggs, roots, vegetables, fruits, etc.). It minimizes foods that would come later through stabilization and development of agricultural advancements such as grains, sugars, and vegetable oils.

This certainly fits the metabolic principles of stress-adaptation and food uncertainty concepts for metabolic flexibility. There is less focus on developing a ketosis state which is mainly concerned about the metabolic breakdown of fat and using that as fuel. However, both paleo and keto emphasize whole food, fiber-rich foods, healthy fats, and high amounts of plant polyphenols. That said, Paleo is more focused on ideology, and keto is more focused on macronutrients and energy metabolism.

Structured Diets

The Redox Lifestyle Diet:

There are many diets that "work" because they in general, to one degree or another, obey the rules of the cells.

Most importantly to a redox lifestyle is a diet that supports a cycling ketosis, metabolic flexibility, hormesis, and predictable autophagy.

These occur because the liver is protected and the gut is properly fed. Refined processed (and over-processed) foods, and fructose and added sugar are eliminated and there is a rich supply of high-fiber foods and phytochemicals. Food preparation is done without high-heat and oil-frying, and due attention is given to intermittent fasting, nutritional ketosis, and managed blood sugar levels.

The Redox Lifestyle Diet can be summarized as being the best from the best – as long as it follows the rules of metabolic health. This is the synthesis and application of the principles presented in this book. All this is owing to a correct understanding of basic metabolic rules and principles – with which the individual can learn to manage their own metabolic health. This is the time-honored principle of teaching correct principles so that people will be empowered to govern themselves.

Thinking through and analyzing the several diets listed above, and by keeping the "rules of the cell" in mind, one can distill out the dietary and lifestyle strategies that fit best with their situation and encourage metabolic health without undue violation of "the rules."

This is why it is so critical to begin the discussion of diet not with what is published by "The Bigs," or according to the headlines on diet and health magazines at the checkout counter, or even with what the advisory councils espouse with loud acclaim, but with knowing the metabolic rules of redox biology. Only then can you successfully consider the effects of personal fitness level, body fat, genetics, microbiome gut status, muscle mass, exercise experience, time of day, frequency of eating, type and mixture of macronutrients, fiber quantity and quality, and more.

Structured Diets

Contrary to many popular diets, the Redox Lifestyle diet is not a weight-loss focused diet. That may happen as metabolic health improves, for weight gain is a symptom of metabolic dysfunction and slowdown.

The Redox Lifestyle diet combines all of the good parts of the best diet strategies together – as long as they obey the rules of the cells. This then all comes together into a sensible formula for health which is kind to the liver and other organs, protects the gut, and activates the redox signaling platform in a way to orchestrate cellular defenses and renewal from within.

The Redox Diet focuses on:

- No processed foods
- No added or artificial sugars; no fructose
- Whole food – Real Food
- Healthy oils and fats
- High amounts of plant polyphenols / phytochemicals
- High fiber carbohydrates
- Periodic ketosis through fasting and / or low carbohydrate eating
- Optimized autophagy
- Metabolic flexibility and fat adaptation
- Increased daily exercise and physical activity
- Living in the "hormetic zone" – each person's "sweet spot" for optimal redox activity
- Use of redox based supplements – both redox signaling and polyphenols

The Redox Lifestyle Diet therefore isn't a specific 'named' diet. It is a formula and a diet strategy that works in sync with metabolic cellular rules. The good diets, the healthy diets, generally follow these rules. It is the rules that matter, not the specific diet. This is a major paradigm shift for many people.

The creation of a mild oxidative stimulus is the goal of all good metabolic based 'redox' diets. Nature's rules rely on and use the redox biology principle of hormesis to stimulate and activate the "Inner Doctor" into action. While we may call these diets and foods "anti-inflammatory," what they really are, are foods that are prepared and consumed in a way to

Structured Diets

activate cellular defense mechanisms – which is what makes them anti-inflammatory and 'anti-oxidant-ory.'

This is the Redox Lifestyle Diet!

From here, to better understand redox-based nutrition, we first need to establish a better working understanding of what constitutes metabolic health and disease.

Part Two – Metabolic Health and Disease

What Does It Mean to Be Healthy?

We have established that many people think of health as the absence of, or at least the better management of symptoms. For example, if someone has a disease or condition, but they can manage it with medications, they consider themselves to be "in good health." An overwhelming segment within healthcare view 'health' this way as well.

> Symptoms of metabolic disease:
> - Weight gain / obesity
> - Visceral body fat
> - Fatty liver disease
> - Cognitive decline & dementia
> - Glycemic control
> - High blood pressure
> - Auto-immune
> - Fatty liver & visceral fat
> - Cardiovascular
> - Heart disease / stroke
> - Lipid problems
> - Blood sugar disorders
> - Neurodegeneration

For example, people with diabetes, high blood pressure, or elevated cholesterol who control those conditions with medications, consider their health well managed and think of themselves as otherwise healthy.

In today's world of healthcare, normalizing health parameters and reducing symptoms and complications (through timely intervention) is considered "health" – and appropriately so, owing to the bad outcomes associated with not managing them. The medical model presently is that health is achieved and maintained when lab values and symptoms are 'kept in check.' This is good. However, it is not the same thing as (also) addressing these problems from the perspective of true prevention – and even reversal - at the metabolic foundation.

The truth is that chronic non-transmittable diseases are symptoms of cellular disorders happening at a deeper level. This may be a hard truth for

What Does It Mean to Be Healthy?

many health professionals to accept. They are very good at what they do – but generally speaking this doesn't include upstream prevention, or correction at the foundational level.

The current medical model is oriented around detection and diagnosis, and risk-factor management. As good as this is, the problem is that screenings and early detection cannot prevent disease. They find it.

Mammograms, stool analysis, blood tests, and ultrasounds, do not prevent cancer or vascular disease any more than dental x-rays prevent tooth decay. These wonderful medical detection and surveillance technologies are wonderful at finding and diagnosing the presence of a problem, which triggers action to intervene. The limitation, however, is that few if any of these address the base redox-level cellular pathology which began the disease process at the fountainhead. Both parts of this equation are needed.

What then does it mean to be healthy? If the symptom isn't the 'disease,' what is?

The answer is located at the foundation level of health, with cellular and mitochondrial dysfunction. Chronic disease *is* mitochondrial dysfunction, and mitochondrial dysfunction *is* chronic disease. They are the same thing![18] The more sick and dysfunctional mitochondria are, the earlier one dies! And – the prelude to that final event is filled with much more medical intervention.

For metabolic health, this core functionality is greatly affected by the health and operation of the liver. Let's dive in and begin this journey by first looking there.

Liver Health

The classic signs and symptoms that the liver is not healthy include:

- Jaundice
- Abdominal pain and swelling
- Water retention (edema) in legs and ankles
- Itchy skin, bruises
- Dark urine

What Does It Mean to Be Healthy?

- Pale stool color
- Chronic fatigue
- Nausea or vomiting
- Brain fog

Even though these signs may appear suddenly, liver cell dysfunction precedes their presentation as symptoms. Long before the signs or symptoms appear, there is trouble upstream which create the downstream problems later.

Aside from the attention given to the liver from the alternative health community (liver cleanses and tonics), the liver doesn't get a lot of attention or popular press. However, it plays a highly important role in digestion, processing energy fuels, fat and protein synthesis and metabolism, and detoxification, and the handling of nutrients.

The liver is important in energy homeostasis[19] and as such is an important appetite regulating organ due to its involvement with hormone balance and how it responds to a state of nutritional ketosis and the presence of ketone bodies (specifically beta-Hydroxybutyrate).

Specifically, hepatocytes are involved in:

- Converting ammonia into urea which is eliminated in the urine
- Producing of bile which helps emulsify and digest fats in the intestine
- Converting blood sugar (glucose) into glycogen for storage and for use by muscles
- Producing cholesterol which is important for heart, hormones, and brain function
- Regulating the amino acid levels in circulating blood
- Storing vitamins and minerals
- Detoxifying medications, alcohol, and toxins.

The liver is uniquely positioned to process and clean all the blood from the intestines and stomach before it travels on to the general circulation. Dysfunction or damage of hepatocytes greatly affect the ability to handle waste by-products from normal metabolism, environmental pollutants, the breakdown of drugs, and which are in processing food. Any persistent

What Does It Mean to Be Healthy?

problems or threats to the liver can and will create a wide variety of health problems.

Many people believe that an otherwise healthy liver accumulates toxins during the filtering process which cause liver disease. They hold that these toxins accumulate and promote serious disease and cause a wide range of often nonspecific symptoms such as itching, skin rashes, jaundiced skin, swelling, vascular problems, gallstones, fatigue, nausea, diarrhea, and more.

While liver failure or disease is a serious health concern, there is little if any evidence to date that toxins accumulate in a healthy liver that has robust cellular defenses and detoxification pathways intact. However, this is different when these situations involve an unhealthy liver – a condition that can gradually and almost imperceptibly manifest.

When liver cells (hepatocytes) have become damaged or diseased to a point where they are not performing well, simply "cleaning" the liver to remove the burden placed upon it, is not enough. Conceptually this would be no different than taking vitamin supplements to off-set a junk-food high-sugar diet and sedentary lifestyle. Cleansing the liver is of marginal benefit if at the same time the lifestyle remains unchanged and metabolic health isn't restored such that natural detoxification occurs consistently.

A healthy liver naturally cleanses itself, but an unhealthy or damaged liver will not get better with a "liver cleanse," as it is popularly referred to. Someone with liver disease – with compromised hepatocyte function – needs to change their lifestyle and diet, and perhaps requires medical attention. The reasons for this are that "cleaning" the liver, to whatever extent possible, does not set in order the proper functioning of a hepatocyte nor does it change the redox landscape that drives detoxification mechanisms. There is a reason why the cells became dysfunctional in the first place.

As a rule, minus an acute poisoning event, the reasons liver cells are compromised are grounded in dysfunctional redox signaling, and abuses with energy metabolism, to include fat accumulation within liver cells. It is

What Does It Mean to Be Healthy?

at this level where the real damage is accumulated over time. This is the core and fundamental "doctrine" of metabolic disease. And health!

This is why "cleanses" only offer temporary help at best. True "cleanses" focus on restoring detoxification pathways through redox-sensitive mechanisms and metabolic health.

This is simply the fundamental axis upon which the cellular world of energy metabolism and the Redoxome spins. Nature has designed the higher way – or shall we say more fundamental way – in which these redox methods operate, and that is upon the axis of redox biology as it relates to cellular health. The reason why an otherwise healthy liver cell can detoxify anything is because it is a healthy cell. The fact that someone needs to detoxify their liver is witness to the fact that their lifestyle does not support cellular health and that they are redox deficient.

The most well-known liver problems are cirrhosis of the liver and jaundice. Cirrhosis happens due to the scaring and damage of liver tissues that results from long-standing dysfunction and damage. Jaundice, also known as icterus, is readily identified by a yellowing of the whites of the eyes, and of the skin generally. It occurs when liver cells can't efficiently process red blood cells as they break down, causing bilirubin to increase in the blood – all outward indicators of an ill-performing liver.

In addition to jaundice, other indicators or signs of liver dysfunction include abdominal pain and swelling, water retention in legs and ankles, itchy skin, dark colored urine, pale stool (feces) color, nausea, migraines, and vomiting.

While the presentation of these signs and symptoms may vary from person to person as well as in levels of intensity, they collectively witness to the fact that the liver is not performing as it was designed to function. Once these signs and symptoms appear, they are evidence of dysfunction that is already occurring. They are the warning signs that damage to the liver has already occurred to some degree.

However, there are other consequences which occur that most people do not readily associate with liver health, and which usually present before overt symptoms of acute liver disease. These include a wide class of

What Does It Mean to Be Healthy?

metabolic disorders such as insulin resistance and blood sugar disorders, elevated blood pressure, weight gain, visceral adiposity and general obesity, cardiovascular diseases, lipid disorders, brain cell dysfunction, neurodegeneration and memory problems, fatigue, personality changes, and etc.

Generally speaking, the distribution of unhealthy fat accumulates differently for males and females. Unhealthy fat deposits for men tend to accumulate around the belly, and for women they are lower around hips and buttocks. This reflects differences in the type of fat being accumulated, with abdominal fat depots being more associated with cardiometabolic risk[20].

Metabolic syndrome

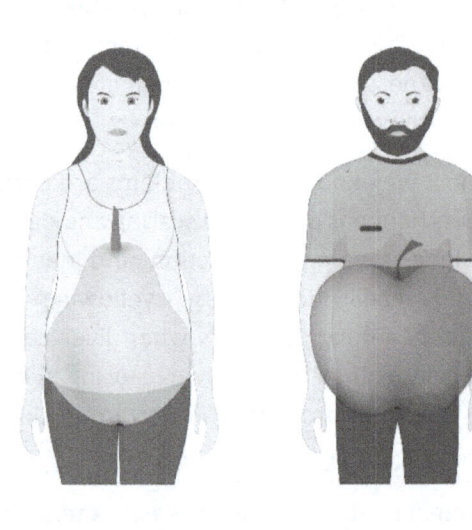

Non-alcoholic fatty liver disease is a new disease that emerged mid-century in the 1900s. Its prevalence is in 20-30% of Americans in general, but rises to 80-90% in obese individuals, 30-50% in those with type 2 diabetes, and approaches 90% in those with hyperlipidemia (high cholesterol). It is 3-10% in children and ranges between 40-70% in obese children[21]. As such it is becoming the most common liver disease worldwide.

In a promising pilot study evaluating the effects of a six-month dietary intervention using a high fat diet on those with stage one and stage two liver disease, found that there was complete reversal of hepatic steatosis[22] (a non-alcoholic fatty liver disease NAFLD - an otherwise incurable condition) in all patients! Notwithstanding the study utilized a moderately high carbohydrate content, and on a small sample group of human patients, the

What Does It Mean to Be Healthy?

fact that low linoleic acid content in the diet produced this effect, is very significant. [See appendix: Fats – for more information on linoleic acid and fat.]

Other studies show the similar effect using ketogenic or low-carbohydrate eating, on fatty liver and liver mitochondrial metabolism in those with NAFLD[23].

Collectively, this assortment of disorders are signs that base-level cellular function is compromised. The liver is a central player in this metabolic landscape which is why it deserves special attention in any redox-based discussion of redox and energy metabolism. Each of these conditions should beg the question about metabolic functionality in liver cells.

Conventional medicine has established that metabolic syndrome is identified by increased blood pressure, high blood sugar, excess body fat around the waist, and abnormal cholesterol or triglyceride levels.

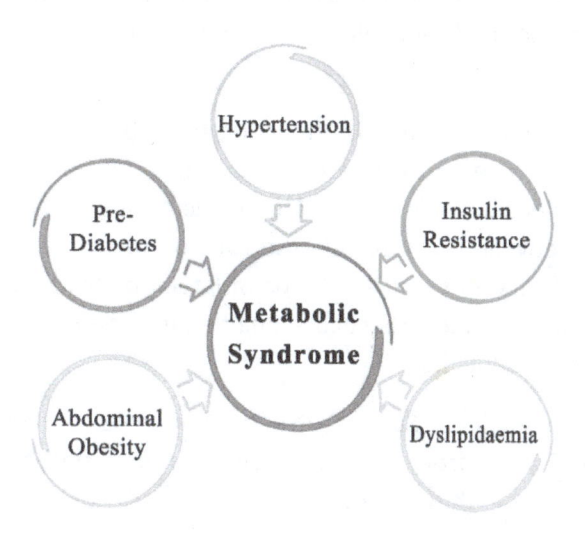

Treatments to deal with the presentations and symptom after the fact, are always advisable. It is not good to leave these symptoms unattended and not corrected, by any means possible. They are associated with further disease and damage, many with very poor outcomes. However, too often that is as far as it goes.

While these are now viewed collectively through the lens of being a "syndrome," the question left unanswered is, where is the disease that ties

What Does It Mean to Be Healthy?

these symptoms together as a syndrome, together? What is the cause that creates the disorders which manifest as this set of symptoms?

Just as fixing leaks in a dam requires more than plugging holes, addressing the root causes, and protecting the functionality of liver cells is extremely important. Answering these questions requires understanding the impact of foods and toxins on cellular function. At the foundational level, this is the essence of metabolic disease.

Fructose, Sugar, and Health

In dealing with the liver, special mention should be made of sugar, and especially fructose. It has an especially notorious and insidious effect on liver cells and can rightly be considered a liver cell "poison."

In today's more 'enlightened' world, everyone knows that sugar is unhealthy. Or do they? There are abundant mixed opinions in the public arena and obviously within the medical health space, and certainly within Big Food.

There are three main types of sugar found in the world of carbohydrates and food, namely lactose, sucrose and fructose. Lactose and sucrose are disaccharides (two sugar molecules) made up of glucose and galactose, and glucose and fructose, respectively. Fructose can also exist on its own as a monosaccharide in various fruits. [I will make the point later that fructose from natural 'real' foods is not a problem for cellular health; but added sugar and fructose during food processing, is.]

Sucrose is produced naturally in plants. Sugar cane and sugar beets contain it in high concentrations (15-20%), from which it is refined and crystalized and converted into table sugar or white sugar.

The consumption of sucrose in typical western diets can be as much as 25% of the total carbohydrate intake. The average person eating a 'Western' diet consumes 22 teaspoons of added sugar a day[24]. The leading voices in nutritional guidance recommend limiting this amount to 6 and 9 teaspoons per day for women and men, respectively. While some of this amount Is added in personal meal preparation, most of it included in processed and

What Does It Mean to Be Healthy?

prepared foods, such as packaged processed foods, beverages, cereals, snacks, and so-called fast foods[25]. What is certain is that there is no nutritional need or benefit for eating 'added sugar.'

Because sucrose is a disaccharide, degradation begins with hydrolytic cleavage which separates the glucose and fructose. This cleavage of sucrose occurs at the surface of intestinal epithelial cells. Sucrase is the enzyme which is responsible for this cleavage. Glucose is then transported across the intestinal wall by the SGLT1 transporter which actively moves glucose through cells against its own concentration gradient[26]. Fructose is passively transported across the intestinal wall by the GLUT5 transporter.

Glucose is generally the preferred form of sugar in cells. It is easily digested and converted to energy through the process of glucose oxidation (glycolysis) which it is broken down and then passed on into Krebs cycle to produce cellular energy.

Despite the fact that these sugars are metabolized (burned) in cells as a source of fuel/energy, they do so in different ways, and each can have a different effect or consequence on cells and the body.

Earlier on, fructose was a minor part of human's dietary sugar intake. Almost all of it (about 16-24 grams per day) came in the form of fruits, honey, and vegetables. Because it is found naturally in plants, many believe that it is healthy to consume when it is added to foods in the diet.

The high amount of daily consumption is from food processing and is estimated to be 55 to 100 grams per day, with an average of about 80 g/day

What Does It Mean to Be Healthy?

in the United States[27][28]. The majority of this comes from high-fructose corn syrup (90% fructose).

The metabolism of glucose and fructose is managed in different ways in the human body. Glucose is a six-carbon ring and is more stable than the five member ring of fructose. Fructose breaks down more easily than glucose and therefore drives the Maillard "browning" reaction which creates 8 to 10 times more advanced glycation end products (AGEs) than glucose[29].

While both are sugars and are found in the food we eat, they are processed differently in the body. Glucose is moved across cell walls with the help of insulin, and nearly every cell in the body is able to break down and metabolize (oxidize or 'burn') glucose and convert it into energy. It does this inside each cell's mitochondria.

However, fructose is handled very differently. The primary cells in the body that manage fructose are hepatocytes – liver cells. The biochemistry required to metabolize fructose, especially if there is too much of it in the diet, is very taxing to the cell and poses dangerous consequences to the liver, the cardiovascular system, the gut microbiome, and the pancreas – to name a few.

High fructose-induced mitochondria dysfunction produces damage to the mitochondria and effects cellular bioenergetics and energy homeostasis and the generation of glucose from non-carbohydrates such as amino acids (gluconeogenesis)[30]. It inhibits three mitochondrial enzymes, AMPKinase, APL, and CPT1 – thereby reprograming and impairing mitochondrial respiration in Krebs cycle and the electron transport chain[31]. Fructose, along with other sugars, has also shown to affect calcium absorption and bioavailability of calcium and other nutrients in the gut, leading to weakened skeletal bones[32].

As will be outlined in greater detail below, metabolizing fructose leads to a loss of phosphates from ATP (ATP is converted to ADP). It also generates uric acid which reduces nitric oxide and leads to elevated blood pressure. The majority of fructose is converted to pyruvate and the mitochondria becomes

What Does It Mean to Be Healthy?

overwhelmed and the excess is converted to liver fat which in turn leads to metabolic disease and insulin resistance.

When carbohydrates are metabolized, excess glucose is converted into its storage form, glycogen. However, fructose does not convert to glycogen and must be stored by other means. Accordingly, it is converted to triglyceride fat. It does this through a complex series of chemical transformations as it metabolizes and clears fructose. This is called *de novo* lipogenesis, or the new creation of a lipid.

With increasing or prolonged fructose ingestion, small fat droplets begin to accumulate inside liver cells – a condition called nonalcoholic fatty liver disease. This condition was for all intents and purposes unknown (except for in alcoholics) prior to 1980. It now affects approximately 30% of adults in countries with a "Western" food culture. Roughly 80% of those with insulin resistance, many of whom are obese, experience this fatty buildup inside liver cells.

In its early stages, this fat accumulation is reversible, but at some point, the forces of inflammation prevail and the fatty inflammation (steatohepatitis)

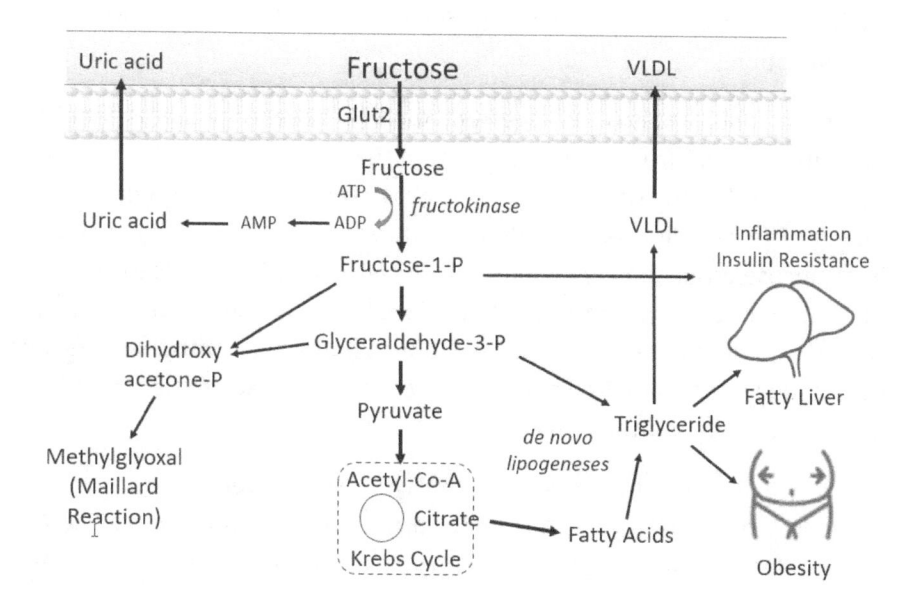

Source: Campbell, Fructose-Induced Hypertriglyceridemia: A Review. 2014

What Does It Mean to Be Healthy?

that results can become more severe and lead to scar tissue forming in the liver – a condition known as cirrhosis, with the naturally attendant reduction in liver function.

Almost all of the fructose consumed is metabolized in the liver, with minor amounts occurring in the kidneys. The kidneys are able to convert physiologic levels of fructose (normal eating of fruits, etc.) to produce glucose/pyruvate. However, sustained excessive amounts induce fructolysis (metabolism of fructose) which results in significant ATP depletion in the cell and inflammation, leading to kidney damage.

While >90% of fructose is metabolized in the liver, glucose is handled differently. The liver will metabolize approximately 20% of the glucose, leaving 80% to be predominantly managed by muscle cells and other cells throughout the body (brain, RBCs, etc.). The effect of healthy insulin levels and lack of insulin resistance on cell walls, allow excess blood sugars to be converted into glycogen first, and then lipids second (via liver cells) which are stored in adipocyte fat cells. The status of low energy need in the body/liver allows the liver to shunt the extra glucose to the systemic circulation where the net result is increased subcutaneous adipose triglyceride accumulation and a decrease in visceral adipose tissue accumulation.

However, when fructose is ingested, there is no energy-status feedback regulation of the fructose metabolism pathway - meaning all of it moves through the fructose metabolism pathway. This results in the creation of new fat (*de novo* lipogenesis), depressed liver insulin sensitivity, increased liver glucose production, elevation in liver cell lipids which leads to increases of systemic LDL cholesterols (bad), and increase in systemic insulin secretion, impaired glucose tolerance, fasting glucose control, and fasting insulin levels. Inflammation and insulin resistance is also created within the liver and throughout the body.

The very first step in the fructose pathway[33] is the conversion of fructose to fructose-1-phosphate. The phosphate comes from the energy molecule ATP which adds the phosphate group to fructose, which converts ATP to ADP

What Does It Mean to Be Healthy?

(triphosphate to di-phosphate), by using the enzyme fructokinase (a "X...kinase" enzyme transfers a phosphate group to a X-molecule).

If the cell is sensitive to glucose and it needs more energy/glucose, it will engage the path towards glycolysis and energy creation. If there is sufficient energy present it inhibits the enzymes that prepare glucose for the glycolysis pathway and shunts it in a different direction.

In the glucose glycolysis pathway, both high energy status and high citrate levels inhibit phosphofructokinase (PFK - the enzyme that forwards the movement of glucose molecules toward glycolysis). While this enzyme (PFK) is inhibited by high levels of ATP energy states and citrate availability for Krebs cycle, it is also regulated by AMP[34]. When ATP and energy levels are low, AMP is increased, and this upregulates glycolysis to create more energy.

PFK enzyme controls the entry of Glucose-6-P into glycolysis. When PFK is slowed, G6P accumulates and is routed toward glycogen synthesis or the pentose phosphate pathway – which is a metabolic pathway parallel to glycolysis moving molecules back to the glycolytic or gluconeogenic pathway. While this may seem like heavy science to some, it matters because this pathway has been shown to be a major regulator for cellular redox homeostasis and biosynthesis.

However, there is no energy-gate sensor to prevent fructose from being metabolized by liver cells. Thus, nature has prepared a way to oversee glucose, but not fructose. And due to the deleterious effects of fructose metabolism on the cell, non-natural or excess fructose exerts a harmful effect on liver cells.

High levels of ATP energy in the liver reduce glycolysis (inhibits PFK), which in turn lowers its enzymatic conversion. Because fructose demands the use of ATP to begin fructose metabolization (thus using up this precious energy molecule) the ratio of ATP and AMP is altered.

This "cost" is significant in the energy equation of the cell. It is 'expensive' to convert fructose to fructose-1-P (because it requires taking a phosphate from ATP and giving it to fructose, thereby converting ATP to ADP / "tri-" to

What Does It Mean to Be Healthy?

"di-"). ATP is consumed unnecessarily (considering that fructose is optional), and as well increases AMP – which further drives the cell's signaling for further energy production. Certainly, the metabolic costs in energy, and the drive it creates for further glucose metabolism, is an unnecessary expense.

The elevation in AMP is also significant because increased AMP levels lead to the creation of uric acid, a significant risk factor for the inflammatory condition called gout. A growing amount of evidence has accumulated to show that sugar intake, particularly fructose, is a major risk factor for gout[35].

With this information one might be prepared to eliminate all forms of processed fructose in their diet (hopefully), as well as eliminate eating fruit, since that is a dietary source of fructose.

However, fruit and veggies that contain fructose are a natural source - and a minor one at that. The good news is that they are "real food." They come with their own natural fiber antidote and an array of naturally existing vitamins, minerals, and enzymes packaged together as nature intended. There simply is no reason to avoid naturally occurring sugars in whole "real" foods – especially when eating a redox-based functional diet that has high levels of fiber and redox-active phytochemicals.

The fructose to avoid is that which is added in processed food. Period. This is done by expunging high-fructose corn syrup and added sugars (which hide by hundreds of different names). This would include any sugar sweetened beverages, processed breakfast cereals, refined carb breads and pastries (missing fiber and the nutrients in the bran), and any and all other processed food products that have been touched by hands in a way that strips food of its natural protections, nutrients, fiber – and which adds sweeteners and preservatives and "essential" vitamins. In other words, anything "processed!"

When in doubt read the label. Sugar, or any of its dozens of other monikers[36] [37], especially when listed as the first two or three ingredients, should be avoided.

What Does It Mean to Be Healthy?

Gastrointestinal Health

Linking the subject of sugar and fructose with gastrointestinal health, is the research that shows that fructose has harmful effects on gut health. In animal models, fructose consumption is a risk factor for inflammatory bowel disorders due to its effect on the intestinal barrier. The proteins responsible for holding intestinal wall cells together is decreased with high fructose diets resulting in a decreased barrier function[38]. As we will see, the happenings and 'goings-on' within the gut, greatly impact the microbial populations that live there, which affect the health and integrity of the intestinal barrier wall and immune system standing guard therewith.

It is a paradigm shift in thinking to consider that much or most of the biological reason for eating is about feeding gut bacteria, not us! Along with everything else food is about, a primary benefit of food is to keep the gut healthy and balanced. Food does this by providing fiber which mitigates the action on metabolic pathways and provides food for bacteria – so bacteria do not feed on you! Food with little or no fiber creates an energy overload to the bacteria which favors a mix of species that produce inflammation, as they quickly digest the food and quickly spike the blood stream with excess glucose.

It is well understood by everyone that the bowel contents contain bacteria. Many understand that there are both good and bad bacteria (healthy and unhealthy), but few understand that they can manipulate and control this population mix by the foods they eat and how metabolically healthy they are. Good diets favor healthy bacteria, and poor nutrition favors unhealthy bacteria – each with their attendant systemic health consequences.

The intestinal mass as it is, is largely a bulk of growing microorganisms representing a broad cross-section of microbial species. What kind they are, and which species dominate to outcompete the other, is largely a function of the diet they are fed and how the gut is respected.

In general terms, probiotics are live yeasts and good bacteria that live in the gut and are very beneficial in digestion. Prebiotics are the food source on which these microbes feast.

What Does It Mean to Be Healthy?

Dietary fiber is considered the 'roughage' of the diet and is found in the portion of plant-derived food that cannot be completely broken down by human digestive enzymes. They are very diverse in composition and structure and are categorized in terms of solubility, viscosity, and fermentability.

The diet provides important sources of soluble and insoluble fiber for bacteria to eat upon and live amongst. Soluble fiber absorbs water and turns to gel during digestion. This slows digestion and very importantly slows the rate at which digested carbohydrates (glucose) leave the gut and enter the blood circulation. Insoluble fiber adds bulk to the stool and helps food pass through the intestine toward elimination.

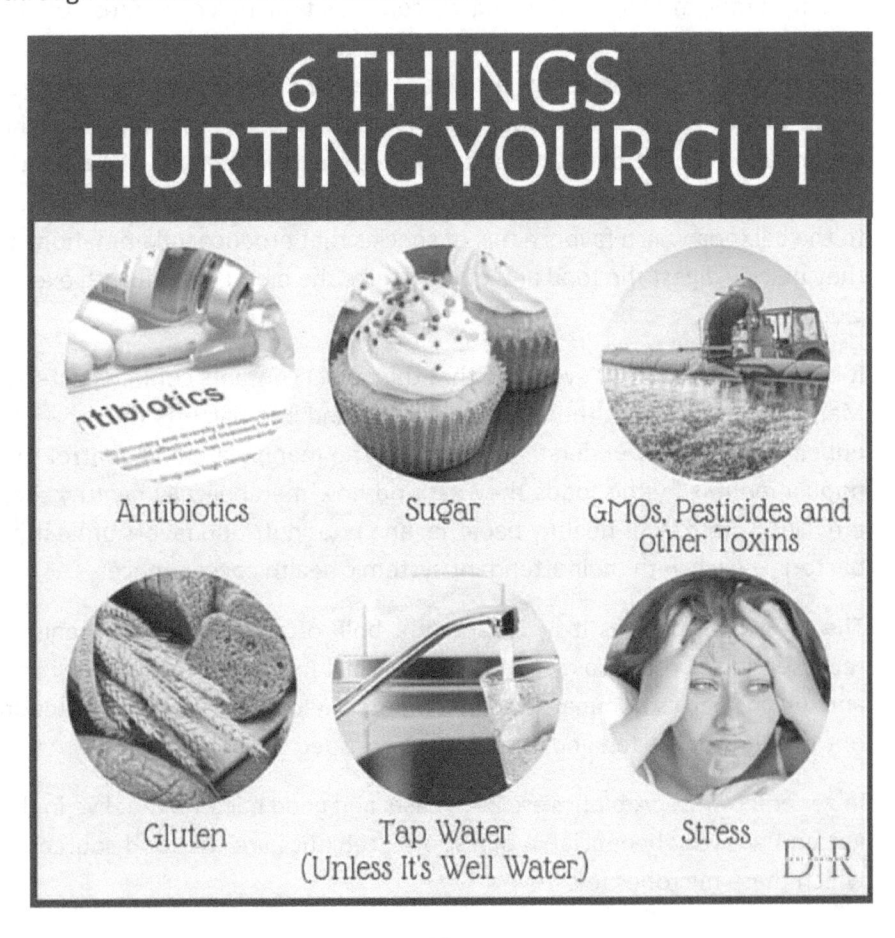

6 THINGS HURTING YOUR GUT

- Antibiotics
- Sugar
- GMOs, Pesticides and other Toxins
- Gluten
- Tap Water (Unless It's Well Water)
- Stress

What Does It Mean to Be Healthy?

These bacteria are not entirely self-serving. Their synergistic benefits are significant. They process and create a large number of vitamins for our use, such as thiamin, folate, biotin, riboflavin, pantothenic acid, vitamin K, vitamin B12, and more. They also produce neurotransmitters and 'brain' chemicals serotonin, dopamine, and GABA. They ferment indigestible carbohydrates (dietary fiber) and create short-chain fatty acids such as acetate, propionate, and butyrate.

Relative to our discussions about metabolic and systemic health, there are important functional differences between the bowels of metabolically healthy and metabolically unhealthy individuals.[39]

Studies have found that gastrointestinal health is a factor in metabolic health. It is a contributing factor in metabolic disorders including insulin resistance, metabolic syndrome, obesity, diabetes, liver disease, cardiovascular disease, and malnutrition. The composition of the intestinal microbiota plays a role in the development of metabolic disease[40]. Those people with obesity and metabolic disease generally have a reduced diversity in bacterial composition, which in turn reduces metabolic energy consumption when compared with lean individuals[41].

Optimum gut health and function require two things: 1) - a healthy and diverse gut microbiome, and 2) - a healthy intact gut lining. Redox signaling plays a central role in all operational facets of this equation and in the biome – host relationship.

Redox mechanisms within the intestine preserve an environment that supports health processes and coordinates networks of enzymatic reactions active against oxidative stress. There, redox sensitive processes regulate epithelial turnover, contribute to a balanced intestinal microbiota, and play key roles in gut biology and many degenerative digestive disorders ranging from inflammation to cell dysplasia[42].

The presence of a healthy commensal bacterial gut biome enhances redox cycles that elevate glutathione content in intestinal epithelial cells, and which help attenuate or lessen mucosal inflammation. When friendly bacteria are diminished, it increases oxidative stress and activates NF-*k*B

What Does It Mean to Be Healthy?

transcription of pro-inflammatory cytokines[43]. Inflammation promotes breaks in the intestinal wall barrier allowing undigested or partially digested food molecules, toxins, and bacteria to "leak" through this barrier and come face to face with the body's immune system, and into the bloodstream. This processes called *leaky gut* is a major reason for food allergy, systemic inflammation, and autoimmune disease[44].

Available evidence highlights the important role of glutathione and redox signaling in maintaining a balance between the intestinal biome environment and intestinal cell survival.

Intestinal bacteria regulate many homeostatic functions. Certain bacterial strains such as Lactobacilli promote healthy levels of redox signaling within intestinal cells[45] including the Nrf2 antioxidant pathway, cell repair during inflammation, and antibacterial action. Additionally, microbes in the gut trigger redox signaling inside intestinal mucosal cells which then produce similar but distinct enzymes to immune cells which can destroy pathogenic bacteria[46].

Both over and under-production of ROS can cause damaging cellular reactions, hence the importance of maintaining redox balance. Indeed, it is the precise control of this redox balance or oxidative state within these intestinal barrier cells that determine the outcome of an inflammatory event. The bottom line is that intestinal epithelium, the gut microbiome, and the body's immune cells all work together because of redox signaling in the intestinal mucosa of the colon - both during health and disease.

A healthy diverse microbiome prevents damage from and to the cells of the intestinal wall, as well as helps maintain the tight junctions that keep intestinal cells "glued" together, thus preserving a healthy barrier wall and preventing the absorption of partially digested food molecules which then trigger and create a hyper-responsive immune system[47].

Unhealthy bacteria are "bad" because they are marked with molecules that identify them as harmful - which provoke an inflammatory reaction in the bowel and immune system. They also help dissolve the cellular glue that hold intestinal-wall cells together and keep it from leaking.

What Does It Mean to Be Healthy?

Contrary to what many might suppose, a normal "healthy" mixture of microbial species in the gut includes a small number of "unhealthy" bacteria. The important point of this is the ratio or balance. The objective is to live and eat such that healthy species outcompete the unhealthy species for resources.

Given this, it is good to remember that pathogenic bacteria also digest food. The rule for gut health, one that gives power to the individual over their health, is to provide the gut with prebiotic foods that favor and select for healthy bacteria - and which diminish bad bacteria.

Generally speaking, this is the mechanism for managing gut health. This means we each can reclaim significant control over problems related to bowel motility (constipation and diarrhea), food digestion, inflammatory disorders of the bowel, systemic inflammation and toxicity, and the ability to better detoxify and eliminate harmful waste products – by changing their diet!

An example of this is SIBO – small intestinal bacteria overgrowth – a condition that is promoted when refined carbohydrates are consumed. Highly refined or simple carbohydrates are quickly processed (digested) in the small intestine and create an explosive surge in pathogenic (bad) bacteria in the small intestine.

These bacteria contain endotoxins and lipopolysaccharides that attach to Toll-Like Receptors (TLR$_4$) and drive the NF-kB inflammatory response. In addition to this quick explosive digestion of simple carbohydrates favoring the growth of bad bacteria, it also quickly elevates blood glucose levels - which in turn drives further inflammation. Like putting gas on a fire, the combustion quickly ignites and consumes the energy, producing massive surges in 'energy' to enter the blood stream in the form of glucose spikes.

As it will be made clear in our discussions about metabolic health and flexibility, the mismanagement of blood sugar levels arising from chronic if not persistent glucose-elevated states (the "fed" state), and has ominous consequences with regard to metabolic disease. This is because metabolic disease is a by-product of the mismanagement of the conversion of food

What Does It Mean to Be Healthy?

energy into biological energy. Chronic lifestyle abuses of this type create mitochondrial dysfunction and disease.

On the other hand, prebiotics and complex carbs are not quickly digested and move deeper into the bowel to experience a slower steady rate of digestion and subsequent slow glucose and nutrient absorption. Prebiotics and healthy anti-inflammatory diets induce the growth and activity of beneficial microorganisms and are responsible for altering the composition of organisms in the gut microbiome.

With poor and pro-inflammatory diets, the gut is set-up to promote unhealthy bacterial populations that out-compete healthy bacteria. With good diets the gut is spared the quick metabolism and will out-compete pathogenic bacteria, creating a favorable condition for health to predominate. With healthy eating, the shift in balance of power to healthy bacteria promotes favorable gut health and protective redox activity.

The microbiome is thus a balancing act – like a teeter-totter – that can go back and forth and be manipulated based on the foods provided and the managed control of the oxidative state within the gut. The current concepts recognizing the role of bacterial balance (probiotic health) is a return to eating styles for which the human organism is natively designed. This means more complex roughage, enzymes, and phytochemicals - and from a variety of sources. This is a proper and natural mechanism for managing energy metabolism within the Redoxome.

In a modern world saturated with processed food choices, shifting one's diet to more prebiotic foods and supplements is an excellent way to help repopulate and shift the biome toward healthy bacteria and a non-inflamed bowel. In a world of disease, the power and effect of improved diets is wildly misunderstood, misstated, abused, and ignored. Yet it is one of the more effective ways of changing one's life.

By eating less processed and packaged foods, and consuming more whole foods, vegetables and fruit, and lacto-fermented and cultured foods, the gut can 'heal' itself – and you the owner! This more friendly support for the gut

What Does It Mean to Be Healthy?

enhances redox mechanisms including antioxidant gene signaling pathways and contribute to stable intestinal epithelial barriers.

A healthy gut microbiome helps create native signaling that improves Nrf2 activation and glutathione production, as well as the inhibition of inflammation via suppression of the NF-*k*B pathway. They do this by improving stem cell proliferation, epithelial cell motility, and dampening of innate immune (NF-*k*B) responses[48]. These mechanisms are a universal and non-discriminating means by which bacterial populations in the gut microbiome can affect a wide variety of signaling and homeostatic processes in our body. This includes the gut-brain axis[49], the epithelial barrier function[50], and the native symbiosis between gut biome and the intestine.

All of this has far reaching positive effects throughout the body systemically. When attention to proper gut health through dietary prebiotic and macronutrient management, and through elevated redox signaling mechanisms, it translates to healthier gut biomes and healthier bodies. The reduced systemic oxidation and inflammation engender a 'ground' state where the redox-sensitive platforms are not overrun with excess oxidation and can operate normally in defense of health.

What Does It Mean to Be Healthy?

Metabolic Disease

Metabolic Disease

Chronic cellular health disorders are related to abuses of cellular energy creation and redox regulation. Referring to them as metabolic disorders correctly identifies the roots and foundation of where chronic disease begins and where it leads.

Metabolism deals with the biological and biochemical reactions within a cell that makes life possible. Without energy metabolism and without the associated redox signaling, life ceases to exist! The degree to which these cellular functions work is the degree to which we enjoy health, or instead suffer with symptoms when they do not function well. When viewed through this lens of metabolic function and dysfunction, all disease conditions can be characterized and described based on cellular function.

At the center of this discussion is how a cell "burns" and "grows." Fundamentally, this is the essence of cellular function. This means cells are either metabolizing and burning and processing fuel for energy, or they are repairing, replacing, and building. Admittedly, this high-level view is simplistic and general because a living cell is always metabolizing and oxidizing a fuel source to produce energy, or it perishes. But in terms of 'roles' it is accurate that there are episodic phases and cycles that cells go through which are functions of many variables.

These 'burn' and 'grow' functions do not happen simultaneously. This is why the cellular repair function occurs during the rest or recovery phase following exercise, for example. While it is an oversimplification, the analogy fits that you can use wood for building furniture or firewood, but not at the same time. Each in their role and turn, both activities are essential. It is all about ATP and energy metabolism. Distress in fuel metabolism or cell signaling threatens stability

---

Signs of Not Being Metabolically Flexible

- Need to snack to maintain energy
- Can't go more than 4-5 hours without eating
- Angry when hungry "hangry"
- Feel sleepy after eating a big meal

Metabolic Disease

(homeostasis) and creates disease. When they are not in balance, disease results. For example, cancer cells don't burn – they grow!

Said more scientifically, when the enzymes mTOR, AMPK, and P13K are in balance and sync, they burn. When not in sync, they grow and move the cell toward disease. One of the major effects of processed foods is the effect it has on this dynamic balance between burning and growing – between energy metabolism and cellular repair.

Energy metabolism strictly defined is the process by which the body converts food into energy. This energy drives all aspects of living and keeps the brain healthy and the heart and all physiological functions working. By burning food as fuel, the calories harvested in the energy reactions are transferred and used at the cellular level. These energy calories are obtained in the form of dietary carbohydrates, proteins, and fats.

At an even deeper scientific level, the transfer of this energy from food to cell, is about the "transduction" or movement of electrons along an energy gradient (electron transport chain) within the mitochondria. How efficiently this occurs is a function of many variables, but most importantly the amount, type, and timing interval of the "fuelings." The underlying health of the cell is greatly impacted by how efficient these metabolic combustion reactions are, and what the body does with the byproducts.

Sadly, these definitions do not translate well in "real life" as experienced by ordinary people in the normal food and nutrition marketplace. Since metabolic disorder shows up as problems with blood sugar, triglycerides, cholesterol (HDL), blood pressure, weight gain, and increasing waist size, metabolic health would be the absence of these - without utilizing medications! This means metabolic disease (cellular dysfunction) is still present even if medications are required to manage the symptoms. Withdrawal of medical intervention worsens the symptoms. Suppressing or compensating for the symptoms does not change the underlying redox deficiencies or metabolic function.

Presently the number of American adults who fit this definition of metabolic health is 12%[51] which is astonishingly low – and even includes normal weight

Metabolic Disease

individuals. This means that 88% of the US population is metabolically inflexible[52].

An interesting side note is that often metabolic health is tightly tied with normal-weight and lean individuals; conversely that metabolic disease is tightly correlated with obesity. Recent research found that the degree of muscle mass is a better predictor of death (all-cause mortality) than is BMI – body mass index[53]. While the exact reasons are still being determined, what is clear is that body composition is a better way of thinking about this than is the time-honored assessment of BMI.

Total body mass (BMI) includes fat and muscles, each of which have different metabolic profiles and effects[54]. As well, obesity itself while having a significant impact on health, has not consistently been associated with higher mortality in aging adults. Being overweight, obese, or morbidly obese (grade 1, 2 & 3 obesity respectively) each have different mortality profiles. In fact, it is understood that overweight people can still be metabolically healthy, due to a variety of factors chiefly associated with their degree of liver and gut health.

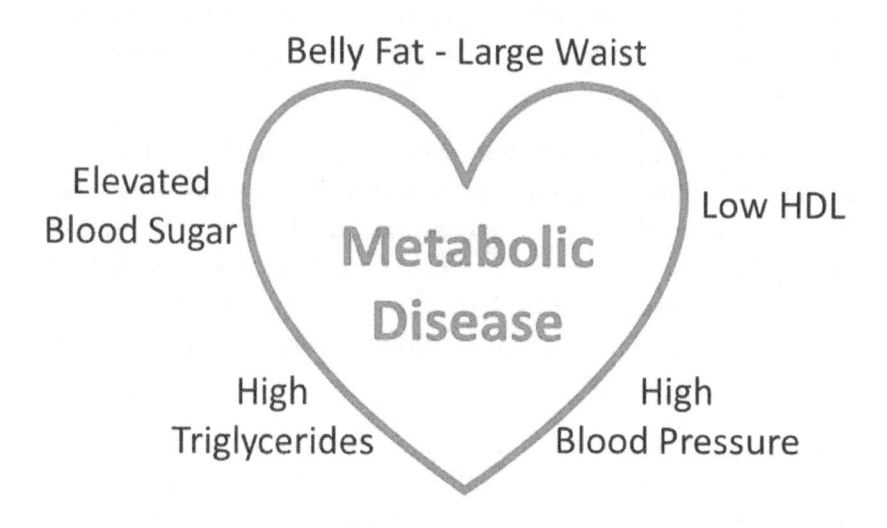

Belly Fat - Large Waist

Elevated Blood Sugar

Metabolic Disease

Low HDL

High Triglycerides

High Blood Pressure

Metabolic Disease

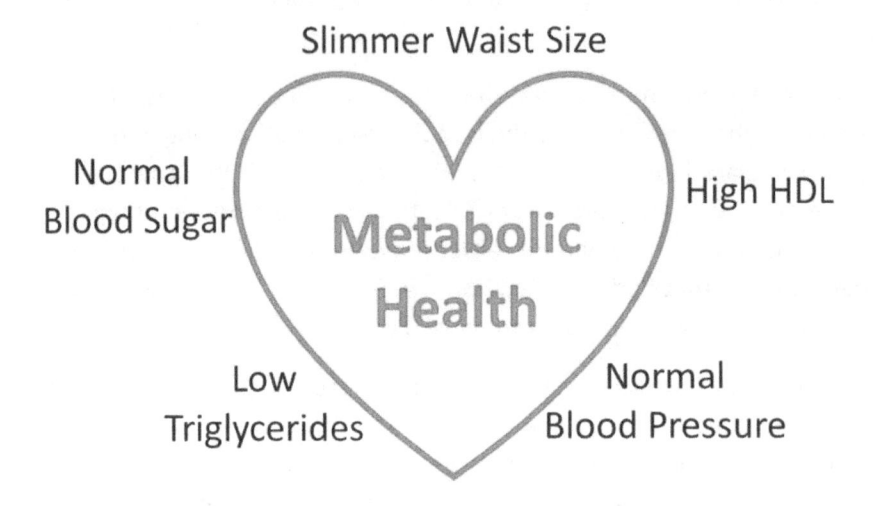

Metabolic Health
- Slimmer Waist Size
- Normal Blood Sugar
- High HDL
- Low Triglycerides
- Normal Blood Pressure

This has given rise to the new descriptor "MHO" – the "metabolically healthy obese" – those who are obese but have no (present) features of poor metabolic health (it has been associated with increased risk of future heart failure). It is not yet clear if it is a transient state on the way from lean to obese, but nonetheless, in all its forms, obesity and weight challenges are a symptom of something amiss at the redox-level foundation of metabolic function, and again highlights the importance of paying attention to the liver, the gut, and the Redoxome.

With that said, still the 12% level of overall metabolic health statistic has serious public health implications, as well as places significant impacts on the lives of these 88%, and all those close to them. This is especially concerning because these conditions relate directly to a person's risk for heart disease, diabetes, stroke, liver disease, and neurodegenerative diseases – conditions that affect and touch every living person on the planet, directly or indirectly.

This number is stunning. It means when looking at a typical crowd of people in a stadium, auditorium, public gathering, concert, or inside your own family, that nine out of ten people you see have metabolic disease – even if

Metabolic Disease

their lab numbers are within normal ranges due to expert medical management.

Insulin Resistance

Diving deeper into the nuances of energy metabolism and metabolic health, this is all closely related to the way the body uses insulin. The functionality and utilization of insulin is center stage in any discussion of cell metabolism and how cells manage and burn their fuel sources. As such there is a sophisticated orchestration that occurs between the various players and conditions within cellular physiology and biochemistry.

Metabolic syndrome is also referred to as Syndrome X, dysmetabolic syndrome, and insulin resistance syndrome. Its incidence increases with age, largely due to the natural decreases seen in metabolic efficiency within Krebs cycle, mitochondrial dysfunction, and lowered redox- and cell-signaling activity.

The attention on insulin resistance has become a dominant focus in dealing with metabolic disease. This is due to its tight connections with how glucose is handled in the digestion and metabolism of carbohydrates.

Insulin resistance means that cells in the body are less able to respond to the energy needs of a cell by efficiently moving glucose from the blood stream into a cell where it can be metabolized. When this occurs, cells become more resistant to the effects of the insulin 'gatekeeper' which opens the door for glucose to enter a cell. The pancreas is then signaled to produce more insulin in an effort to overcome this resistance, meaning that both blood sugar and insulin levels rise. This process of resistance can proceed for years and years, slowly increasing damage and inflammation.

As blood glucose and insulin levels rise, and as inflammation increases in the pancreas further slowing insulin production, the combined effect can eventually lead to matured blood sugar disorders. At this point there is an obligate need for medical intervention to compensate for this resistance and deal with elevated sugar levels that resist normalization following eating, and which have a powerful effect on inflammation.

Metabolic Disease

Secondary to this inflammation and metabolic dysfunction, other complications can occur when endothelial and nerve cells become damaged, and proteins become damaged ("sugared" or glycated) due to elevated glucose levels. This adds to the burden of cellular damage and debris which must be dealt with in order to maintain cellular balance. With a symptom-only focus, the metabolic disorder is often not addressed as it should be to correct the root-cause.

The Metabolic Healthcare Cliff

Unfortunately, too many people are 'victims' of their own ignorance or of a medical system that ostensibly fails to educate them (and the public) about how metabolic dysfunction starts - long before symptoms and laboratory signals present. It is the metabolic disorder that is the root-cause precursor to the syndrome!

If these problems are so pervasive and grave, why does a system – and even a society – not do more to protect its citizens with prevention, at least in the form of education? Too often, little if anything happens until after the disease symptoms emerge. Why would the occurrence of diabetes, or a heart attack, or Alzheimer's be a surprise to anyone? Obviously, we don't live in a perfect world! After a diagnosis, retrospective analysis should teach us about what should have been happening all along – to prevent it.

Consider what happens within the realm of everyday life and healthcare at the moment a sign or symptom presents. Whether it is a vascular event such as a stroke or heart attack, or a lab value that has 'suddenly' risen above a certain level - what is the discussion? All diagnoses are attached to the occurrence of the event, sign, or symptom. Thankfully, everyone springs into action to provide cardiovascular care and even rehabilitation, diabetic care, surgical care, and any and all other needed medical intervention - for a metabolic disorder that no doubt preexisted for many years. But was there deep concern or a serious discussion about metabolic function and a redox lifestyle in the months and years ahead that would prevent the event or sudden appearance of symptoms?

Metabolic Disease

This is not to disparage any group of healthcare workers. Both those at the top of the cliff and those at the bottom are needed. However, is needs to be acknowledge that there is a difference between working at the bottom of a cliff to pick up injured bodies after-the-fact, and working at the top of the cliff to erect fences and keep people away from the edge.

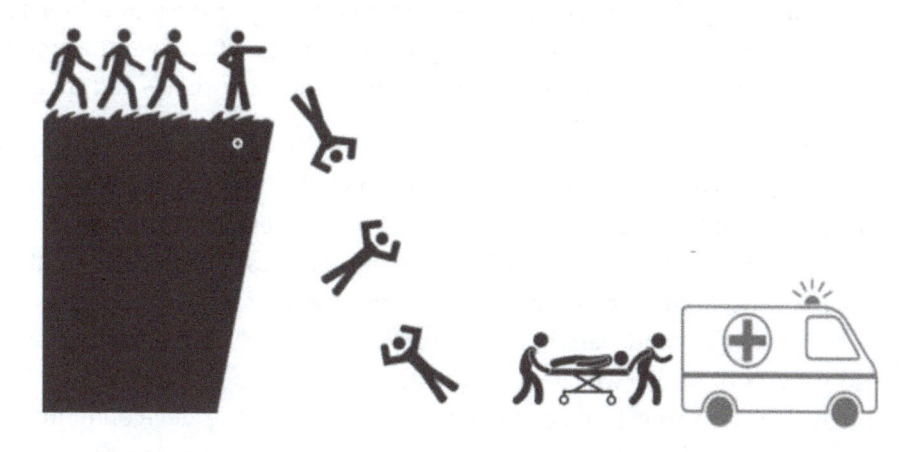

The point is that heart attacks do not happen in healthy blood vessel walls unaffected by the effects of oxidation and inflammation. Diabetes is not "caught" by a weekend stay in the hospital! And cognitive decline doesn't suddenly appear out of nowhere!

Insulin resistance or untoward weight gain or cognitive decline or blood pressure problems do not occur in metabolically healthy people. If any of these or other conditions are happening, it is a hallmark sign that something is amiss with metabolic health.

When these conditions begin to occur, it is due to unchecked metabolic dysfunction – usually occurring over considerable time. It is human nature to spring into corrective action once an event occurs or when an unwelcome diagnosis is given – and there is nothing wrong with that. Redox principles thankfully still apply to those who tumble down the healthcare cliff and then work to get back on top and anchor themselves in safe territory behind the protective redox fence. These situations are all too common for every person, and it is reassuring that health can be positively impacted and that cellular dysfunction can become healthy cell function once again.

Metabolic Disease

What makes this confusing to many is that the spectrum of metabolic symptomology is just that – a continuum. As far as what is observable, it is not as simple as on-off, healthy-not healthy, diabetes-not diabetes. The emergence of metabolic signs and symptoms themselves (consequences of dysfunction) occur over time and along a continuum. This is due to the body's amazing ability to compensate and adapt, and because of its ability to protect vital functions. However, there is no question that eventually the adaptive capacities and compensatory abilities will wear thin – and then it is too late.

This ability to adapt and compensate is evidenced in the fact that with type 2 diabetes, between 25 and 50% of beta-cell loss (where insulin is made) has occurred prior to diagnosis, (70-80% for type I diabetes) [55]. In cardiovascular disease, considerable collateralization of new blood vessels will reroute new blood vessels around narrowing or blocked arteries[56] well ahead of any heart attack or stroke which would produce a symptom or event. Similarly, it is well known that brain cell dysfunction predates the development of cognitive decline and dementia by as much as a decade or more before symptoms appear[57]. Ponder that!

Contrast this disease side continuum with the rather simple metabolic health paradigm where a cell is either functioning in a healthy way, or it is not – regardless of the many compensatory mechanisms that enable the body to keep moving.

What this means is that during the elapsed time where dysfunction occurs, even while showing no detectable symptoms, there already can be slow progressive cellular dysfunction occurring.

Taken together this is why education, prevention, and intervention are collectively important. They all have place together in our healthcare environment. The difference is that redox measures work upstream – at the foundations of a problem – not as a drug or procedure to intervene after-the-fact. Redox is prevention and as such is the fence at the top of the cliff.

Metabolic Disease

The Modern Pill Mentality & Metabolic Disease

A practical point should be made about the medical treatment paradigm we live in and which many embrace in their thinking. People who believe and behave like high blood sugars are a problem of insulin mis-management, often believe they are treating their disease through well supervised medication usage (the "pill mentality"). The same is true for blood lipid management, or any number of other diseases.

Viewing diabetes as simply mismanaged blood sugar levels, mistakes the symptoms for the disease. Believing that treating diabetes is about having the right amount of insulin to cover the effects of dietary food consumption, shifts the focus to carb counting, insulin units, blood sugar levels, and managing other associated complications. This focus entirely misses what is going on at the metabolic cellular level.

This illogical mindset accepts the distorted idea that insulin resistance occurs due to poor medication usage - that if they simply manage blood sugar levels with better precision they then are properly 'treating' diabetes. If this is true, then the same rationale applies to almost all other disease issues – that health is achieved through proper medication usage and the elimination of symptoms, regardless of the disease – instead of addressing the cellular dysfunction that is at the foundation of the problem.

For example, by taking the right cholesterol drug at the proper dosage, that cardiovascular disease is managed. The risk factor should not be just with the lipid level, but with the energy metabolism and metabolic dysfunction occurring in the 'basement' that is producing the dyslipidemia condition. Suppressing the lipid levels with drugs may help lower the risk for a heart attack, but it doesn't necessarily stop the metabolic dysfunction that arises from depressed redox functionality within the Redoxome of the body.

Fortunately, increasing numbers of people are taking more interest in their own health at earlier stages, and are understanding the redox-based importance of prevention and redox-based lifestyles. Many physicians are also doing more to help their patients take proactive steps in the areas of wellness and anti-aging. Whether they realize it or not, when they make

Metabolic Disease

these proactive steps, they are focusing on the redox landscape. While "pills" for some may still be essential to maintain stability, more health professionals and their patients are recognizing that if they stay entrenched in the "pill mentality" and do not emphasize lifestyle and dietary changes, they will continue to suffer the effects of metabolic disease – regardless of their devotion to "pills."

The surging rates of non-communicable metabolic disease witnesses that that redox-based lifestyle has not been addressed in a serious or proportionate manner. It is certainly not being addressed by the institutional "Bigs!" Metabolic disease is surging as confirmed by the rising levels of chronic disease - despite the modern advances and good treatment platforms.

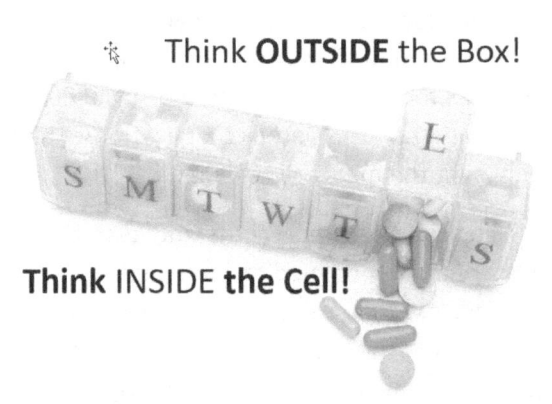

Think OUTSIDE the Box!

Think INSIDE the Cell!

A closer look at statistics for heart disease and cancer provide some interesting nuances to how modern medicine is better in these areas.

Again, it may be a fine nuance, but we should not be misled by statistics that say that diseases such as heart disease and cancer are declining. There is a difference between declining mortality and the overall incidence of these diseases. The former has to do with better "treatments," while the latter still speaks to the metabolic foundation.

This is confirmed by none other than the American Heart Association (AHA) in their statistical analysis in 2021[58]. While the incidence of heart attacks in the US was 805,000 (605,000 new and 200,000 recurrent), the death rate declined 27.9%, and actual deaths declined 9.8%. Even with these declining numbers and trends, the AHA notes that "the burden and risk factors remain alarmingly high."

Metabolic Disease

One has to ask, why? What is the relationship or correlation between a stubborn and "alarmingly high" rate of risk and burden, and the fact that fewer are dying? Would the alarmingly high rate of "risk and burden" remain high if the root-causes of the problems were being dealt with effectively? While this speaks to the effective use of medication and intervention to manage the problems, it says little about the base of metabolic health.

While the improvement in management witnessed by the decline in mortality is wonderful (especially when it is you or your family), this still means that there are 800,000 heart attacks per year – a solid indicator of the level of ongoing metabolic disease being inadequately addressed. It's a bold statement to make in today's health landscape, but this 800,000 level of activity would or could be dramatically decreased in a world focused on metabolic health, which would have an astonishing effect on these statistics.

Without saying it in so many words, the AHA's own statistical review is an admission that they recognize that the foundational issues related to metabolic disease are not being addressed as well as they could be.

A similar conclusion from analyzing improved 5-year cancer survivability could be reached due to improved early detection and treatment – but the real question is why the cancer occurs in the first place.

Whether it is cancer, heart disease, neurodegenerative decline, insulin resistance, or other metabolic conditions, it is not really so much about the management of the risk factors, as it is about the reasons why those risk factors are present in the first place – especially those brought on by poor lifestyle and nutrition choices. An absent risk factor trumps a managed risk factor – where possible.

While avoiding health complications and death through good management of the disease processes is good, those efforts must be complimented and improved upon with healthy redox-based prevention – focusing on reestablishing good metabolic function and cell-signaling capabilities, through lifestyle corrections.

It is all about metabolic lifestyle!

Metabolic Disease

The Metabolic Redox Machine

The Metabolic Redox Machine

Before extrapolating or extending what we have learned thus far, we must first restate the disclaimer that redox-based nutrition is not a treatment for non-communicable disease, in the context of how the healthcare establishment considers treatment. Nutrition and redox "treat" metabolic cellular function precisely because metabolic disorders are amenable to nutrition and redox correction - meaning they deal with energy metabolism and redox pathways.

Without question there is a wide disparity of opinion and advice as to how best to implement lifestyle measures. Much of this is heavily swayed by medical/nutrition consensus, Big Food interests, and Big-Media driven health pundits - all zealously defending their ideologies, commercially vested interests, and profit margins. This is often done with reckless disregard for how cells actually function.

With a better understanding that "real disease" is the upstream metabolic-level dysfunction and not the resulting pathologies, and that drugs cannot 'fix' dysfunctional metabolism or cellular communication at the foundation level, the role of an improved redox lifestyle becomes clear. It is to resolve problems of energy metabolism and redox-level mechanisms through lifestyle measures.

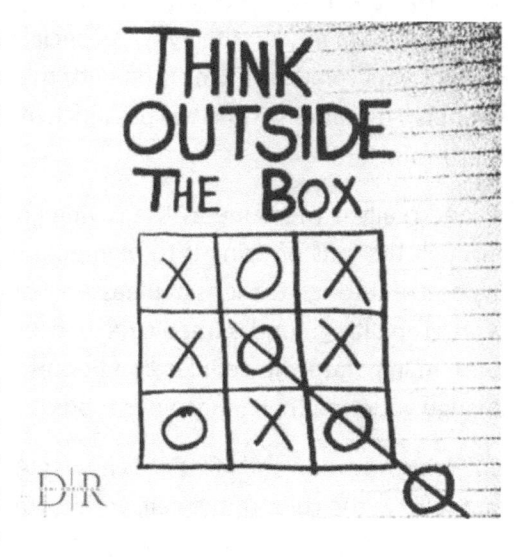

This is an important paradigm shift that forces one to think outside the box. Playing the 'game of health' by the wrong rules is an exercise fraught with frustration and failure. Defining health by any other parameter or standard than what cellular redox biology dictates, is a quick way to frustration and

The Metabolic Redox Machine

false security. Health and wellness is much more than the mere absence of symptoms!

Dr. Robert Lustig MD (author of the book *Metabolical*) has stated that chronic metabolic diseases are symptoms, and as such are not "drugable." However, he argues they are "foodable"[59]. The reasons for this relate to the fundamental nature of energy metabolism, and how this impacts cellular function.

This means that the "we are what we eat" maxim is true! Additionally, because they are also grounded in redox principles, physical activity, stress management, quality of sleep, and the existence of oral and gut dysbiosis (infection), each impact metabolic pathways in substantive ways, and are intimately tied into the Redoxome's control of pathway genes - for good or for bad.

All of this taken together argues that if you want to change your disease, you must change your lifestyle – especially food. The latter is true because of the direct relationship of food with the innate cellular blueprints related to energy metabolism and the presence of the reactive molecules generated therefrom.

If food really is medicine as the saying goes, then it needs to be looked at through the lens of using it to manipulate and manage the cellular state – instead of through the lens of pleasure, comfort, or sociability. This is a point worth repeating: food is 'medicine' because it has the power to manage and even manipulate the cellular condition for good (and bad). If you want to change your health, change your food!

Changing nutrition and lifestyle is how to *Awaken Your Inner Doctor*. It obeys and follows the rules of the cell, as laid out in nature. Therein lies the power to clean the garbage out of cells, to rescue mitochondria, and re-engage metabolic pathways that are critical for health and anti-aging. Therein is the power to change the course of disease and dysfunction - at the base metabolic level. Therein is the power to modulate and tame hungry hormones, lose weight and to turn on fat burning, to reduce inflammation, to enhance protection and preservation of brain cells and nerves and so

The Metabolic Redox Machine

much more. In this regard from a metabolic health perspective, more drugs are not needed; better food and eating practices are!

Identifying and following these rules leads to better health outcomes – better healthspan and better lifespan.

It is this focus on "how cells function" that should be the guiding dictum in both professional healthcare and in every-day personal living. The clues and guidance for which diet is best comes from knowing the rules of cellular function, the principles of redox signaling, and of applied functional nutrition. This must come from the perspective of how a cell would view it and not in how our taste buds, appetite hormones, or even 'expert' guidelines would dictate.

Cells do not think in terms of which popular diet strategy works best. They are not thinking Atkins, Mediterranean, South Beach, Weight Watchers, or Eastern or Western philosophy. They don't even know about vegan, vegetarian, paleo, carnivore, or high- or low-carb.

Instead, they "think" and behave in terms of redox sensitivity and energy metabolism. They "think" in terms of fuel availability (type and source) and the timing of its consumption, as well as the redox sensitivities and nutrients that are within the environment.

The effect of this nutrition on the cell can be very predictable, which is what gives food the ability to 'act like medicine.' While it really is not "medicine" the effect of food can manipulate cellular function very predictably. These effects combined with the redox state, affect the way mitochondria burn food for energy and how the cell utilizes nutrients to support its own defense mechanisms.

While genetic factors cannot be overlooked, and while it remains obvious that urgent disease symptoms and conditions may need attention through conventional medicine, the emphasis in every-day health and wellness should focus on addressing metabolic function. Fortunately, that is almost entirely within the realm of lifestyle! Both health and disease are the outcome of how cells function. Pure and simple!

The Metabolic Redox Machine

Supercharging metabolic health demands a focus on an improved redox lifestyle. This does not require expensive intervention, complex measures, or difficult over-promising diets. What it does require is a mindset to be well and to follow the only rules that matter – the rules of the cell.

This places wellness and anti-aging squarely within the realm of the Redoxome - and squarely within reach of anyone possessing the will to obey those rules.

Energy Metabolism, and Functional Ketosis

When diets and lifestyle match up with the cellular rules, health is favored. When they ignore these biological laws, regardless of their popularity or support, health is not favored. Individual variability and degree of burden from existing dysfunction and pathology may vary the responsiveness and the amount of redox sensitivity involved. However, there is no other way to *Awaken Your Inner Doctor* than to abide by these rules.

As we explore deeper into redox metabolism and the way cells create energy and execute signaling, we discover that cells respond differently to different dietary fuel sources. This in part explains why food can be used to manipulate how cells conduct their business. Cellular metabolism and the dynamics of energy and cellular communication are influenced by such factors as the relative concentrations (mixtures) and quantity of these fuels, and the timing of how/when they are consumed.

The factor of relative concentrations and "mixture" refers to the macronutrient mix of food (carbohydrates, protein, and fat). The 'timing of eating' variable relates to the patterns and timing of eating and the resulting effect on blood glucose concentrations over time.

The controlling issue is the amount of free glucose in the blood stream and its ease of access to the inside of the cell. This is why both the amounts and timing matter.

Cellular energy metabolism is also impacted by the effects of physical activity and stress on glucose levels, and the effect of systemic inflammation on the cell's ability to uptake glucose. Taken together each of these variables

The Metabolic Redox Machine

impacts hormones, blood sugar levels, fuel selection, and how mitochondrial function creates signaling molecules.

The way that these dynamics relate to disease is that metabolic disease occurs progressively along a function-dysfunction continuum. When dysfunctional energy creation creates too much oxidation, or inflammation, or prevents cellular defenses from operating naturally, the results are injurious to cellular function and disease eventually results.

This happens with too much oxidative stress or from not having enough oxidative stress to activate the hormetic redox-switch that drives redox-sensitive pathways. This science principle called *hormesis* is a grounding redox biology principle that forms the basis for all redox signaling mechanisms. A later section will expand on this very important principle of redox biology.

How a cell 'selects' and metabolizes fuel (food) is a fundamental determinant of how cellular energy metabolism proceeds. This pertains to both the quantity of glucose in the blood stream available as fuel (carbs in diet), and the relative mixture of other dietary fuels (proteins and fats). While that may sound complex, it is actually a simple concept.

The rules that govern energy metabolism are 'hard-wired' biochemically into how cells respond to the presence of glucose and fats. Altering the relative ratios or mixture of food source between the three macronutrient fuel sources (carbohydrates, fats, and proteins) determines what happens at a cellular and hormonal level when food is metabolized.

The first of the basic metabolic rules is that (with some minor but notable exceptions by organ), glucose is the primary fuel and the first preferential fuel to be metabolized in Krebs cycle - if it is present in the blood stream. As long as there is glucose (and insulin) in the blood stream, little if any fat will be metabolized to produce energy[60], nor will any follow-on cellular repair happen (autophagy). This is nature's way of preserving protein and fats for the proverbial "rainy day."

However, when blood glucose levels fall, becoming less available for cellular energy metabolism, fats and proteins become the primary source for energy

The Metabolic Redox Machine

metabolism. It is an absolute given that energy requirements of the human body must be met regardless of the fluctuations in nutrient availability. Without an energy source, or the presence of oxygen which enables its combustion, life ceases to exist.

Minus glucose, fats become the dominate fuel source. They are converted to ketones (primarily in liver cells) through a process called beta-oxidation. Ketones then convert to acetyl-CoA and enter Krebs cycle as a fuel source.

Amino acids can also be converted into pyruvate or acetyl-CoA and enter Krebs cycle via acetyl-CoA or a Krebs' intermediate, but the body does not maintain official reserves of protein for use as fuel. Protein is preferentially used to build, maintain, and repair body tissues. Fat, however, is readily stored in the body and is an efficient fuel per unit of weight compared to carbohydrates.

It is also true that different organs and tissues have their unique preferences for fuel type. For example, heart muscle cells prefer fatty acids, and skeletal muscle, and brain cells, and red blood cells prefer glucose. Brain cells utilize

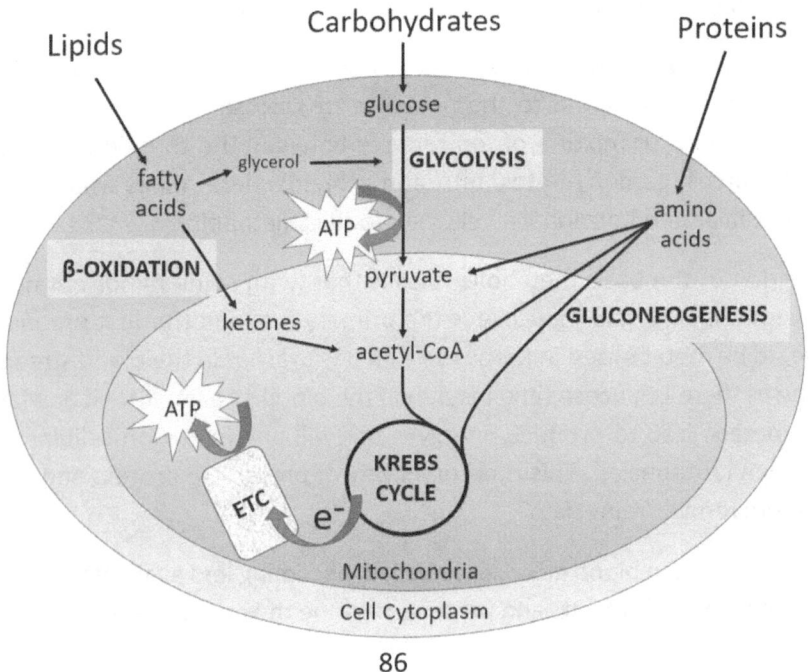

The Metabolic Redox Machine

glucose and ketones because fatty acids are not preferred in the brain due to limitations crossing the blood brain barrier. Thus, there is a dynamic adaptability throughout the body based on cell type and fuel availability, as to which fuel source is utilized for energy needs.

The dominant result of glucose un-availability (when carbohydrates are restricted) is that cells switch to fatty acids for their energy supply. This is especially true in the liver. The adaptation for switching between energy sources is a dynamic and responsive process.

Consider what happens during fasting. During times of fasting (and between meals) available blood glucose is depleted. This activates glucagon hormones which work to liberate more glucose from glycogen storage. Once these sources are exhausted, two things happen. First, hunger hormones are affected and tell the brain that the now-deprived glucose state needs rescued through additional dietary consumption. Secondly, cells shift to a different fuel supply to provide their energy needs. If this shift is difficult or not flexibly practiced, the hormone drive to increase the "rescue" food supply is intensified.

These needs are particularly critical in brain and heart cells, so adaptive mechanisms are at play in these organs so as to maintain needed energy sourcing. As total glucose is depleted, fatty acids are taken from stored triglycerides (adipose) and are oxidized to provide the raw ingredients that fuel Krebs cycle. Liver cells are particularly good at taking fats and converting them into *ketone bodies.* These molecules are a cleaner-burning energy source in Krebs cycle. Ketone bodies provide improved energy efficiency and helps to restore dysregulated energy metabolism[61].

Since fats are challenged in crossing the blood-brain barrier, ketone molecules become an important source to maintain brain cell function during glucose restriction. They have the added benefit of being very 'clean burning' in that they produce less oxidation by-products in nerve cells.

The ability of a cell to switch from using glucose to fatty acids as a fuel source is termed *metabolic flexibility*. Being metabolically flexible means that one is flexible or "fat adapted" – i.e., able to utilize fats easily and comfortably

The Metabolic Redox Machine

as a fuel source inside the cell. Flexible also means able to go back to glucose, and then again to fat, and back to glucose, with efficiency and without undue stress.

Not being metabolically flexible means that one is "carb-addicted" or dependent on an ever-present source of glucose as a fuel source. Due to the activation of hunger hormones, carb-addicted cells (and their owners) have a difficult time adjusting to not having glucose readily available. When cells are not flexible and are more dependent on carbohydrates, the physiology is punishingly harsh on the brain and the body - demanding carbs be consumed to rescue the carb-energy imbalance.

This is a survival mechanism, where the body is programmed through hormone control to signal the need for more glucose. Falling blood sugar levels and rising glucagon levels drive the hunger hormones which tells the brain that cells need more glucose quickly. As the body experiences the hypoglycemic "sugar crash," hormones quickly demand a quick dietary "fix." This ghrelin/leptin-driven hormone cascade powerfully drives food intake and the reward centers in the brain by altering the dopamine receptors in brain neurons and brain synapse plasticity[62] - thus conditioning the brain to seek a solution and reward. This can become the essence of 'food addiction' where food is eaten in quantities beyond homeostatic energy requirements.

However, eventually, without carbs, cells do shift to burn fat and create ketones. These are the body's fourth energy source – made from within. As ketones accumulate in the blood, a state of ketosis occurs. As this state occurs, it is viewed by the cell as a "nutritional stress" and a litany of cellular mechanisms activate and initiate cellular repair and defense processes via a hormetic stress-adaptive mechanism. Again, these health-associated mechanisms will be discussed in more detail hereafter.

This biochemistry describes an innately brilliant cellular mechanism which utilizes fat as fuel when the right dietary conditions prevail. This means we have the ability to intelligently manipulate metabolic function through macronutrient consumption and the time-management of eating (alternating fed and fasted states). This result is reached with the dietary and lifestyle manipulation of glucose levels. This then is the determinant

The Metabolic Redox Machine

that selects which fuel is used in cellular energy metabolism. This is a key point. This is nature's design for initiating "fat burning." This is one reason why working against this design through "fat-burning pills" and herbs, while not managing the glucose load in the body, is counter-productive.

There is more to this than simply reducing food and or calories. While reducing caloric fuel load can drive down glucose levels, the levels must be low enough to trigger the switch to fat metabolism. If this doesn't happen, then the body stays in a 'rescue mode' hungry state. A caloric reduction strategy which focuses on 'energy in - energy out,' may cause weight loss even without addressing metabolic function. This is because carbs may be still at the level to make flexibility difficult and eating frequency is enough to suppress hunger drive. Regardless, it can make the redox-flex and fat burning a challenge.

This is a common finding with meal replacement diet strategies which lower calories, but still disrespect these basic cellular rules. There is more to metabolic health than burning more calories than one takes in.

The point to be made from a metabolic health perspective is that being metabolically flexible and able to make this shift, improves metabolic function and health at all levels – especially as the food protects the liver and respects the gut.

In this state of *nutritional ketosis*, fats are removed from storage and metabolized ("fat burning") and a state of ketosis is more easily achieved and maintained. Researchers have found that cycling in and out of ketosis increases the cells' ability to be redox-responsive. This powers the many redox-sensitive mechanisms that support cellular repair and renewal and homeostasis[63]. The evidence is mounting that nutritional ketosis enhances mitochondrial function and endogenous antioxidant defense mechanisms[64], again via the redox-sensitive principle of hormesis.

Taken together, increased metabolic health means that there is more "flexibility" in choosing and using fuel sources within a cell. The state of being metabolically flexible is by definition a result of being metabolically

The Metabolic Redox Machine

healthy, fat-adapted, and less carb addicted. Metabolic health equals metabolic flexibility.

With this flexibility and the disciplined practice of entering a fat-burning metabolism regularly, comes a host of health benefits to the cell and the overall body. Specifically, these benefits translate to the role of redox signaling on transcription factors and the activation of a wide range of pathway genes, including antioxidant genes and cellular renewal mechanisms (autophagy) – all of which are redox-sensitive.

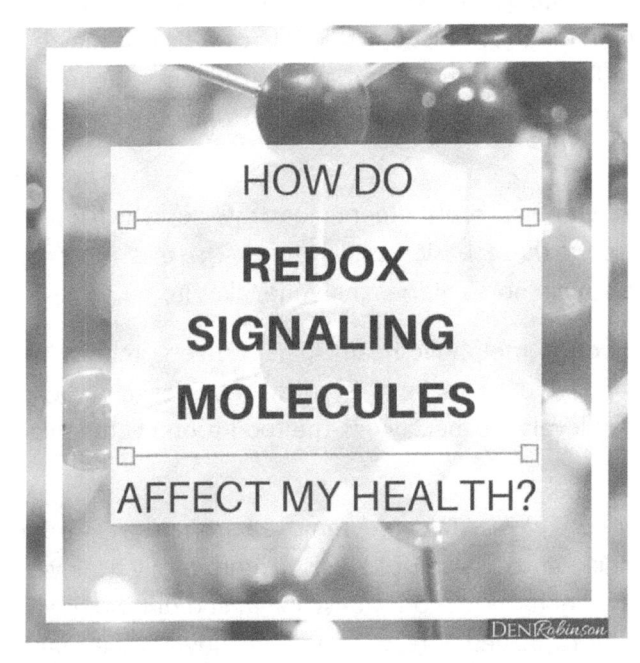

With this basic energy-metabolism information in mind, one can begin to understand the impact that various diets have on health.

An interesting side note is to consider the effect of dietary supplements and vitamins on the flexible shift in fuel source choice - and can mimic the effect of ketosis while even in a "fed" state. The extensions of this are significant. This begins to explain their parallel effect on redox-sensitive, hormesis-driven cellular health mechanisms.

Knowing the basis for these rules will begin to make this new phenomenon more understandable because they highlight the power of manipulating the Redoxome with mild oxidative stimuli via food selection and supplements, to drive healthy pathway gene activation.

The Metabolic Redox Machine

With this introduction to the rules of cellular energy metabolism, ketone bodies and ketosis, we can now explore the relationships between metabolic flexibility and nutritional ketosis.

Metabolic Flexibility, Krebs Cycle, and Energy Metabolism

As we have learned, the ability to switch fuel sources is called *Metabolic Flexibility* [65]. This is an adaptive response that happens with low glucose and insulin levels in the blood. Metabolic flexibility or "fuel switching" is the ability of a cell to switch between glucose and fatty acids as an energy source. The inability to do this is metabolic inflexibility.

Being "fat adapted" is metabolic flexibility. There is an increased ability to use fats for energy. This means that there is an enhanced ability to switch between carbs and fats. This increases metabolic efficiency – something that occurs with practice and metabolic conditioning.

The new redox-based science helps explain the phenomenon of insulin resistance, along with cell mechanisms that control the selection of fuel source between glucose or fatty acids. These concepts are central to metabolic disease because the development of almost all chronic diseases is a consequence of having metabolic in-flexibility and mitochondrial dysfunction. This also helps explain the importance of liver health because it plays such a significant role in energy metabolism physiology.

Damaged or dysfunctional liver cells contribute to the development of insulin resistance[66]. Insulin resistance likewise causes damage to liver cells. It can be a vicious cycle.

Glucose is the primary energy source for the brain and body. Carbs are utilized first because of the quickness and ease in utilizing them as fuel in the glycolysis pathway. Fats activate when glucose is depleted. Thus, carbohydrates and fats are the main fuel sources.

These fuel sources exist in a reduced state awaiting the biochemical reaction that begins an oxidative process. The oxidation of these fuels transfer electrons through a series of reactions which harvests and transfers energy, thus generating the power to drive life. However, not all of the oxygen is

The Metabolic Redox Machine

reduced, leaving a small amount of it oxidized, which is the source for "reactive oxygen species."

As an aside, this is similar to the burning of wood in a campfire. Wood as a fuel source exists in a "reduced" state (has all of its electrons) and becomes oxidized or "burnt" during combustion with oxygen in a process that gives up those available electrons to oxygen, which in turn becomes reduced. The water that is created in this reaction is evaporated into the atmosphere.

In principle, this is the same type of biochemical reaction that occurs in human cell biology when glucose and fat and protein is "burnt" in the combustion process we call "oxidative phosphorylation" within the mitochondria. In all forms, "redox" (reduction – oxidation) is the movement of electrons from one molecule to another, resulting in the creation of energy in the process. These molecules also have various electrical charges which is what affects the oxidative state of its environment.

Returning to the discussion of biological energy sources, fats are stored as triglycerides in adipose tissue. A triglyceride is composed of three fatty acid molecules held together by a glycerol backbone. After glucose is depleted, triglycerides are broken down or hydrolyzed into their four component parts – three free fatty acids and one glycerol molecule.

Glycerol is an intermediate in the glycolysis reaction which is converted to pyruvate and continues on into Krebs cycle. The three fatty acid portions are oxidized and converted to ketone bodies which then also continue into Krebs Cycle.

In all of this, delivering the Acetyl group to Krebs cycle is the key factor and starting point in all Krebs-based energy metabolism reactions. Creating it from the breakdown of fats (lipolysis & beta-oxidation), sugars (glycolysis), or proteins (proteolysis) is a function of many enzymes that are driven by the metabolic demands of a cell and the availability of an energy source.

The balance and direction of these metabolic reactions are in general dictated first by the availability of carbohydrate, and its relative amount compared with the other fuel sources. With less carbohydrate fuel available, ketone bodies are produced which then become the dominant fuel. This

The Metabolic Redox Machine

results in a glucose-sparing effect for organs which otherwise depend on glucose as their primary energy source (such as the brain and red blood cells).

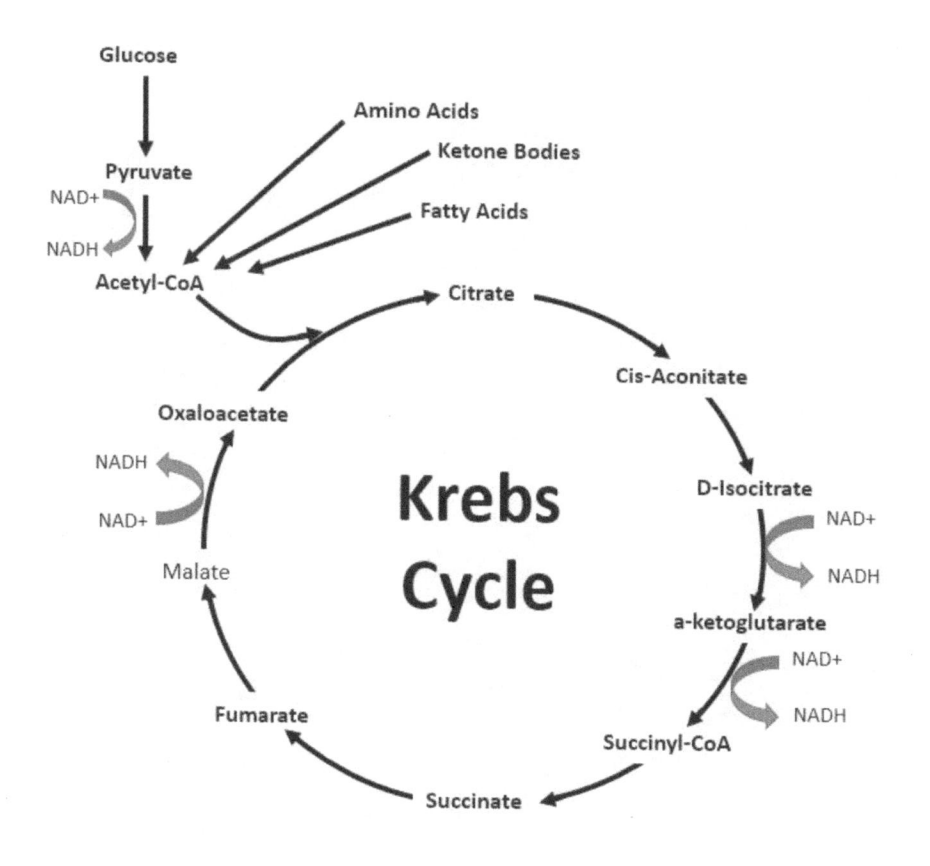

Krebs Cycle

- Glucose → Pyruvate (NAD+ → NADH) → Acetyl-CoA
- Amino Acids → Acetyl-CoA
- Ketone Bodies → Acetyl-CoA
- Fatty Acids → Acetyl-CoA
- Acetyl-CoA → Citrate → Cis-Aconitate → D-Isocitrate (NAD+ → NADH) → α-ketoglutarate (NAD+ → NADH) → Succinyl-CoA → Succinate → Fumarate → Malate → Oxaloacetate (NAD+ → NADH) → Citrate

The Metabolic Redox Machine

Part Three – The Functional Redoxome

Nutritional Ketosis

With a better understanding of basic energy metabolism engraved within the mitochondria and Krebs cycle, let us now take a closer look at the health principle of ketosis.

As we have learned, ketosis is the metabolic response to an energy "crisis" and is used by the body as a mechanism to sustain metabolism (life) by altering the source of fuel for energy metabolism. There are many distinct biochemical advantages that are realized during the state of ketosis.

The ability to utilize various fuel sources is a wonderful adaptation built into the human body to assure survival during lean times. This allows the body to access and fill energy demands from stored fat during periods of starvation or fasting. It also provides fascinating benefits to the human experience and in improving the body's ability to stress-adapt and be responsive to changing conditions.

Along with the deprivation of oxygen, perhaps the most stressful form of environmental stress to a cell is the restriction of its energy supply. Of course, there are other stresses that affect a cell such as transient hypoxia, persistent toxicity, and injury, but the day-in and day-out threat seen through all of time is the demand for metabolic energy and the disruptions to that supply.

Fortunately, cells and organ systems have acquired the ability to adapt to decreasing fuel supplies. They do this by switching to, or manufacturing, other energy sources. When carbohydrates become scarce, cells switch to fats and proteins, and even make new fuels (ketones) upon demand. They do this as redox-sensitive "switches" recognize the mild oxidative stress imposed by declining glucose levels (nutritional stress) which activates signaling pathways that trigger the oxidation of fats and proteins as needed.

Ketones provides an alternative fuel to facilitate electron transfer within Krebs cycle[67]. Because of the different fuel sources and the unique entry

Nutritional Ketosis

points of each into Krebs cycle, burning ketones decreases muscle glycolysis and plasma lactate concentrations. This is an important feature that many are beginning to recognize as it reduces recovery time after significant exercise and physical exertion.

There is a certain 'biologic magic' that is built into these processes. In times of limited nutrition and energy availability, a stress-adaption phenomenon is activated. This happens as glucose and insulin levels fall, which enhances insulin signaling and overall protein production. During these periods, cells experience growth and repair. These processes when appropriately cycled, improve the body's ability to be metabolically flexible and to deal with systemic and cellular stresses, as well as to adapt to changes in bioenergetic and metabolic challenges.

As it turns out, all of this is grounded on finely tuned biological science that utilizes the stress-response adaption phenomenon in ways to improve survival and fitness. Today we call this the Redoxome.

This Redox "ome" is the newest category of healthcare. It isn't the reinvention of something already known about. It is new! Or, at least, our

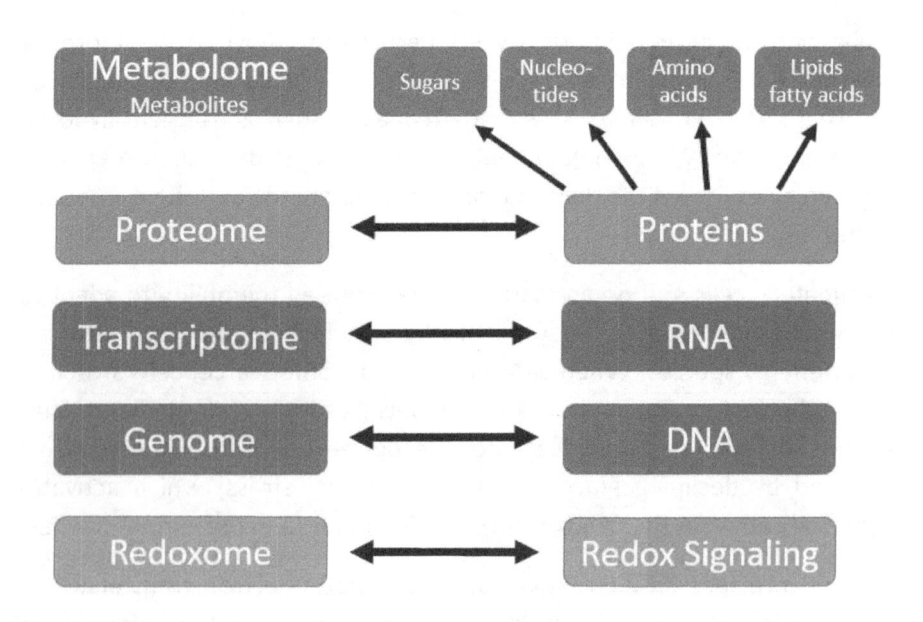

Metabolome (Metabolites)	Sugars	Nucleotides	Amino acids	Lipids fatty acids

Proteome	⟷	Proteins
Transcriptome	⟷	RNA
Genome	⟷	DNA
Redoxome	⟷	Redox Signaling

Nutritional Ketosis

understanding of it is new since. The truth is that it has always existed – for it is Natural Law – the way the cells are programed.

The Redoxome is the grounding epigenetic level that instructs the genome (DNA) what to do and when to do it – the "overlay" on our genes. The fact that nutritional ketosis has the ability to influence redox states and play in the landscape of redox-sensitive transcription, is what makes ketosis such a powerful ally for health.

Even though the principle of ketosis has also been around for eons, the understanding of its science and how to use it for health is also new - and there is much yet to be clarified.

This practice has its detractors, and much about what it is, has been misrepresented over the decades. Certainly, a persistent fasting and ketogenic state that is long-term or unended caries risk and uncertainty and is seldom recommended. There is a valid concern for "keto" diets that are not well executed as this can overly stress the body with long duration, as well as to diminish fruit and vegetable consumption with their phytochemicals and fiber.

Exercising caution to compensate for this and to cycle in and out of ketosis to enhance flexibility (which is one of the main objectives of 'keto'), and to assure optimum levels of dietary fiber and phytochemicals, has become a wise recommendation for those experienced in this area. Such "keto cycling," (which means alternating between low and normal carbohydrate levels through a week) often occurs in a 5:2 pattern - 5 days in ketosis and 2 days out. The rate at which one can comfortably cycle is a function of how metabolically flexible they are and can at least be an indirect indicator of one's metabolic state. (A quick indicator of how "flexible" one is, is to see how easy it is to skip a meal or fast.)

As always, diets which manipulate energy metabolism should not be abused or used carelessly, especially where there is preexisting metabolic pathology or disease – without the supervision and oversight of a health professional familiar with your health, and with energy-based biochemistry and physiology. We should always have a healthy and generous respect for the

Nutritional Ketosis

multi-variable impact of metabolic problems when it comes to energy metabolism. As mentioned previously, this is especially so for people with insulin resistance, as well as for others with significant metabolic disease.

Nonetheless, the ketogenic arena has taken on new life in the medical and wellness / anti-aging landscape. What gives life to these strategies is that a ketosis state can be reached through a variety of avenues, including fasting, macronutrient management, exercise, and utilization of pathway gene activators such as redox signaling molecules.

Early Beginnings of Functional Ketosis

To date, ketosis has been poorly understood outside of starvation modes and diabetic crisis (diabetic ketoacidosis). Early interest in the subject of ketosis began in the 1920s when it was discovered that it was particularly beneficial in managing the condition of epilepsy, especially in drug-refractory cases, and especially in children.

It was found that the state of glucose deprived ketosis provided such dramatic benefits to the brain that it possessed powerful abilities in quieting the brain, reducing the oxidation excitement and subsequent seizures.

However, the interest in ketosis as a viable strategy for health has not always been positive. While it enjoyed some positive regard and the medical press in the early 1900s, the practice of using fasting as a method to induce a state of ketosis was sidelined with the introduction of the anti-seizure drug Dilantin, in 1953. Prior to this time, it was discovered that extended fasting affected brain cells in a way to control extreme epileptic seizures. However, with appearance of a pill to treat seizures, it became a much-preferred modality over subjecting people to lengthy periods of fasting each day.

During this same general time period much was also being learned about diabetes, especially type 1. It was understood that those with Type 1 diabetes (and even for those with uncontrolled type II diabetes) could slip into a state of "ketosis" called *diabetic ketoacidosis*, a dangerous and life-threatening complication of uncontrolled blood sugar levels and altered blood pH balance problems.

Nutritional Ketosis

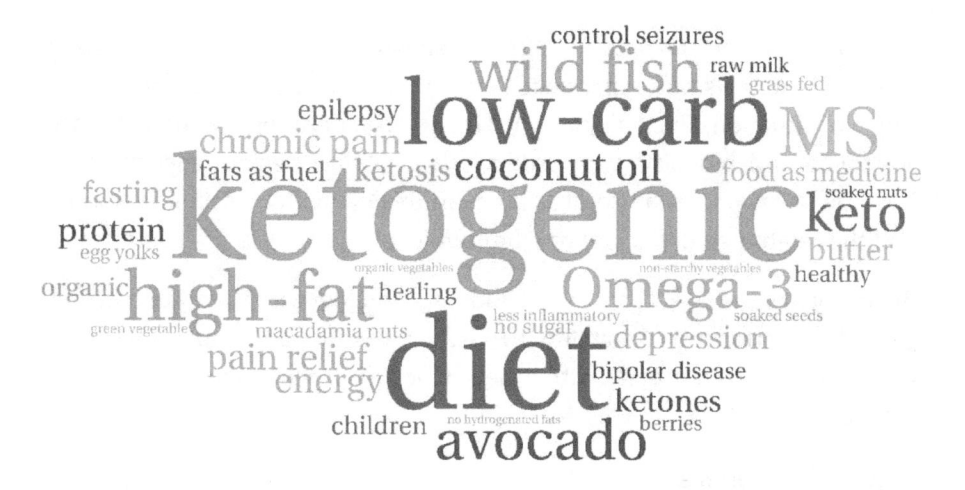

Word cloud: ketogenic, diet, low-carb, high-fat, wild fish, coconut oil, Omega-3, avocado, MS, control seizures, raw milk, grass fed, epilepsy, chronic pain, fats as fuel, ketosis, food as medicine, fasting, soaked nuts, protein, keto, egg yolks, butter, organic, organic vegetables, non-starchy vegetables, healthy, healing, green vegetable, macadamia nuts, less inflammatory, no sugar, soaked seeds, pain relief, depression, energy, bipolar disease, ketones, children, no hydrogenated fats, berries

At this point it is important to emphasize that diabetic ketoacidosis is not the same thing as nutritional ketosis, although some of the same principles of glucose metabolism apply to both.

Diabetic ketoacidosis occurs when cells that are unable to, or are resistant to, moving glucose across cell walls, sense their own state of fuel starvation and begin making ketones as a backup fuel source to compensate. These ketone acids are then released into the blood stream which adds additional levels of fuel to the already high levels of glucose in the blood. Because of their acidic nature they have a profound effect on acid-base balance in the blood. Unchecked and unmanaged, this condition can quickly escalate and progressively create a serious medical emergency.

In this early era, the increasingly negative concerns about 'ketones' (due to diabetic ketoacidosis in people with type 1 diabetes) combined with a quicker and easier solution for controlling seizures using Dilantin, caused the medical and health world to turn its attention away from ketones. Overnight it seemed, "ketosis" became a dirty word!

In very recent years as ketone biochemistry has become better understood, the purposeful use of nutritional ketosis to trigger redox-driven cellular repair has become popularized. This has found its home in wellness and antiaging healthcare, and within the area of diabetes management.

Nutritional Ketosis

Due to the powerful health benefits linked with improved cellular function, interest in ketosis has expanded. Today it is used with effect for a broad range of situations, including but not limited to neurodegenerative disease, weight control, blood sugar disorders, and even high-performance athletics. It is now emerging as a useful strategy in dealing with metabolic disorders and the related epidemic of non-communicable disease so prevalent today.

Achieving a state of ketosis through fasting and low carbohydrate diets has gained attention for its ability to reduce weight, and improve several parameters often seen with metabolic disorders, including insulin resistance.

Ketosis for Diabetes

As a sidenote specifically about diabetes, low carbohydrate or ketogenic diets are attractive options for helping those with blood sugar disorders and have the added benefit of often helping people adjust their requirements for medications. Prior to the advent of insulin, low carbohydrate dietary management was the primary modality utilized to help diabetics manage their condition. While it appears to be safe and effective for most diabetic patients, it should always be pursued with the consent, advice, and awareness of your physician.

The good news is that nutritional ketosis happens at much lower and safer levels of ketones in the blood than ketoacidosis – and for very different reasons. Nutritional ketosis happens during fasting and dietary restriction of carbohydrates. It also occurs in the course of nighttime "fasting" each and every night while sleeping, going without food for several hours. It is, after all, a function of the amount and timing of carbohydrates that are eaten, which provides an effective way to help induce weight loss and to better manage A1C levels[68].

The redox biology of ketosis and metabolic flexibility is intriguing. The possibility of using nutrition to deal with metabolic disorders and to realize improvements in overall health, and neurological disorders, is tantalizing, if not incredible.

Nutritional Ketosis

While ketogenic diets and fasting do work for improving metabolic flexibility and ketosis, they can require extra amounts of management and discipline. By understanding the principles, and applying a "cycling" strategy, going in and out of ketosis, it can help discipline the "flexibility" part of the process, and make life easier in the psychological aspects of the practice.

Redox Biology of Ketosis

Nutritional ketosis occurs when glucose is relatively unavailable in the blood stream. This forces the cell to use fatty acids as a fuel substrate. These fatty acids are derived from stored triglycerides and are metabolized and converted into ketone bodies. The actual "ketone bodies" (molecules) are the ketone acids named β-hydroxybutyrate and acetoacetate. They are converted to acetyl-CoA which is the primary energy molecule that enters Krebs cycle for complete oxidation.

Because ketones enjoy an enhance energy profile and avoid glycolysis and issues with lactate production, they are considered a "cleaner" fuel in making cellular energy[69]. They are used as an energy source by many cells throughout the body during times of glucose deficiency. This is especially beneficial to various cells and tissues throughout the body, especially brain neurons.

We have learned that under normal physiologic conditions the brain's primary energy fuel is glucose. However, ketone bodies are an important source of energy for the brain during times of glucose deficiency. Ketones readily cross the blood brain barrier and are used in the mitochondria of brain cells. This ability appears to ameliorate the energy crisis that occurs during neurodegenerative diseases which is characterized by a deterioration in glucose metabolism and increased oxidation within brain neurons[70]. This helps explain the benefit of fasting and ketones on brain health.

Ketones are reported to be helpful in traumatic brain injury cases where compromised energy deficits are seen. At the same time, they reduce inflammation and oxidative stress and subsequent neurodegeneration and are associated with improved recover following injury[71]. This lessens the amount of oxidative stress imposed in brain cells and improves their energy profile and the neuro-protective qualities.

Furthermore, evidence exists that ketone bodies play neuro- and cell-protective roles[72][73] and are active in upregulation of genes involved in protection against oxidative stress and the regulation of metabolism[74]. This means that ketones bodies are not only a better energy source for neurons, especially after injury or during neurodegenerative processes[75], but they offer many advantages for cellular health generally.

It is this universal beneficial effect on all cells, and the impressive ability to activate redox-sensitive mechanisms, which gives ketones the ability to play in the redox wellness landscape.

Thus, ketones play a major role not only as an energy source, but also within the Redoxome itself. Due to its unique energy dynamics, the breakdown of ketones (ketolysis) produces a mild oxidative stress in the mitochondria. This is beneficial over the long term because it initiates an adaptive (hormetic) response in the cell. This activates and positively influences many pathways and cellular functions. This signaling function from ketones has a significant effects on cells[76]. Their roles on these cellular metabolic pathways are impressive, as they have an impact on:

- Nrf2 activation[77]
- FOXO1 (Forkhead Box O1) gene[78]
- Hypoxia inducible factor (HIF1)[79]
- Atg - autophagy genes[80]
- Sirtuins[81]
- BDNF production in the brain[82]
- AMP-activated kinase pathways[83]
- mTOR inhibition[84]
- Peroxisome proliferator-activated receptor γ coactivator 1α (PGC-1α), responsible for activating the fasting response in liver cells which includes fatty acid beta-oxidation[85]
- Fibroblast growth factor 21[86]
- ADP ribosyl cyclase (CD38)[87]

Nutritional Ketosis

- NAD+, nicotinamide adenine dinucleotide[88] and metabolic switching
- Enhanced redox state[89]

These actions and influences collectively resolve oxidative stress through increased antioxidant production, improved mitochondrial function and growth, DNA repair, and enhanced cellular renewal mechanisms[90] (autophagy). Clinically, this translates to improved glucose regulation, blood pressure and heart rate, reduced inflammation, improved sleep and cognition[91], and reduced abdominal and organ fat. Additionally, and gratefully, the presence of ketones directly suppress appetite hormones[92].

When ketosis is not in effect, the dynamic effects of glucose levels are profound. High glucose levels decrease Nrf2 transcription activity which suppresses the expression of antioxidant enzymes[93]. This can have profound effects in cellular health and healing - especially in those people with metabolic disease such as diabetes[94]. High glucose levels also increase inflammation via NF-*k*B transcription factor activity[95].

Fasting and ketosis can be a significant factor in metabolic health[96]. Clearly, ketosis and metabolic flexibility (fat adaptation) are among nature's powerful mechanism for activating cellular repair and renewal. These are among the many powerful health applications that are activated due to redox-driven biochemistry.

In fact, those familiar with redox biology will recognize the redox overlay in all of these pathways and systems. They are all a part of the vast Redoxome and derive their effect from induced mild levels of redox oxidation.

With a better understanding of the principles of redox biology, one can begin to connect the dots in applying these principles to daily living. This allows for the informed and wise manipulation of these variables to improve cellular health. This is ultimately the essence of the redox lifestyle.

These variables and redox-based factors include:

- macronutrient quantity (the glucose trigger)
- macronutrient ratios (low carb, high fat)
- timing of eating

Nutritional Ketosis

- fed and fasting state
- phytochemical content
- fiber - presence or absence
- liver cell function and liver health (toxins)
- existing state of metabolic disease
- genetic background – gene defects
- supplementation practices
- ketosis cycling
- exercise.

[For more information on the effect of exercise in creating a state of ketosis, see Appendix: Ketosis and Exercise.]

Due to its effect on metabolic flexibility and redox health, we will now discuss some of the practical applications of fasting in more detail.

Intermittent Fasting

Fasting is more than just going without food, starving, or being 'hangry.' From a metabolic point of view the strategy is about managing frequency, types, amounts, and quality of food consumed – precisely for the effect this has on cellular function.

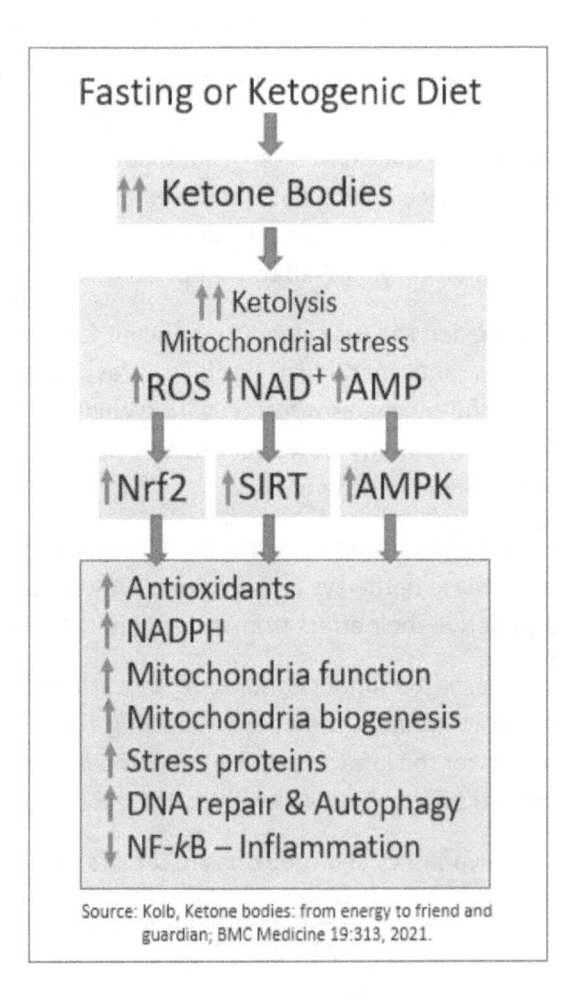

Fasting or Ketogenic Diet
↓
↑↑ **Ketone Bodies**
↓
↑↑ Ketolysis
Mitochondrial stress
↑ROS ↑NAD⁺ ↑AMP
↓   ↓   ↓
↑Nrf2 ↑SIRT ↑AMPK
↓   ↓   ↓

↑ Antioxidants
↑ NADPH
↑ Mitochondria function
↑ Mitochondria biogenesis
↑ Stress proteins
↑ DNA repair & Autophagy
↓ NF-kB – Inflammation

Source: Kolb, Ketone bodies: from energy to friend and guardian; BMC Medicine 19:313, 2021.

Nutritional Ketosis

Simply going without food is not the point. It doesn't make any sense nor is it physiologically helpful to skip meals if the follow-on meal is a banquet at the local buffet. The point in exercising this level of control over food consumption is to activate metabolic processes that improve physical, mental, emotional, and physiological health.

To know what that means for each person requires a better understanding about the innerworkings of how cells function or "think." This impacts one's ability to 'play the game' by the correct set of rules - in fact the only set of rules that govern true metabolic health.

Intermittent fasting, otherwise called "time restricted eating" is gaining in popularity and is receiving its due recognition in scientific literature for what it is able to do at the cellular level. Frequent eating is not a healthy practice. The historical advice to *always* eat three 'square' meals a day defies cellular health principles and is not wise.

It is recognized that too much and too frequent eating, and consuming excess 'energy,' promotes obesity and excess body fat. However, few understand the impact of how eating 'too much fuel' and too frequently, affects hunger regulation hormones, impairs brain function, increases metabolic disease risks, affects blood sugar control problems, creates dysfunctional cell signaling, affects the gastrointestinal tract, disrupts brain health, and sleep – to name a few.

Always being in a "fed" state is correlated with metabolic disease and periodically abstaining from food consumption yields significant health benefits.

Early researchers believed the health and lifespan benefits derived from reduced food availability (caloric restriction) occurred due to a passive reduction in harmful free radical oxidation. Currently, research points out that the health benefits are not simply from a reduction in reactive oxygen species being generated, or even from caloric weight loss. Rather, the main health benefits are now understood to occur due to adaptive cellular response to dietary stress and the healing processes this activates.

Nutritional Ketosis

This is due to improved glucose regulation, decreased insulin levels, improved stress resistance, and the suppression of inflammation[97]. These cellular mechanisms are directly under the control of redox sensitive pathways, and these in turn are affected by the quality of the redox lifestyle.

The intermittent fasting strategy calls for restricted food consumption to a 4-to-8-hour window of time through a 24-hour day, with the remaining 16-20 hours being without food consumption. Ideally, the last meal of the day would be no sooner than three hours prior to bedtime. This better assures that glucose metabolism is minimized during sleep, and that the body is actively transitioning into an autophagy mode – (i.e., cleaning the brain and 'taking out the garbage'). Variations of this strategy may include eating every other day ("alternate-day fasting") or with some ratio of on/off days eating.

The crucial point in fasting is the time spent without food, not that calories are restricted. This is because during fasting, the changed state of energy metabolism activates pathways that are cell protective and defend against metabolic stress. This is the essence of the stress-adaptive response. This describes those processes that repair or replace damaged molecules and cell components (autophagy and apoptosis).

Dietary, cultural, and half-truth practical considerations often sabotage the widespread adoption of these healthier eating patterns. The cultural notion of three meals per day with snacks in between is so deeply ingrained in our culture that the idea of intermittent fasting is seldom if ever seriously contemplated by people. And then there are the pesky hormones! Usually fasting is seen through the eyes of pain and discomfort – physically and mentally.

The fact that carb-addicted individuals 'cannot' tolerate abstinence from food due to the relentless driving of hunger hormones is a very real deterrent to people's willingness to move their metabolic physiology to a healthier plateau. This hormone-driven irritability and impact on concentration are powerful factors, even though these side effects subside within three to four weeks.

Nutritional Ketosis

Those who are practiced with fasting remark that they may feel hunger, but it is very manageable (if present at all), and that the increase in overall energy, clear thinking, and improved health far outweigh any temporary inconvenience.

Fasting requires a paradigm shift from old rules, a new mindset, and careful planning (socially and with the calendar) - and a healthy nutritive diet plan. To repeat, this isn't about going hungry. It is about becoming metabolically healthy!

While there are many health benefits derived from weight loss as a result of fasting, several benefits linked with fasting are dissociated from weight loss. These include improved blood sugar regulation, blood pressure, heart rate, athletic endurance, and visceral and organ fat loss.

The three most studied fasting practices are alternate day fasting, 5:2 intermittent fasting (2 days each week), and daily time-restricted eating. Single day fasting or days with serious calorie restriction (500-700 calories) result in increased ketones on those days.

We have previously outlined the redox biology affected with fasting and nutritional ketosis. In review, the salient points are that lowered glucose and insulin levels initiate important cellular repair process inside cells (autophagy). The benefit of this phenomenon happens because of the cell's ability to respond to mild nutritional stress (a principle of hormesis), which yields a redox stimulation of cell defenses. This results in the prevention of premature aging and neurodegeneration and provides general disease resistance[98]. This is why and how fasting as part of a redox lifestyle, is healthy!

Over time and with practice, the body and brain and mitochondria adapt to fasting because they become more flexible. Fasting done right yields long-term adaptive metabolic benefits. These include:

- Increased Nrf2 signaling and antioxidant gene expression
- Antioxidant defense
- DNA repair, translation, and protein controls
- Mitochondrial biogenesis,

Nutritional Ketosis

- Autophagy and apoptosis
- Decreased inflammation

These processes protect against cellular stress that would otherwise lead to metabolic disease, chronic oxidation and inflammation, ionic and osmotic threats, cellular damage, and protein-toxic stress.

What might the foregoing cell physiology teach us? If there was a bottom line, summary, take-home message that could fit this science to one's personal life, what would it be?

Summary

Better understanding the redox landscape involving energy metabolism, ketosis, and metabolic flexibility, empowers better lifestyle choices and practices which create and maintain metabolic health. This enables the ability to activate redox-sensitive cellular health mechanisms at will which support metabolic health.

The ability to enhance and manage the redox-sensitive mechanisms that are hardwired into our genetic and epi-genetic blueprints is vastly improved when the eons-honored rules of cellular health and energy metabolism are followed. The native abilities to detect and respond to threats, to "repair and replace," and to combat disease and premature aging, are positively affected.

This means each person has within their capacity the ability to improve their health and to correct disease processes and to slow down aging, by adopting and following a redox-based lifestyle. This produces lasting and profound effects on cellular metabolism and provides significant advantages for brain and organ health, growth and repair, psychiatric well-being, and overall health.

This knowledge will affect all points of the Redox lifestyle including food production, shopping, and cooking, and eating. It will affect activity levels and physical exercise decisions. It will affect sleep habits and patterns, oral health, and stress management. It will influence the selection of quality

Nutritional Ketosis

redox-based supplements which facilitate and leverage the health effects derived from a redox lifestyle.

The Redox Lifestyle takes all this into consideration because of the ability to reverse engineer diets, exercise, recreation, and vocations to respect the rules of the cell.

All of these cellular health mechanisms are activated because of the redox-sensitive principle of hormesis. We will look at that in depth, next. It is one of the important foundational principles of redox biology and the very bedrock of redox stress adaptation and health.

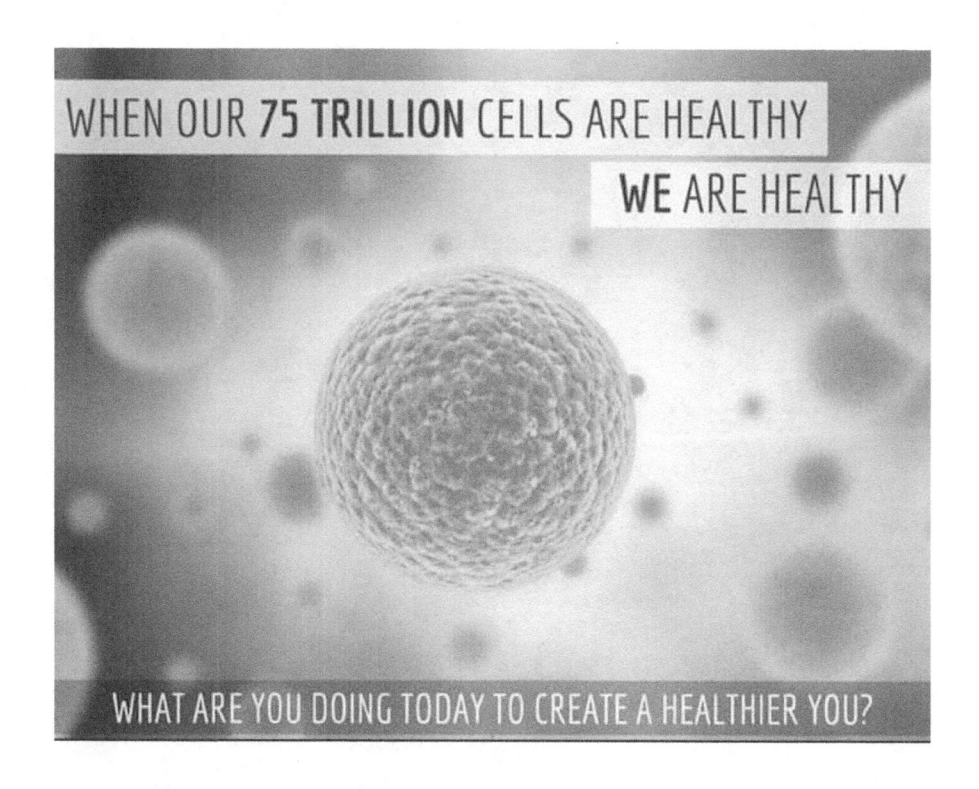

WHEN OUR **75 TRILLION** CELLS ARE HEALTHY

WE ARE HEALTHY

WHAT ARE YOU DOING TODAY TO CREATE A HEALTHIER YOU?

Hormesis – The Dual Nature of Redox

Hormesis – The Dual Nature of Redox

Introduction

What do vitamins, antioxidants, exercise, vaccinations, sunshine, cryotherapy, allergy treatments, heat therapy, hyperbaric treatment, oxygen deprivation, high-altitude training, cognitive exercises, and fasting ... have in common? The Answer - hormesis!

This is a powerful principle of redox biology because its effects are so far reaching within the Redoxome. The benefits of hormesis include:

- Enhanced cellular repair and healing
- Improved behavior and learning
- Cognitive and neurological health
- Disease and injury resistance
- Quicker athletic recovery
- Anti-aging and healthspan
- Healthy immune system
- Reproductive health
- Reduced systemic inflammation
- Reduced age-related metabolic disease
- Increase in hormonal balance

This process of hormesis is broadly witnessed in the modest improvements seen in cognition, growth, longevity, bone density, immune function, cell defense, and other biomedical endpoints. The consistency and broad landscape over which hormetic findings present throughout nature, witnesses that hormesis is responsible for biological plasticity and adaptability. This would explain why this principle is broadly selected for and highly preserved in nature and enhances survival and biological stability.

The History of Hormesis

The understanding of hormesis is a relatively recent development. It was first described in the late 1800s by a German pharmacologist who discovered that a very small amount of a poison helped yeast to grow[99]. This adaptive response phenomenon was later (1943) given the name "hormesis". Soon thereafter, the concept fell into disfavor. It has remained

Hormesis – The Dual Nature of Redox

marginalized within the medical and biomedical communities until recently. Today it is receiving robust attention in both the medical research and healthcare community.

From the early simple observations related to a single yeast sample, today there are 5,600 hormetic functions which have been identified and attributed to nearly nine hundred different agents representing a diversified spectrum of chemical and physical agents. This rich database of literature argues for the validity of this biological principle. This spectrum of diverse endpoints documenting the hormetic dose response is vast and broad. It includes the areas or topics of growth, aging/longevity, metabolic pathways, disease incidence, psychological and cognitive function, immune and antioxidant response, and inflammation.

While the science grew out of the observations that bacteria, insects, plants, and animals all show enhanced ability to respond optimally to minor environmental and nutritional stresses, the last fifty years has produced a new health paradigm around the principle of hormesis. Earlier concepts have been reconstructed and promise to reshape the future of healthcare and prevention - as well as our understandings of redox signaling biology.

This new focus has occurred due to a convergence of research in the fields of pharmacology, chemical toxicology, radiation biology, and nutrition. Because of the advancing research which has laser-focused on the bi-phasic model of hormesis, the biological and redox phenomenon of hormesis has gained new traction. It is now producing new and exciting applications within the biological and biomedical arenas. It is upon this principle that nearly everything within the redox landscape operates, as well as the mechanism by which many nutritional supplements and new redox supplements operate.

What is hormesis?

The ability to respond to stress is and always has been an essential part of survival and thriving in challenging environments. The principle of hormesis is founded on the idea that living systems initiate a series of survival mechanisms to offset, adapt, and survive otherwise threatening conditions.

Hormesis – The Dual Nature of Redox

Cells have been brilliantly designed to respond to 'common and ordinary' stresses of daily living. These are the insults experienced within their environment. These stresses function as two-sided swords with a dual function and effect, depending on the intensity of stress which is experienced. Hormesis is the principle that low doses of a toxin or an activity that produces stress results in a stimulation of cellular health. High doses produce an inhibitory response, or in other words an up-tick in inflammatory response.

Such "common" mild oxidation stresses come from exercise, calorie restriction, blood glucose reduction, shifts in energy metabolism, mental-cognitive stimulus, fasting, vaccinations, allergen immunotherapy, cryotherapy, radiation, sunlight, and even plant-based nutrients (polyphenols and phytochemicals).

If there were a word that characterized these stresses as they relate to their effect on cellular and mind/body health, it would be 'balance.' Never too much, and never too little! Old adages like "if a little is good, a lot is better" do not fit this model. Others such as "what doesn't kill you makes you stronger" are much more apropos to this discussion of hormesis. The Goldilocks description of the middle zone of "just right," also fits.

If we accept that physiological hormesis leads to beneficial health outcomes by exposure to stress, then hormesis is an everyday reality for every person. Interestingly, it is all anchored in redox principles at the most foundational level. It is these redox principles and activity which modulate these mechanisms of action which induce and initiate healthy responses to stress.

It is important to qualify and even quantify what the word "stress" means. It is nigh to an axiomatic law that almost all stressors imposed on the human condition, directly or indirectly, cause changes in the redox state. This means there is an increase in the oxidation level within a cell or body system to one degree or another.

This occurs when the level of oxidants increase beyond the ability of available reductants (antioxidants) to neutralize and stabilize the oxidants

Hormesis – The Dual Nature of Redox

and to keep the cell in homeostasis. When this happens, the cell becomes 'oxidized' and experiences oxidative stress.

The important distinction for the principle of hormesis is that the degree of this stress can be mild (physiologic) or it can be high – and the difference between those two degrees is physiologically significant.

There is also a temporal aspect to it in regard to duration. Long-term oxidation damages the cell and creates chronic low-grade inflammation which contributes to metabolic disease and accelerated aging.

Note that the degree or amount of oxidation is a relative variable based on 1)- the amount of oxidants being produced with a cell, and 2)- the amount of opposing antioxidants available within a cell to counter-act and neutralize the oxidation. A poor or deficient antioxidant response combined with an increased presence of oxidants is problematic, to say the least.

Redox Biology Basics - Review

Before proceeding further with hormesis specifically, a quick review of the details related to the production and effect of these oxidant molecules may prove helpful. These redox molecules are central to the story of how hormesis works!

As we have learned, the "side-effect" or by-product of cellular energy creation is the creation of reduction-oxidation molecules called reactive oxygen species (ROS). Converting food calories to energy occurs within mitochondria. The 'smoke' of this metabolic combustion consists of reactive molecules that are generated as electrons are moved along the energy path, transferring energy from one molecule to the next in a sophisticated electron transport chain.

Because oxygen is central to this process, it is often referred to as "mitochondrial respiration" and "oxidative phosphorylation." The words 'respiration' and 'oxidative' highlight the is vital role of oxygen. In these reactions, oxygen acts as an oxidized agent accepting electrons from the metabolizing fuel source, and from molecules all along the cascading electron transport chain, thereby becoming reduced and leaving the

Hormesis – The Dual Nature of Redox

fuel/energy substrate oxidized. This is the 'burning' or combustion reaction which liberates energy from the food/fuel, to be used as metabolic energy.

As an aside, burning wood in a campfire or fireplace follows the same principles of redox physics - as electrons are transferred from the (reduced) wood to (oxidized) oxygen, and while doing so, releasing energy from the reaction. The same principles apply in a biological cell. Oxygen delivered from the lungs through red blood cells is the driver of these reactions and is the final electron receptor, due to its electrical charge (i.e., the most electronegative). Its vital role explains why the "fire" goes out without oxygen.

However, as nature has designed this reaction, inside mitochondria not all of the oxygen is reduced. A small percent remains oxidized and highly reactive. This oxygen derivative is called *superoxide*. Superoxide is converted to a less reactive molecule called *hydrogen peroxide*, which in turn is converted to water and oxygen, by the reducing action of antioxidant enzymes.

Beyond the dynamics of their involvement in energy metabolism these oxidants serve important roles in the immune system. They are a biocidal killer of microbes (white blood cell phagocytosis), and function as redox signaling molecules within and throughout the Redoxome.

This brief review highlights again the basic redox biology which is foundation for biological life and energy metabolism. The amount of these oxidants increase with cellular dysfunction, and with failed cellular defenses.

Any perturbation or stress or assault or insult on the mitochondria, either through abuses with energy metabolism, and/or through any toxic environmental agent, increase the amount of ROS molecules within the system. The important distinction about this is, 'how much?'

Hormesis and Mitohormesis – A Stress-Adaptive Response

Normally in health, cells enjoy a homeostasis and balance. This is not about having zero oxidation; it is about having well managed oxidative states. As oxidation levels increase, nature's solution is to use antioxidants supplied

Hormesis – The Dual Nature of Redox

from within the cell (glutathione, superoxide dismutase, and catalase) and from plant-based sources to rebalance the cell.

However, when this process does not proceed optimally, problems occur. The question must be asked – how does the cell know its redox state is out of balance? How does it detect that there is a problem, and what does the cell do about this situation?

The answer to this is found within the Redoxome, the presence of redox-sensitive molecules, and the principles of hormesis.

The reason a cell knows something is wrong and out of oxidative balance is because it has mechanisms in place which are sensitive to changes in oxidation (i.e., the degree or amount of oxidative stress). Molecules which are sensitive to mild states of oxidation are able to sense these changes and trigger a response which in turn activates defensive responses.

This stress-response ability sets in motion various mechanisms to repair damage within the cell and to rebalance the oxidant-reductant balance. Dysfunction or mismanagement anywhere along these pathways results in

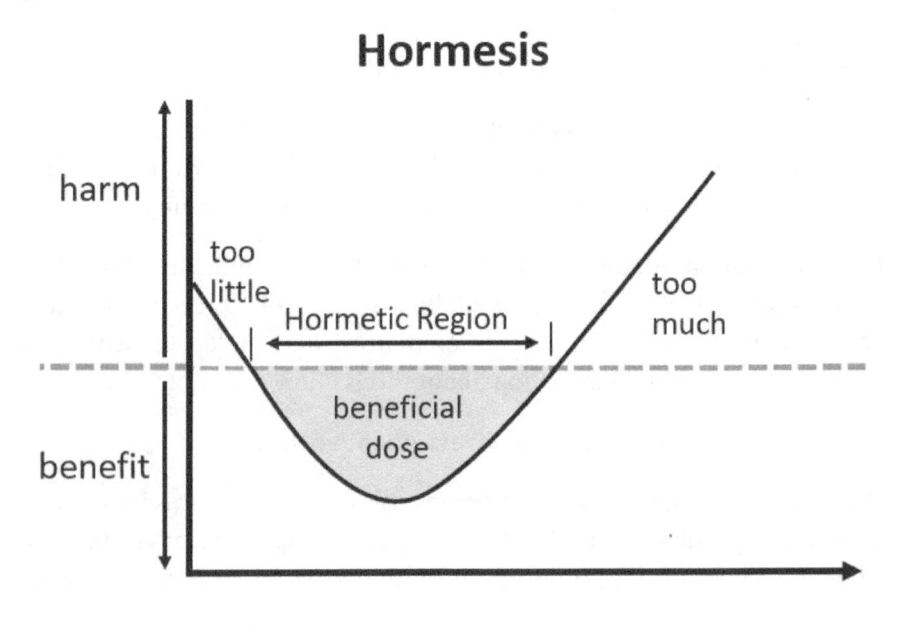

Hormesis

Hormesis – The Dual Nature of Redox

diminished response and leads to ongoing oxidative insult and chronic inflammation and disease.

However, a timely and adequate response leads to corrective action and restored health. This is the essence of awakening the Inner Doctor! This response or stress-adaptive feature is hard-wired into cellular redox biochemistry and occurs because of the universal biology principle called hormesis.

In science terms, hormesis is a "biphasic dose-response to an environmental agent" or condition[100]. In common language it is that a low-dose stimulation from an 'agent' or condition produces a beneficial biological effect, whereas a high-dose of the same agent or condition yields an inhibitory or toxic effect. This is how the body uses the presence of oxidation with both good and adverse effect. This defines its dual role.

In other words, there is a beneficial "dose" or amount of oxidation (or of any activity or agent which produces such oxidation) that is 'just right' and falls within the hormetic zone for stimulating healthy responses.

This means that notwithstanding the dangerous consequences of elevated oxidation generally, there is a universal benefit which arises from experiencing mild oxidative stress. Hormesis is thus an important part of nature's design to activate protective measures which protect and heal the body.

In addition to the functionality within the cell cytoplasm, hormesis also functions within mitochondria. *Mitohormesis* is the term used to describe this phenomenon occurring inside mitochondria. This is the biological response which occurs when a mild or physiologic amount of oxidative stress occurs in the mitochondria, which then leads to an improvement of health and viability within the cell and the body[101].

The principle of hormesis is causing many in the aging-research community to begin to realize that the 'free-radical damage' model for aging needs to be updated. The emerging research shows that reactive oxygen molecules at mild doses are actually protective throughout the body and are not

Hormesis – The Dual Nature of Redox

something that should be categorically extinguished (as has been the effort for decades using plant-based antioxidants).

The free-radical theory of aging traditionally holds that any degree of free-radical oxidation is damaging to the cell and promotes inflammation – "inflammaging." A current and correct understanding of the role ROS plays would require recognizing that the relationship between ROS exposure and aging is a non-linear dose response - and is in fact moderated via the hormetic response. This is because mile levels of oxidation are required to activate redox-sensitive cellular defenses which work to slow aging and maintaining health.

The "devil-in-the-details" is that there is an art and a science to hormesis. It's operations and variables are slightly unique to each person's condition – influenced by the weight of genetics and the gravity of pre-existing disease and the degree of medical interventions.

This mitochondrial response to mild stress coordinates its communication with the cell's nuclear DNA, by a process called "mito-nuclear

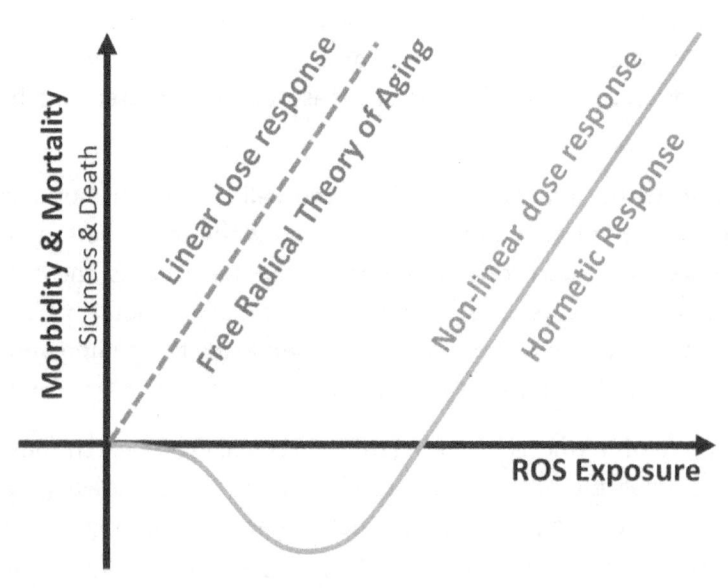

Source/Adapted: Ristow. Dose Response, May 2014.

Hormesis – The Dual Nature of Redox

communication"[102] – otherwise known as "redox signaling." There are many vitamins and enzyme cofactors which participate in this process and which collectively affect and work through redox-sensitive pathways to coordinate and choreograph this cellular response. There are a number of primary and secondary messengers involved in this communication, but the dominant messengers are the redox signaling molecules created from the energy metabolism process itself (i.e., reactive oxygen species – ROS).

The activation of these *mitohormetic* redox signaling pathways increase lifespan in various animal models from worms to mammals. It also improves healthspan by making substantial improvements in energy metabolism and cellular defense and repair mechanisms. The cellular mediators responsible for activating these mechanisms are redox molecules throughout.

The source of "physiologic" stress in day-to-day living comes from lifestyle practices. These practices are called "bio-oxidative" due to their effect on energy metabolism in the mitochondria. This creates a mild inhibition in the electron transport chain, the net effect of which is to bump the production and action of redox messengers. This means that a slight amount of mitochondrial dysfunction 'lives and breathes' on the hormesis platform and produces the mild elevation in oxidation needed to produce the adaptive stress.

In this paradoxical manner, mild oxidative states created through the influence of "lifestyle," produce a redox feedback or retrograde signaling within the cell, which activates redox-sensitive pathway genes to dial-up an adaptive stress response which instruct and guide the cell to improve its defense and healing posture[103].

Thus, each person experiences the effects of the hormesis principle every day. Exercise increases free radical formation, as do plant phytochemicals and intermittent fasting and glucose deprivation and ketosis. The mild oxidative stress produced from these activities protect the body from infection, diseases and neurodegeneration[104] - all validating the hormetic principle that "less is more."

Hormesis – The Dual Nature of Redox

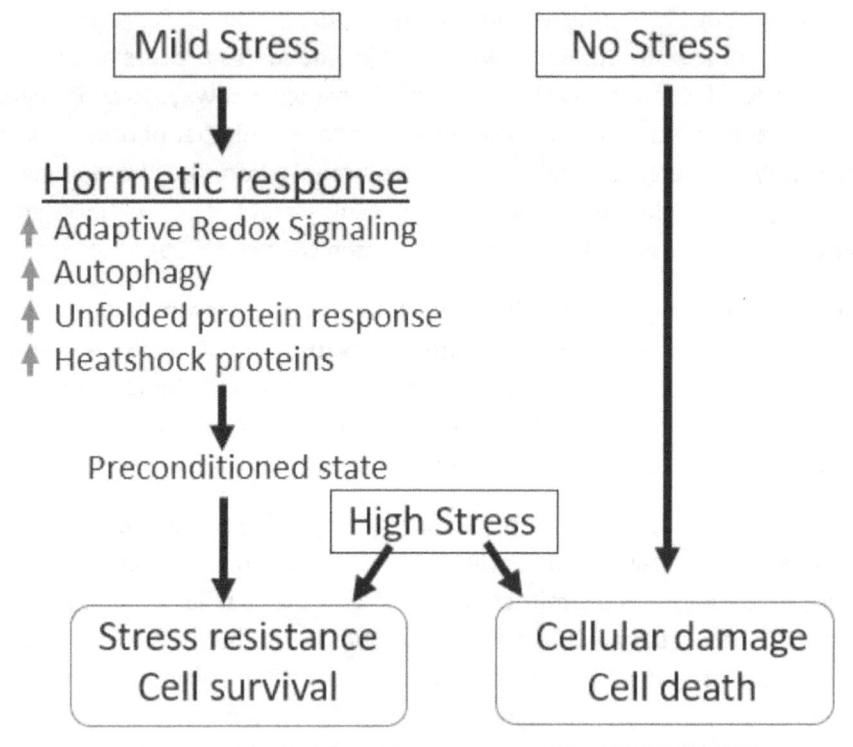

```
    Mild Stress                    No Stress
        ↓                              │
  Hormetic response                    │
  ↑ Adaptive Redox Signaling           │
  ↑ Autophagy                          │
  ↑ Unfolded protein response          │
  ↑ Heatshock proteins                 │
        ↓                              │
  Preconditioned state                 │
        │      ┌─High Stress─┐         │
        ↓      ↙             ↘         ↓
  ┌──────────────────┐   ┌──────────────────┐
  │ Stress resistance│   │ Cellular damage  │
  │  Cell survival   │   │   Cell death     │
  └──────────────────┘   └──────────────────┘
```

Source: Adapted from Zimmermann, Microbial Cell 2014.

The additional value of this principle is seen in the ability of "conditioned" cells to withstand the perils of high stress. Cells which are "practiced" and pre-conditioned through the effects of hormetic challenges (exercise, food restriction, good nutrition, etc.) are able to tolerate the effects of high stress better than those cells which are not so conditioned[105].

These new understandings are beginning to reshape the old scripts relative to free-radical damage and aging, by recognizing the role and relative contributions which mitochondrial redox molecules serve – namely for activating antioxidant defenses, clearing damaged proteins (autophagy), stimulating cell biogenesis (mitosis), removing damaged cells (apoptosis), and cellular DNA repair and renewal[106]. This core principle of hormesis and redox-sensitivity sit at the very foundation of the Redoxome.

Hormesis – The Dual Nature of Redox

This in its most simple construct explains the reason why fasting, nutritional ketosis, exercise, good nutrition, stress management, gut health, and improved sleep are so important and effective in cellular health. It also explains the role and mechanism-of-action which various supplements have in manipulating this redox state such that these desired outcomes can become modulated and enhanced.

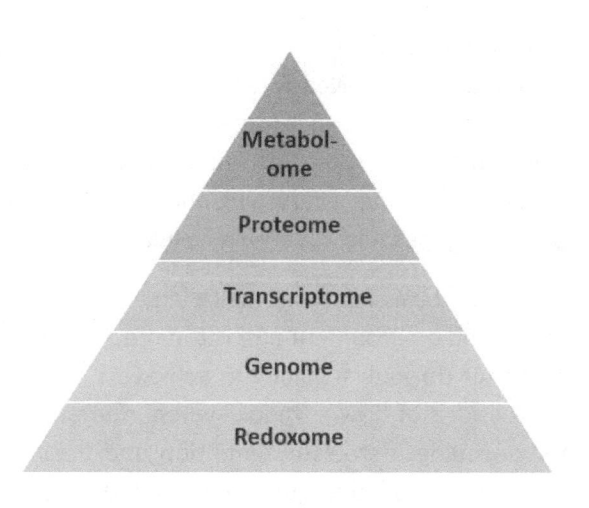

(Pyramid, top to bottom: Metabolome, Proteome, Transcriptome, Genome, Redoxome)

The "low-dose stimulation / high-dose inhibition" model of hormesis varies with each person. There is not a universal set-point which is the same for every person. Each person has their own "sweet spot" or hormetic zone relative to the amount or dose of stimulus that is required to activate a healthy cellular response.

Factors such as mitochondrial health and dysfunction, preexisting state of metabolic health or disease, processed foods in the diet, the quality and quantity of food consumed, the timing of eating, family history and genetic predispositions, and a myriad of other factors all weigh in on this complex formula as to what determines the best dose or "sweet-spot" for each individual. Nevertheless, the principle remains true that when a small or mild doses of what would otherwise produce a toxic effect at higher levels, is experienced, there is an almost magical response from the body to protect and enhance health.

Simply put, hormesis is the dose-specific response to a condition, state, stressor, or toxin which stimulate cells to be more response-able and adaptable to their environment.

Hormesis – The Dual Nature of Redox

The state of oxidation thus becomes the most basic and universal stimulus within the body. Nearly anything and everything that impacts a cell's homeostasis or balance does so by affecting its state of oxidation. This places the "Redoxome" at the foundational level for cellular function and support. It impacts everything and serves as a universal lever for activating pathway genes and governing cellular function.

This is the basis for how a cell – any cell – knows how to interpret its own status and environment and is the mechanism through which it adapts and responds through signaling to activate a healthy response. This is the basis for the idea of how a 'redox switch' operates. This is the cell's mechanism for decoding a stressful condition and activating transcription factors to respond through upregulation of pathway genes.

Because the stress-induced shift in oxidation status is the trigger that sets in motion the adaptive response, and since the responsive effect is determined by the degree or amount of oxidation, the questions arise, how much is "enough?" What constitutes a mild physiologic level of stress sufficient to stimulate hormesis?

While researchers are continuing to learn more about hormesis, all indicators and an amazing amount of emerging research, points to the

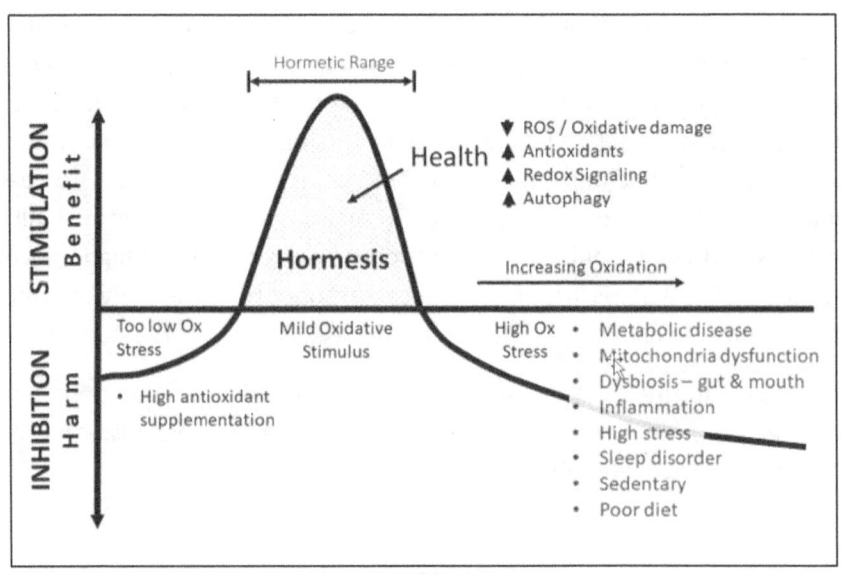

Hormesis – The Dual Nature of Redox

manipulation or activation of redox-driven transcription factors as the biological redox switch mechanism. This is due to the fact that transcription factors are highly sensitive to even mild changes in oxidation. The fundamental principle here is that a mild shift in oxidation status is the triggering mechanism for initiating meaningful action – all a function of redox signaling.

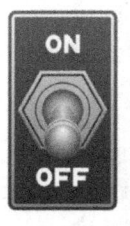

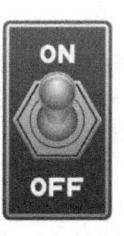

A common model used to illustrate this principle is that of a "redox rheostat" – a sliding scale illustrating a concentration gradient of oxidation – from mild to high along an oxidation continuum. The resulting outcomes or output from differing concentrations of the same oxidative source, determine and drive the cell's varied response toward healing or destruction. Willful manipulating the cell's status toward mild physiologic levels of oxidation, results in the activation of cellular defenses and repair, while allowing excessive or chronic levels of oxidation to occur, produces inflammation and disease.

Mild Oxidation   **High Oxidation**

The Redox Rheostat Scale
ANTIOXIDANT DEFENSES
OXIDATION LEVELS

In fact, all good health - reverse engineered - begins with the activation of antioxidant and cell repair mechanisms. These occur through redox-sensitive hormetic activity using a mild oxidative stimulus. This means that anything which produces and supports optimal health does so because it stimulates cellular defense and repair through direct effect on redox-sensitive transcription factors.

A prime example universally used to represent this phenomenon is the Nrf2 antioxidant gene transcription factor. When mild oxidation separates the Nrf2 transcription molecule from its inhibiting partner (Keap1), Nrf2 moves to the nucleus and up-regulates antioxidant gene expression. This activates antioxidant genes which are cell protective. The same oxidative system activates autophagy gene activation (ATG4) operates by these same principles. Other cellular response pathways such as the Sirtuin and Forkhead box protein (FOXO1) pathways are also activated with these same methods.

The redox application of this hormesis principal lays with the ability of mild oxidative stress to activate healthy cellular defense signaling pathways. They are all part of the cellular programming which allows for low doses of drugs, toxins, plant polyphenols, thermal stress, sunshine, radiation, and more, to elicit positive cellular responses in terms of adaptation to, or protection from, environmental stress.

Nutrition and Hormesis

Plants are the mainstay of life. Regardless of one's dietary practices, what grows as plant material is always 'upstream' in the food chain and provides essential nutrition and energy for animals and humans.

It is well known that plants provide fuel for biological energy, as well as many vitamins and antioxidants and phytochemicals and structural components necessary for healthy living and cellular repair. These have profound effects in restoring mitochondria homeostasis and activating the cell-clearing systems related to autophagy[107]. What is less well known is that many of the plant phytochemicals have toxic qualities which are vital to producing their hormetic effect in the body. Ironically, this is what makes them nutritious[108].

This means that dietary phytochemicals and plant-based polyphenols are "nutritious" precisely because they are in small measure a bio-toxin to humans[109]. Phytochemical nutrients exert their healthy effect because they are just toxic enough to stimulate redox-sensitive responses in cells.

Plants contain both nutrients and antinutrients. That plants contain (sub)toxic compounds should come as no surprise. Plants produce "antinutrient" biochemicals which are useful to them in their own defense in their growing environment.

These include lectins, trypsin inhibitors, alpha-amylase inhibitors, protease inhibitors, tannins, phytates, goitrogens, raffinose oligosaccharides, saponins, oxalates, and exorphins[110]. Of this group, phylates, oxylates, and lectins are a few of the well-known antinutrients.

As a group, they are highly bioactive and are capable of producing deleterious effects, as well as some beneficial health effects in humans. Their negative effects relate to their interfering with absorption of nutrients, and their effect on digestion and the comfort of the gastrointestinal tract.

Their positive effects relate to the effect they have when presenting a mild stress to the body, which stimulate stress-adaptive responses in cells. When consumed in low levels, phytic acid, lectins, and phenolic compounds as well as enzyme inhibitors and saponins, have shown to exert many positive health benefits related to insulin resistance, cardiovascular function and lipid levels, liver function and fatty-liver disease, and platelet agglutination[111].

Plant-derived phenolic compounds such as phytic acid, protease inhibitors, saponins, and lignans have shown benefit with cell dysplasia through its effects on cell signaling and alterations in cell cycle[112], and tannins have shown favorable results in targeting viral infection[113].

Phytochemicals in plants are there in the first place as a self-defense mechanism, defending against insults in their growing environment (oxidation, bacterial parasites, insects, and other pests that forage on them)[114]. While the levels of these biotoxins are suitable for their own defensive purposes, they are generally "sub-toxic" to the animals and humans that consume them, when consumed wisely.

At low concentrations, the residual (sub)toxicity provokes mammalian cells to maintain a state of adaptive stress which provide mechanisms for counteracting oxidative stress[115]. Phytochemicals at sub-toxic doses use the principle of hormesis to activate gene pathways which provide this healing and protective response in cells[116] [117].

This twist on traditionally viewed nutritional understanding is counter-intuitive. One might think to ask, how can a "healthy" and nutritious food be "toxic" in any degree? While this may challenge mainstream health paradigms and worldviews, it is nonetheless a true principle. In elevated

Hormesis – The Dual Nature of Redox

amounts these "antinutrients" can create disease and discomfort but used wisely they prove useful in managing various diseases and metabolic processes – precisely because of the principle of redox-based hormesis.

The most important aspect is the amount and dosage, and in finding the right balance between hazardous and beneficial effects of the plant's bioactive compounds. In this regard, they can be considered as an 'antinutritional' with negative effect, or a 'non-nutritive' compound with beneficial health effect. The consumers' awareness of these differences is important.

An example of nutritious foods activating redox pathways has been noted in the scientific literature related to the popular and health-associated Mediterranean diet[118]. This diet has been shown to prevent a variety of age-related diseases where low-grade chronic inflammation plays a role. Low carbohydrate Mediterranean diets have shown to produce weight loss, A1C levels and reduce triglycerides, while increasing HDL cholesterol[119]. The question to the inquisitive mind should be, why and how?

This diet emphasizes eating fish, fruits, vegetables, beans, fiber-rich breads and whole grains, nuts, and olive oil. While meat per se is de-emphasized, oils from fish and olives and from nuts, are emphasized. Likewise, high fiber foods are emphasized and by implication the reduction or elimination of refined grains, are focused upon. (Sidenote: reducing oils from processed seed would be an improvement in this diet).

Based on redox principles, the Mediterranean diet can be thought of as a form of chronic hormetic stress arising from phytochemicals, similar to that which occurs through moderate exercise or fasting (which utilize a parallel principle of ketosis and fat-burning). There are a variety of phytochemical compounds capable of exerting hormetic influence and which support "neuro-hormesis" and which help explain the neuroprotective properties and mitochondria support available with this particular diet[120][121]. This includes its ability to provide a homeostasis balance between pro- and anti-inflammaging factors and the increased ability to better manage the inflammation response.

Hormesis – The Dual Nature of Redox

This is not to particularly favor the Mediterranean diet over any other similar approach, only to say that utilizing rich vegetables and fruits and healthy oils along with a healthy respect for energy metabolism and a properly-fed bowel, should expect to return a healthier result – and it does. Why? Because it follows the rules of hormesis, antioxidant support, and properly feeding the gut. Again, there are similar diets that accomplish similar outcomes utilizing a different approach such as low-carb / high-fat, etc. which have a different respect for energy metabolism and glucose biochemistry. The point, however, is that from a metabolic perspective, the cell's rules, rule!

This helps explain the positive effect of plant polyphenols on health which go beyond their value as enzymes, antioxidants, and as cellular building materials. In addition to these time honored effects, emerging research is explaining additional mechanisms of action regarding their effect on cellular redox-based hormesis.

Hormesis Biochemistry

The question to be asked is whether plant polyphenols obtain their beneficial health effects *indirectly* due to the effect of polyphenols bumping mitochondrial ROS levels which in turn impact Nrf2 activation, or with *direct* action on the Keap1/Nrf2 complex itself to trigger antioxidant gene expression. The answer appears to be both, and more.

Regarding the former, there are two plausible mechanisms to explain how plant antioxidants can increase levels of reactive oxygen species.

First, once plant antioxidants donate their available electron to reduce an oxidant, they themselves become oxidized[122] and produce a pro-oxidant effect. They also have a hormetic effect on mitochondria helping them create redox molecules which increases oxidation. This means plant antioxidants can function as a secondary messenger stimulating mitochondrial activity to generate ROS. This is called the bio-oxidative effect upon mitochondrial function.

Furthermore, as a class, phytochemicals influence mitochondrial biogenesis, mitochondrial autophagy, and apoptosis, reduce dysfunction, inhibit

Hormesis – The Dual Nature of Redox

mitochondrial fragmentation and cytotoxicity, protect mitochondrial membranes, and generally support the mitochondria electron transport chain[123]. The net effect of improved function and resolved mitochondrial dysfunction, is to increase functional support and efficiency and create native redox molecules for redox signaling purposes. In this way, plant based chemicals stimulate cellular redox processes which upregulate the more powerful antioxidant endogenous mechanisms.

Secondly, there is a proposed indirect action beyond antioxidant activity. This is significant since it is suggested[124] that due to cellular kinetic considerations, the effects of plant flavonoids and polyphenols are limited within cells - even though they may have significant antioxidant effect in vitro (i.e., in test tubes and in extra-cellular environments outside cell walls). What then could explain the significant nutraceutical effect of these dietary compounds?

One of the most significant signaling pathways related to cellular defense and homeostasis, is the Nrf2 antioxidant pathway. Nrf2 regulates the expression of phase 2 antioxidant and detoxifying enzymes in response to noxious stress.

It has been proposed that the healthy effect of dietary antioxidants occur indirectly by upregulating this endogenous antioxidant pathway – i.e., to activate the Nrf2 pathway[125]. Thus, while acting as free-radical antioxidants outside the cell, they function as a stimulus to induce enzymatic systems inside the cell – in vivo – which generate enhanced protective enzyme efficiency.

Plant chemicals themselves affect the thiol or Sulphur containing cysteine molecules on the Keap1 molecule which keeps keeping Nrf2 inactive. When this occurs the shape of this inhibitor is altered, and Nrf2 is free to move to the cell nucleus. When it arrives in the nucleus it interacts with cellular DNA to upregulate gene activity, which produces antioxidants[126].

What is certain in this secondary indirect model is that plant polyphenols do play a role in Nrf2 activation[127], sometimes by their effect through the Nrf2/Keap1/ARE gene pathway, and in other cases through their effect on

Hormesis – The Dual Nature of Redox

upstream kinases (such as PI3K, p38, ERK, PKC, JNK which causes the activation of Nrf2 from the Keap1 inhibitory complex[128]).

Nevertheless, it is not as straightforward as some suppose. Notwithstanding the foregoing, still, a majority of phytochemicals (including phenols, monosulfides, furans, and indoles) acquire this ability (through biochemical processing or metabolic action) by increasing mitochondrial-produced ROS[129]. This means their primary effect on Nrf2 activation is not a direct action[130], as seen with redox molecules such as superoxide and hydrogen peroxide, whether native or supplemented. This means that while there is some evidence that plant phytochemicals can have an effect to upregulate antioxidant pathways, their ability to do so is indirect and not as efficient as through direct redox upregulation.

This means that while antioxidants in fruits and vegetables (exogenous sources) do provide protective effects, they do so through additional redox mechanisms aside from what most are accustomed to think.

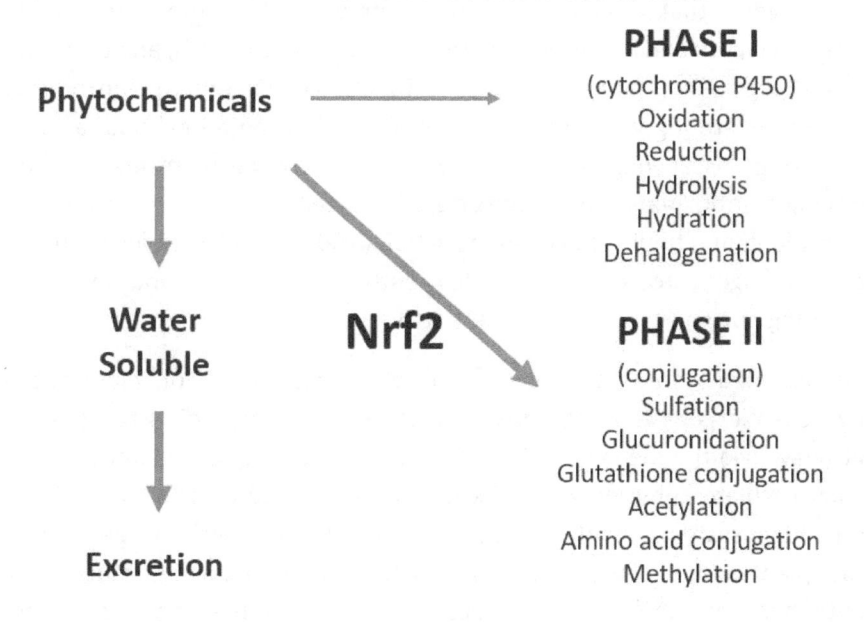

Phytochemicals → **PHASE I**
(cytochrome P450)
Oxidation
Reduction
Hydrolysis
Hydration
Dehalogenation

↓

Water Soluble   **Nrf2**   **PHASE II**
(conjugation)
Sulfation
Glucuronidation
Glutathione conjugation
Acetylation
Amino acid conjugation

↓

Excretion   Methylation

Adapted: Son, Hormetic Dietary Phytochemicals, Neuromolecular Med, 2008

Hormesis – The Dual Nature of Redox

Notwithstanding the widely popular view that fruits, vegetables, and vitamin supplementation provide direct antioxidant support to protect from free-radical damage, there are new concepts emerging[131] that describe the sub-toxic effect of plant chemicals to produce beneficial cellular stress adaptation.

This means that the important effect of plant antioxidants occur because they either function as a mild sub-toxic stimulus themselves, and/or as an electrophile oxidant after being modified - which then reacts with the Nrf2/Keap1 complex.

Taken together, the antioxidant effect of plant phytochemicals thus occur through both direct antioxidant reduction of oxidants (their most noted role), as well as indirectly through enhanced mitochondria activity which increases redox oxidants, and/or through their modified indirect effect on Nrf2 antioxidant genes, indirectly.

This suggests that their direct antioxidant effects are more within the intestinal lumen and in the extracellular space outside of cells, and that their intracellular role (as far as "antioxidant" function is concerned) is an indirect function, operating via a redox mechanism within the mitochondria - and then to a lesser degree with transcription factors themselves. Their dominant antioxidant role is outside of the cell as a non-enzyme-based antioxidant, and their intracellular function inside the cell is to function as a hormetic agent to stimulate redox pathways, thereby and indirectly triggering enzyme-based antioxidant activation.

This has led some researchers to label this effect of plant-based phytochemicals as the "paradoxical oxidative activation of Nrf2 signaling pathway," via the mechanism called "para-hormesis' (*para* = alternative) – which regulates physiologic redox molecules and stimulates intracellular antioxidant systems and the mechanisms for cellular repair[132]. It seems clear that plant-based phytochemicals function as redox-active nutritional phytochemicals, at least in part because of their sub-toxic hormesis effect within a cell[133].

Hormesis – The Dual Nature of Redox

Hormetic phytochemicals (sometimes referred to as *xenohormetic nutrients*) include resveratrol[134], isothiocynates such as sulforaphanes[135][136], curcumin[137], the organosulfur compounds allium and allicin (present in onions and garlic)[138], capsaicin[139], quercetin[140], epigallocatechin gallate (EGCG – green tea)[141], and many other substances seen in common vegetables and herbs[142]. They each help protect cells against injury and disease by stimulating the production of intra-cellular antioxidants and aid in cellular 'repair and replace' mechanisms (autophagy) – all via redox signaling pathways utilizing hormesis principles.

One of the reasons why research has shown conflicting outcomes when measuring the claimed health benefits from taking dietary supplementation with antioxidants such as Vitamin E and Vitamin C, is that the evidence suggests that activation of Nrf2 pathway, rather than direct free radical scavenging activity (functioning as a reducing agent), better explains the health benefit of phytochemicals.

Whereas direct antioxidant action from plant-based antioxidants have a very short half-life, the activation of the endogenous antioxidant pathway genes have long-lasting effect because their action is based on the activity of transcription-based signaling[143].

Some of the better studied compounds which activate the endogenous antioxidant pathways, include[144]:

- Carnosic acid, containing hydroquinone and catechol (found in rosemary - *Rosmarinus officinalis*)
- Sulforaphane, containing the isothiocyanate sulforaphane (found in cruciferous vegetables)
- Fumaric acid / dimethyl fumarate (found in shepherd's purse - *Capsella bursa-pastoris*)
- Resveratrol, has strong antioxidant and hormetic profile, contained in over 70 plants (found grape skins)
- Curcumin, antioxidant, and strong neuroprotection (found in spices and turmeric - *Curcuma longa*)
- Carnitine transports long-chain fatty acids into mitochondria for energy use and removes short- and medium-chain fatty acids to

Hormesis – The Dual Nature of Redox

prevent toxic accumulation within mitochondria (found in red meat and dairy products).

In summary, and to translate this, a "healthy diet" is healthy because it contains mild low-dose levels of plant-toxins which serve to activate hormetic pathways, which activate stress-adaptive mechanisms deep in the cell. This means that a healthy diet consists of consuming mildly toxic (sub-toxic) polyphenols (found in whole plant food and quality whole-food supplements), which create a mild oxidative stimulus – enough to activate

Mild Stress
(dietary phytochemicals)

↓

Hormetic Response Pathway
(Ion channels, kinases, deacetylases, transcription factors)

↓

Stress Resistance Proteins
(Heat shock proteins, antioxidants, growth factors)

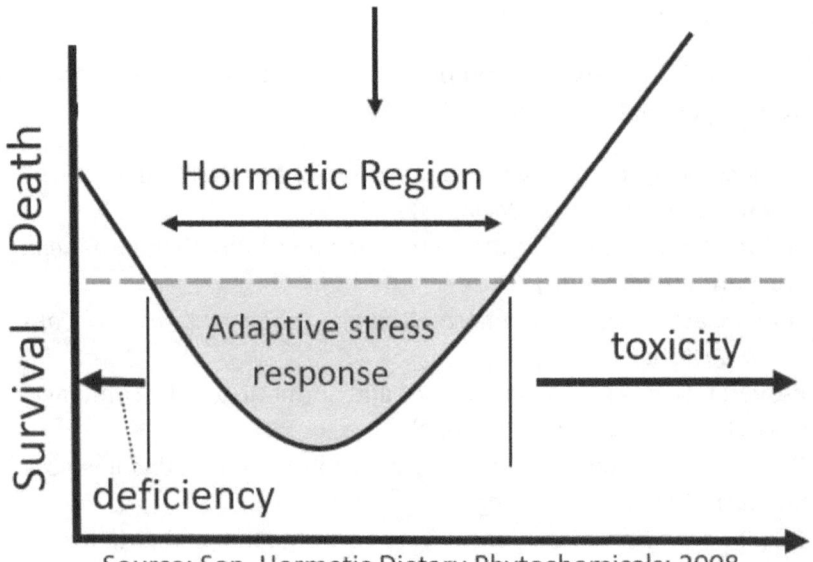

↓

Source: Son. Hormetic Dietary Phytochemicals; 2008.

Hormesis – The Dual Nature of Redox

cellular defense and repair mechanisms. This primarily happens through their effect on transcription factor activation available within the Redoxome landscape. Both Nrf2/ARE antioxidant and autophagy gene (Atg) activation are notable examples.

In other words, the "noxious" chemicals which plants use to defend themselves, are actually a sub-toxic dose for humans (and animals), which serve to stimulate and precondition mild cellular stress-responses through the hormetic effect[145].

It is important to understand that aside from onboarding fuel for energy metabolism and consuming vitamins, enzymes, and cellular building materials, the objective of healthy eating is to create sufficient nutritional stress which creates mild oxidation – either through periodic glucose deprivation or through plant phytochemicals and polyphenols. The end point is to activate transcription factors which upregulate cellular defense and repair mechanisms.

All of this must happen in an environment as clean and free from contamination from processed foods and environmental toxins (which harm these pathways and processes) as possible. (Note that the consumption of clean and plentiful water through all this is a given and can be researched independently).

All things considered, this redox-based nutrition science solidly anchors nutrition as a redox phenomenon and an essential component of the redox lifestyle and the Redoxome.

Exercise and Hormesis

We have learned that hormesis mechanisms increase cellular stress resistance[146]. This is also referred to as "preconditioning." It applies to a wide variety of stresses that when properly experienced help condition an organism to better weather future stresses. Better stress adaptation has powerful health benefits. Exercise and fasting are important working examples which illustrate this principle.

Hormesis – The Dual Nature of Redox

It is widely and universally believed that moderate exercise upregulates the immune system, while physical inactivity as well as over-strenuous exercise has the opposite effect. But why?

We know that regular exercise decreases the oxidative challenge to the body, whereas excessive exercise and overtraining lead to damaging oxidative stress. But again, why? And how?

The principle of hormesis is that biological systems respond to stress with a bell-shaped curve. This "low-dose stimulus / high-dose inhibition" phenomenon manifests itself in either a J-shaped or an inverted U-shaped dose-response curve.

The effect of exercise on mitochondria is to increase energy production and reactive oxygen species. The beneficial effects of exercise occur because regular exercise generates mild increases in ROS levels which are in the hormetic range of redox-sensitive transcription factors. Exercise-induced redox stimulation results in activation of transcription factors which play a key role in antioxidant production, enhancement of cellular repair

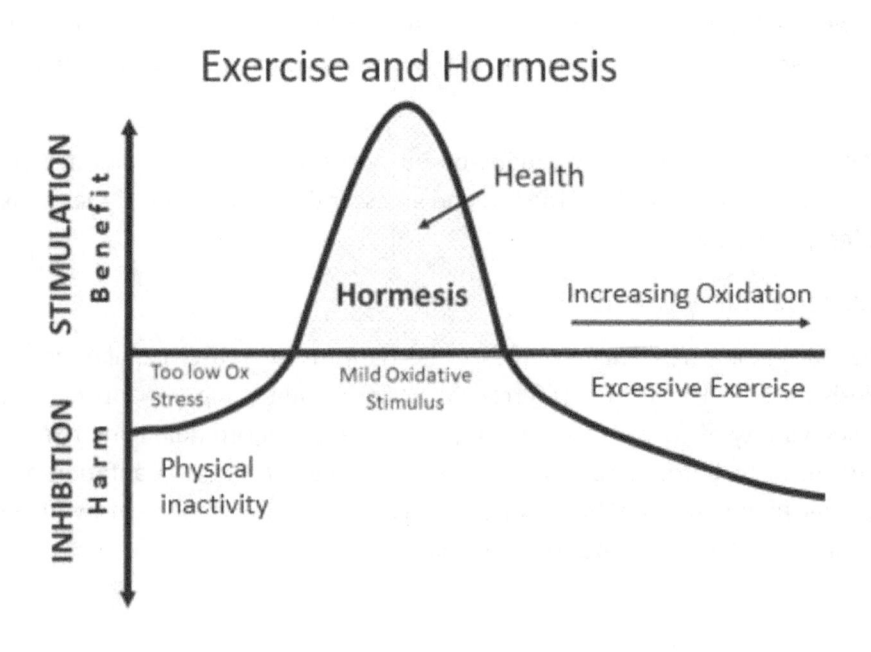

Hormesis – The Dual Nature of Redox

(autophagy), and DNA maintenance – all of which result in diminished incidences of disease and accelerated aging[147].

Balanced exercise seems to be the key point. Both of these two endpoints, too much and too little exercise, each represent different ends of the hormetic curve and effect, at least at the cellular and mitochondrial level.

During exercise, there are various forms of stress experienced by the body. These include thermal, metabolic, hypoxic, oxidative, and mechanical. These stressors collectively produce the mild stimulus which activates signaling messengers and gene pathways which govern adaptive responses.

Signaling messengers play an important role in muscle cells in adapting to exercise-induced stress. These include ROS (oxygen species), RNS (nitrogen species), calcium ions, growth factors, inflammatory cytokines, and eicosanoids (signaling molecules made from arachidonic acid or fatty acids such as omega 3) [148]. The endpoint of this messenger mobilization is to activate stress response which promotes adaptation. This includes an increase in the number of mitochondria (biogenesis), muscle cell growth, and the creation of muscle protein.

Because protein synthesis is a function of DNA/RNA (transcription/translation) and depends on the activation of transcription factors which initiate this process, it is reasonable to assume a linkage to the effects of redox molecules with this process. In fact, this is true. This is because increases in the rates of protein synthesis are under translational control and are enhanced with exercise[149].

Conversely, with excessive exercise stress, the continuous production of reactive molecules (ROS) overwhelm the cell's native defense mechanisms and destroys proteins (proteolysis), while at the same time inhibiting protein synthesis – thus diminishing muscle remodeling and health[150]. This means that a dysfunctional and unconditioned overproduction of ROS (from either mitochondrial dysfunction or overly strenuous exercise) resulting in increased oxidation, serves as a signal to depress protein synthesis throughout the body[151]. This happens because there exists a universal

Hormesis – The Dual Nature of Redox

mechanism that controls protein production through changes in cellular functions that are dependent on the redox status.

Chronic exercise stress from long and repeated endurance exercise or heavy physical activity, can be injurious without adequate rest. The rest phase following exercise is a critical piece within the redox playbook, for this is where recovery and stress-response occurs. This is true even in well trained individuals, especially if they do not properly undergo redox-specific support and recovery strategies. When appropriate redox support is obtained, it lessens the impact of strenuous exercise and speeds recovery.

Stated earlier in this book was the principle that metabolically, cells are either burning or growing. While that may be a generalization, the rest and autophagy phase between exercise periods, allows muscles to grow and become stronger and better stress adapted. During this rest phase, exercise-induced autophagy is initiated. This process removes the metabolic end products (lactate and free radicals/oxidants) and damaged proteins created during exercise.

The time in, and to, recovery, is an important variable which can be accelerated with proper recovery support (massage, compression, cold water immersion, stretching, electrostimulation, etc.)[152] and redox supplementation.

A powerful strategy that has been suggested and demonstrated by leading researchers in metabolomic science, is to replenish the pre- and post-exercise hormesis environment with redox supplementation directly. Doing so has shown to positively shift Krebs metabolic intermediates sufficiently to help offset the cellular demands that arise from intense exercise and further aid with recovery and cellular redox support. It also decreases the lactate formed by helping to shift the fuel being metabolized from glucose to fatty acids[153][154]. [More information on this is available in the Appendix: Metabolomics Study – The Supercharging of Krebs].

The shift from glucose metabolism to enhanced fat oxidation creates both an amino acid-sparing and a glycogen-sparing effect in the energy metabolism of the body, and with no apparent adverse effect on biomarkers

Hormesis – The Dual Nature of Redox

of inflammation and oxidative stress or the immune system. This strategy is about using redox replenishment to create a metabolic state of nutritional ketosis, without the normal requirement of fasting or of using a ketogenic diet – (albeit the blending of these strategies is a perfect tactic within the redox lifestyle!).

At the opposite end of the exercise continuum (little or no exercise), it is noteworthy that lack of exercise and low or no physical activity are also linked with redox signaling – but in a negative health and inflammation manner. Too little physical activity promotes inflammation rather than health[155].

In the extreme (such as microgravity conditions and prolonged bed rest) muscle disuse atrophy is known to upregulate the NF-*k*B inflammation pathways and change the signaling pathways related to protein synthesis[156]. These findings reveal clues to the impact of physical inactivity in as short a time as two days of disuse[157]. These clues extend to less severe forms of "disuse" such as simple inactivity because inadequate redox stimulation produces a diminished antioxidant and autophagic response, along with an increased level of inflammation[158].

The key point is that disease happens at both ends of the hormesis curve - with too much oxidation, as well as with not enough oxidation to stimulate cell-protective pathways. Having low physical activity and being lethargic, creates a state of insufficient oxidative stimulation, and misses living within the hormesis zone.

With too low or suppressed, there is less transcription and translation activity and less protein formation. Physical inactivity, along with excess food-energy consumption is associated with elevated systemic oxidative stress and the sustained activation of redox-sensitive inflammation (transcription factors - NF-*k*B)[159]. This validates the rule that proper diet and proper exercise are equivalent variables in the redox lifestyle equation. This is because they help keep the body balanced within the hormetic zone, and responsive to challenging environments. This is the scientific justification and rationale for the redox lifestyle!

Hormesis – The Dual Nature of Redox

The point of this as it relates to the principle of hormesis and exercise, is that there is both an overuse/disuse effect, and a "Goldilocks" hormesis effect – where the latter represents the "just right" amount of exercise. Dialing in the right amount of exercise is different for each person but is key to optimizing and activating the redox-driven hormetic effect that explains the health benefits which arise from exercise. This is why intense endurance activity is not necessarily better than walking, as is evidenced in literature showing effects on metabolic disease[160][161].

As it relates to cellular and metabolic health, the focus here is on clean energy metabolism and metabolic fitness and flexibility - not calorie reduction or boosting the metabolism. This is why knowing the rules of the cell and energy metabolism is so helpful. If one is favoring the "energy in – energy out, diet-and-exercise paradigm," but is still using carbs as the main energy fuel source, it will be difficult to manage the related endocrine and hormone challenges, let alone improve metabolic health. This is true notwithstanding that successful weight loss occurs. The full advantages that come from autophagy and cell renewal will be shortchanged without metabolic flexibility and periodic nutritional ketosis. Still, exercise across the board – works! And hormesis-driven signaling is the key – at least from the redox and metabolic health perspective.

In regard to hormesis and exercise, the result of exercise is to increase cellular conditioning, by placing "just enough" stress on the body to encourage flexibility, improved energy production and utilization, and the better management of metabolic pathways.

The "Goldilocks just right" effect using a mild oxidative stimulus, activates the hormesis response in cells, which in turn drives cellular function and protection. This redox supported recovery strategy optimizes the autophagic rest-and-recovery phase post-exercise and enhances the translation-driven protein repair process to proceed more optimally.

Nullifying the Hormetic Effect

There is a final point to be made regarding the principle of hormesis as it relates to exercise and nutrition. We learned earlier that the hormetic effect

Hormesis – The Dual Nature of Redox

in mitochondria is called *mitohormesis*. The mitochondria is intimately involved with exercise[162]. It participates in the health-promoting effects of exercise. Paradoxically, the use of plant antioxidants has shown to nullify the hormetic ROS-antioxidant effect in mitochondria and impair the health-promoting capabilities of glucose restriction and physical exercise, respectively[163].

Because of the required redox stimulus needed to activate hormesis (as shown in animal models), taking antioxidants prior to exercise serves to neutralize ROS and diminishes the ability to activate the necessary redox signaling which ultimately upregulates antioxidant enzymes (specifically SOD), which in turn affects a cell's ability to benefit from exercise[164].

This means that the benefits from mild oxidation created through exercise, which is "just enough" to activate and make the cellular antioxidant system stronger (conditioned) and more responsive, can be sabotaged and undermined with antioxidant consumption proximate to the time of exercising. Providing excess outside plant-based antioxidants coincident with exercise, risks suppressing this mechanism, and diminishing or muting the hormesis effect.

Summary

What the science of redox signaling biology and hormesis teaches is that mild levels of reactive oxygen species are necessary to signal and activate cellular defense and repair mechanisms. The principle of hormesis is a fundamental component of the redox platform for cellular health. The very same oxidative molecules which in higher quantity produce inflammation and disease, in low or mild or physiologic amounts produce a healing stress-adaptive conditioning within the body to recover and survive. This is an essential and fundamental principle of redox health, and it helps explain the redox biology and physiological effects of exercise, stress reduction, good nutrition, healthy sleep, and glucose restriction (fasting) [165].

Each of these bio-oxidative and redox-based processes induce or increase mitochondrial metabolism – producing more ROS – which amongst everything else happening in real time, has a degree of action on redox-

Hormesis – The Dual Nature of Redox

sensitive transcription factors. This increase in cellular respiration produces an increase in reactive oxygen species, which yields a mild oxidative stress within the mitochondria which leads to an adaptive stress response which results in improved resistance to stress - which conditioning is paradoxically believed to result in a long-term reduction in oxidative stress[166].

The sophistication within these metabolic and physiologic principles is stunning and taken together are the essence of what it means to "Awaken Your Inner Doctor!"

Before concluding the topic of hormesis and nutrition, it is important to acknowledge and address the emerging role, good and bad, of "anti-nutrition."

Redox, Hormesis, and 'Anti-nutrition'

Within the world of hormesis and redox biochemistry, the reduction of reactive oxygen species (ROS) by endogenous antioxidants, and in their absence the action of secondary plant-based metabolites, is an important aspect of the hormetic cellular effect. The many associated redox reactions which plant phytochemicals are associated with are characterized by the non-linear effects of these secondary metabolites within the human hormetic zone. These compounds, otherwise known as plant polyphenols, include a class of plant chemicals known as "anti-nutrients" and because of hormesis, play both sides of the redox-sensitive spectrum. These compounds are considered "non-nutritive" as they are not directly involved with energy metabolism. However, as we will see, they are intimately involved with the Redoxome at large.

All of this operates on the hormesis principle where low levels of an agent or condition produce stimulation of cellular health, and high levels produce cellular damage and dysfunction. This is due to the redox-sensitive stimulation which occurs from mild physiologic levels of oxidation which initiate cellular defense, cell cycle differentiation, and adaptive stress resistance – as well as the opposite effect of inflammation occurring from high levels of oxidation producing inflammation and disease.

Hormesis – The Dual Nature of Redox

These secondary compounds and plant metabolites participate in this redox chemistry and is the most important reason and function for these secondary metabolites[167], notwithstanding their sometimes notorious downsides. These non-nutritive downsides have gained wide attention and are often misunderstood and improperly focused upon, largely due to a misunderstanding of their role in supporting and playing within the broader Redoxome – something that involves the ubiquitous world of atmosphere, soil, the plant kingdom, and finally animals and humans.

There is longstanding evidence in life and literature that a diet that is rich in plant-based content plays an important role in prevention and reduction of disease. In addition to their supplying important micro- and macronutrient nutrition, they contain concentrations of bioactive plant compounds which clearly demonstrate positive health benefits.

Within the many various dietary patterns today including the Mediterranean, DASH (dietary approaches to stop hypertension), vegan and vegetarian, ketogenic, paleolithic ('hunter-gather') - all provide emphasis on whole foods which include vegetables, fruits, legumes, nuts, and whole grains. The positive health benefits are generally attributed to the synergistic effects of anti-inflammatory and antioxidant phytochemicals including polyphenols, alkaloids, organosulfur compounds, terpenoids, and phytosterols[168].

However, many have questioned the healthfulness of these phytochemicals, noting their association with blocked absorption and bioavailability of minerals (iron, calcium, zinc, etc.), gastrointestinal distress, altered gut function, inflammation, limited calcium absorption, kidney stone formation, and more. In this regard, these polyphenols have been labeled as "anti-nutrients." Specifically, this class of polyphenols include[169]: lectins, lathyrogens, oxalates, phytates, phytoestrogens, saponins, tannins, and alpha amylase inhibitors.

[See Appendix: Anti-Nutrients, for more information on antinutrients.]

If these plant chemicals are found in nature, the question must be asked – why would they be harmful? The answer is that plants synthesize a number

Hormesis – The Dual Nature of Redox

of secondary metabolites and phytochemicals called polyphenols, which help protect them against attacks from plant-eating animals, insects, and pathogens – within their own growing environment. To avoid predation, these chemicals function to help plants survive in adverse conditions. This toxicity and how it is experienced by humans, is the essence of this discussion.

From a nutritional point of view, because antinutrient compounds interfere with digestion and absorption, and can contribute to gastrointestinal distress and inflammation, they should be considered as toxic and harmful when unwisely ingested[170]. This is concerning because the plants/foods that contain them comprise a significant part of the modern diet, especially in the form of legumes and grains – of all varieties. These are important food groups because they contain important starches, proteins, fibers, saccharides, polyphenols, minerals, and other micronutrients – all of which contribute significantly to human health. Therefore, understanding the role of the so-called "antinutrients" as a special class of phytochemicals, should be understood better by all, and especially how to reduce or neutralize them in the diet to safe levels.

While much research continues about their effects, their health benefits are generally thought to outweigh any potential negative nutritional effect[171]. What is being learned is that their mechanism-of-action for producing these beneficial health effects is due to the stress-adaptive redox

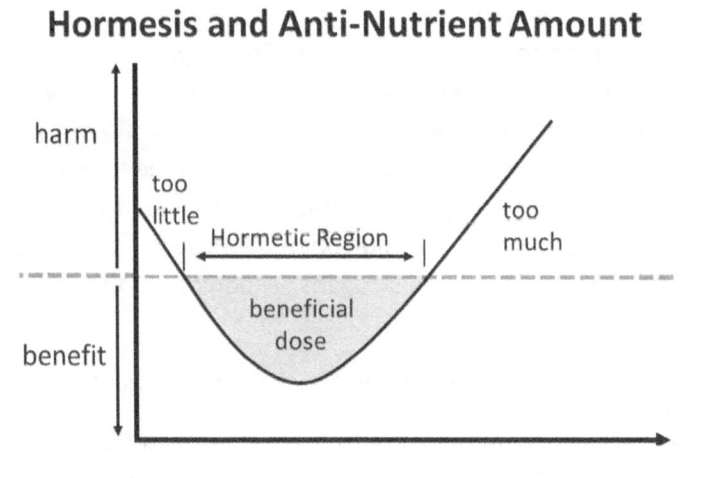

Hormesis and Anti-Nutrient Amount

Hormesis – The Dual Nature of Redox

principle of hormesis and redox cell signaling. (For further information, refer to the section "Nutrition and Hormesis" in Part 3 of this book.)

Is Wheat Bad?

Wheat has particularly come under fire in recent decades for its emerging relationships with these issues, especially as it relates to gut function, coeliac disease, gluten sensitivity, allergies, and its disproportionate linkage with obesity and type 2 diabetes[172]. The increasing awareness of these issues has caused many to eliminate or reduce wheat (gluten) in their diet ('gluten-free'), something that obviously deprives them of an important protein source, B vitamins, minerals, and many bioactive compounds.

There is evidence that the predisposing haplotypes (genetic predispositions) were in existence as early as the first century AD[173], and that its autoimmune basis dates back thousands of years. Although the symptoms are similar, celiac disease is different from gluten intolerance (sensitivity) and the latter does not have the full negative impact on overall health that the autoimmune celiac disease has.

Celiac disease affects 1% of the U.S. population, while non-celiac gluten sensitivity affects 6%. Yet combined they have created immense public awareness about all-things "wheat & non-gluten" in the dietary marketplace. Our purposes here are not to explore or resolve all aspects of gluten sensitivity or celiac disease, but to suggest that a significant part of this is related to "antinutrients," plant phytochemicals or polyphenols.

Notwithstanding that wheat remains a staple in the modern diet, it has become a controversial 'hot-topic.' As such, it begs the question, why after thousands of years with wheat as the "staff of life," has wheat and the associated gluten sensitivity it can create, become such a dominant issue for many people's health? All things considered, with its increasing prevalence, it appears to be a modern problem. But why?

Gluten is a protein found in rye, barley and wheat and acts as a sticky glue to hold food together structurally. Bread makers routinely knead and agitate their wheat dough to 'develop the gluten' for this purpose.

Hormesis – The Dual Nature of Redox

Various theories have emerged about the causes of this emerging and heightened sensitivity, and include changes in gut bacteria, too much wheat in the diet, overuse of antibiotics, collateral digestive issues that impact gluten issues, and the impact that processed foods and oils have on the body and the gut. Intolerance occurs when the body cannot properly digest gluten. However – gluten itself is natural! It remains an interesting thought to consider why this problem appears to be a modern condition, along with the surging interest in eating gluten-free.

An emerging explanation for the role of wheat in producing these conditions is the role of phytic acid and other "antinutrients" that are in high(er) levels in dormant seeds - high enough to be problematic for some people. Because grains contain anti-nutrients and phytochemicals, they deserve careful consideration and preparation.

Many seeds and grains contain phytates, lectins, oxylates and other antinutrients. This includes the wide class of legumes. A common method for removing these preservative plant chemicals from these seeds and grains is by soaking. This mimics what happens in nature when a seed or nut is planted in moist soil, where soil moisture removes and disables the chemicals, thereby allowing the sprouting process to activate and for germination to begin.

The important take-away is that "anti-nutrients" can be modified and dramatically lowered to safe levels by something as simple as soaking prior to cooking[174]. Soaking and dehulling of seeds improves digestibility (protein and starch) and contributes significantly to the reduction of phytate and anti-nutrient content by nearly 75%[175]

Plant chemicals are created and used by seeds as a means of preservation – both as a defense while growing, as well as to prevent sprouting until the right conditions occur. Modern agricultural and farming practices interrupt these processes and as a result certain compounds in the grain fail to go through the natural processes used through ages past, which lessen their presence and effect in the diet.

Hormesis – The Dual Nature of Redox

Prior to modern agricultural industrialization, grains were soaked (sprouted) or fermented before making them into cereals, breads, and cakes. Sprouting deactivates these antinutrients (polyphenols), making them less toxic – sufficient enough to make them easier to digest and to remove the majority of ill-effects and causing them to have a positive hormetic effect.

Soaking or increasing the moisture for 12-24 hours is the first natural step which reduces the enzyme inhibitors and the starch content. (Longer soaking caused fermentation which is a more complete way to pre-digest the grain and neutralize these antinutrient chemicals and hard-to-digest proteins. This is the essence of sourdough bread.).

This sprouting of grain is the process of seed germination which biologically transforms the seed, just as happens to it in natural wet soil. This process increases the protein and amino acid composition and the B vitamin content. As well it releases the stored phosphates, minerals, and enzymes within the seed to begin its initial growth phase out of dormancy. These are the nutrients needed to begin the early plant growth prior to its establishing a root system and drawing its own nutrition from the soil. This process transforms dormant (resting) seeds into active, germinated, and growing plant life.

These principles were unknowingly utilized with early harvesting practices. In former times, grain was harvested in the fields and sheaved. The *sheaves* were bundled into *shocks* and left standing in the field awaiting gathering while the fields were harvested. The sheaves of cut grain stalks were arranged in teepee like fashion called a shock or stack, in such a way that the grain heads were kept off the ground while still in the field and prior to threshing. During this time the grain was exposed to the elements of weather – alternating dew, rain, humidity, moisture, wind, sunshine – and then later were taken to threshing floors where the wheat berries were separated from the chaff and made ready for food preparation by milling or grinding.

During the time the shocks of wheat stood in the field awaiting gathering, they were exposed to the effects of weather, which moisture functioned as a form of sprouting or initial germination which remove the high levels of

Hormesis – The Dual Nature of Redox

phytates and antinutrients from the wheat berries prior to food preparation.

This weathering process created conditions that were ideal for favoring a degree of germination (sprouting) and enzyme multiplication in the grain, as the antinutrient chemicals were neutralized and removed. The resulting wheat and the milled flour coming from this was thus much richer in vitamin and enzyme content and had lowered antinutrient levels. Knowing redox and hormesis principles, today we would say these levels fall to be within the safe(er) ranges of the hormesis zone for promoting health and improved cellular function.

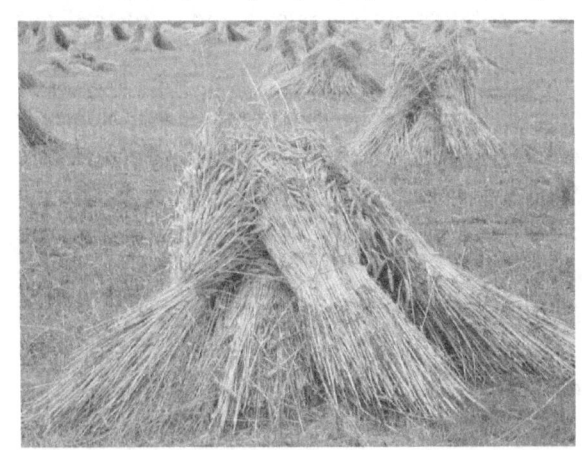

Contrast this with the modern methods using combine harvesting where grain is removed immediately from the stalk and transported immediately to storage. There is no weathering or moisture conditioning, and no enzyme development. The result is a mature but still dormant seed with high levels protective of 'antinutrients,' and lacking the nutrition qualities as seen with grain that is otherwise weathered, germinated, and made safer by reduction of excess toxic antinutrients.

An important point to keep in mind when considering the effects of modern diets compared to the effects of ancestral diets, is the consideration about the levels of so-called "antinutrients," (polyphenols or plant phytochemicals), in today's grains and flours and food products. These antinutrients and higher levels of phytochemicals are presented to the human diet in thousands of ways.

The degree of involvement as an etiologic explanation for modern food sensitivities and immune system irregularities is intriguing, but yet to be fully explained. However, the merging of these points of redox science and

Hormesis – The Dual Nature of Redox

practical living, go a long way to explain why the food sensitivities, gluten intolerance, and depleted nutrition seen with modern food processing, may be of such high significance.

The historical records which assert that wheat was the "staff of life," had good reason to so attest. Their natural harvest techniques differed considerably from what happens today with massive agricultural methods designed around expediency and volume. The modern aversion to wheat / gluten on many fronts, is in part explained by the agricultural methods used today. These methods shortcut the wheat harvest in a way which leaves elevated levels of anti-nutrients in place in a dormant seed and processes them to completion where they are then consumed without nature's involvement in making them safer.

Combine this with processed foods throughout the diet, and the collective insults on the gut, inflammation, and high toxic stimulation for cellular oxidation dramatically impacts the risk for diseases common to this situation.

As a practical note, the early practices which allowed grain to weather and begin and then stop the germination/sprouting phase can be readily accomplished today by pre-soaking grains, legumes, and nuts, prior to food processing and eating. Simply sprouting, and then using sprouted or pre-soaked wheat (then dried and milled to flour), produces a food product that is full of enzymes, vitamins, and reduced levels of (toxic) phytochemicals / antinutrients. The same is true for beans and other legumes.

Extended, this discussion can also expand to embrace the merits of soaking of all seeds, legumes, nuts, prior to food preparation and consumption. This is the principle behind the practice of sprouts/sprouting, microgreens, and pre-soaked grains prior to milling - all of which dramatically boosts nutrition, enzymes, vitamins, and redox-active qualities of the food.

A common and sometimes humorous example of these principles in action is in eating beans that have not been soaked overnight prior to cooking and eating. The phytates and chemicals (alpha-galactosides) are present in mature legume seeds (beans), which when consumed, produce

Hormesis – The Dual Nature of Redox

gastrointestinal 'distress' as bacteria struggle to digest the beans, starches, and their associated saccharides. Soaking overnight removes the excess of these protective (to the seed) chemicals rendering the food more digestible and less irritating to the gut (and to those around the 'unsoaked-bean' eater!).

The topic of Redox Nutrition must acknowledge and factor-in this discussion as it relates to *modified* antinutrients, polyphenols, and plant phytochemicals from across the spectrum, and their effects upon the cellular Redoxome. It is an awakening and a maturing of nutritional thinking whose time is now – because it is based within the redox landscape. The principle of redox-driven hormesis applies centrally to secondary plant-based metabolites which affect the redox status both directly and indirectly due to their effect upon redox status, transcription factors, and pathway genes.

These 'awakenings' result in the operation and management of many pathways working in serial and parallel (vertically and horizontally) throughout the redox landscape. Collectively they contribute to the vitally important role which autophagy plays in cellular renewal.

Autophagy – Redox Driven Cellular Repair

Autophagy – Redox Driven Cellular Repair

In 2016 the Nobel Prize in Physiology and Medicine was given to Yoshinori Ohsumi for his discoveries in the mechanisms for autophagy. This recent event witnesses the 'newness' of this discovery as well as to its importance in cellular biology and health.

Autophagy is a natural cellular mechanism our cells utilize to perform its internal housekeeping role in removing damaged, misfolded, aggregated proteins, damaged DNA, and cell membranes, and eliminating intracellular pathogens. This includes the process of mitophagy which is the selective degradation and turnover of mitochondria following damage or stress[176].

Literally the term auto-phagy means "self-eating." It is an important homeostatic process where damaged and degraded cell components are pushed toward cellular lysosomes where they are degraded and recycled. This is such an important process that if it is absent or interrupted the effects of cell degeneration and cell damage accelerate to the point of producing excess oxidation, inflammation, disease, cellular dysfunction, and accelerated aging.

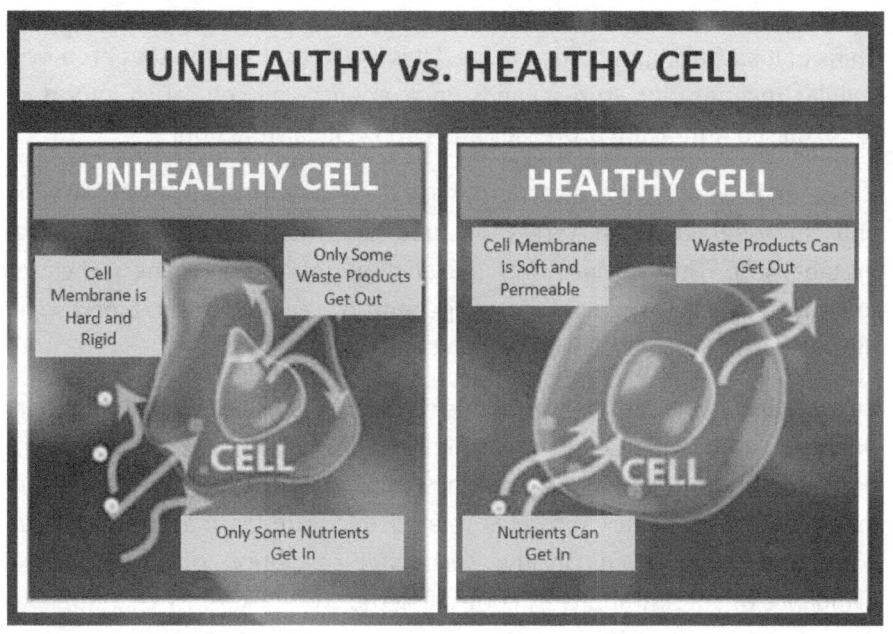

UNHEALTHY vs. HEALTHY CELL

UNHEALTHY CELL
- Cell Membrane is Hard and Rigid
- Only Some Waste Products Get Out
- Only Some Nutrients Get In

HEALTHY CELL
- Cell Membrane is Soft and Permeable
- Waste Products Can Get Out
- Nutrients Can Get In

Autophagy – Redox Driven Cellular Repair

The process of autophagy is that damaged cell components are degraded, decomposed, and cleared by lysosomes inside the cell. These "parts" are then recycled and reused as building blocks for cell repair, new protein synthesis, and as a new fuel source in the mitochondria. In the extreme and during periods of starvation, autophagy provides an internal source of nutrients and energy generation which enables prolonged periods of fasting.

Autophagy is a powerful force in metabolic homeostasis and serves as one of nature's prime methods in prevention of degenerative disease[177]. It is an emerging anti-aging mechanism and strategy[178].

In 'ancient' days this is how our ancestors survived periods of starvation, as it was the body's adaptive mechanism in surviving from season to season with varying levels of food availability. While some of that may be considered conjecture, it certainly fits with the known science of how the body works, regardless of whether it came to be by adaptation or design.

This cleaning and clearing of cellular and molecular debris is the path to better cellular functioning – the essence of "repair and replace." Through this process cells recycle and dispose of "spent" and damaged components. Think of it as "taking out the garbage." It is like a reset button that promotes cellular regeneration, repair, and replacement – all central to important redox-based anti-aging processes and good cellular function.

However, like everything else, autophagy declines with age, chronic disease, and improper diets in terms of food-fuel management (i.e., energy metabolism). This decline and dysfunction intensifies aging-associated metabolic diseases such as neurodegeneration, cell dysplasia, blood sugar disorders, and vascular-based disorders to name a few[179].

Because this is the primary mechanism which cells use to deal with cellular debris created with cellular metabolism, it is important to have well-functioning autophagy. This especially applies to the proper handling of inflammatory cytokines (proteins related to the inflammatory response). The latter feature aids in the successful resolution of infection and avoidance of autoimmunity by controlling the crosstalk between autophagy

Autophagy – Redox Driven Cellular Repair

and the inflammatory signaling pathways, essentially balancing the cell defense pathways and homeostasis[180].

When it comes specifically to the mitochondria, "mitophagy" or mitochondrial autophagy, is the only known mechanism for the turnover of damaged or poor performing mitochondria[181]. Therefore, if the autophagic process is compromised or is not activated for any reason, it can result in abnormal mitochondrial function and the increase of further oxidation.

These adaptive autophagic responses (meaning they are not automatic and must be activated) are a primary mechanism for restoring cellular homeostasis and balance. Not only does this recycling of spent cellular components provide the cell with recycled nutrients and new energy sources (useful in starvation, fasting, or limited carbohydrate consumption), it also serves to eliminate toxic components from the cell that arise from cellular dysfunction[182] and from daily living.

Because of this, autophagy is emerging as one of the foundational mechanisms and targets that regulate aging. The ability of a cell to perform this function is a quality control measure which affects disease management, aging, and cellular turnover. It plays a key role in protecting against the instability of DNA, and prevents against chronic diseases such as cancer, neurodegeneration, heart disease, diabetes, liver disease and autoimmune diseases and infections[183]. Thus, it can be thought of as a survival mechanism that is called upon to help protect and prepare us for diseases of aging and in restoring cellular health.

> Autophagy induction is correlated with glucose levels and inversely correlated with insulin levels in the body. This correlates with the "fed" and "fasting" states. Elevated insulin levels thus suppress autophagy, and low glucose levels stimulate autophagy.

Given its central role in health, important questions about autophagy relate to what initiates it, maintains it, and even what happens when this process is defective or sabotaged – and how.

Autophagy – Redox Driven Cellular Repair

The signaling pathways that lead to autophagy are sophisticated and varied but can be summarized as being regulated by redox-based nutrient sensors. These sensors are responsive to the presence and mixture of macronutrients and their responsive hormones within the blood stream. All of this in turn, affects the redox state of the cell. It is to this central thesis that we will direct our attention.

The induction or initiation of autophagy occurs as redox-sensitive "switches" activate in response to the mild oxidation produced from nutritional stress imposed by ketosis, which happens when glucose levels decline. These redox switches or nutrient sensors are molecular switches (transcription factors) that are sensitive to and respond to specific nutrient states. They do this through hormone-based physiology and redox states created in the body. Better understanding the processes that up- and down-regulate metabolic pathways and knowing the relationships that exist between what is eaten and their actions on various chronic metabolic diseases, is an important place to start in any journey toward better health.

Nutrient sensing and the hormonal regulation from feeding behaviors related to our "fasted" and "fed" states, are all central to this discussion. By and large, these mechanisms and capabilities define our degree of health, amount of cellular energy, the rate of aging we experience, and the effect which disease processes have on our body.

At a higher level, the nutrient state is the predominant and general controlling regulator for autophagy activation and inactivation. This has to do with the amount and mix of macronutrients available as a fuel source for energy metabolism.

Generally speaking, and with regard to energy metabolism, carbohydrates, are the preferred fuel source in mitochondria. The energy in glucose comes from the chemical bonds between the carbon atoms in the 6-member (hexane) carbon ring of a

Alpha-D-Glucose

Autophagy – Redox Driven Cellular Repair

glucose molecule. The energy in those high-energy bonds was created originally through the process of photosynthesis in plants when glucose is originally formed and locked into the carbohydrate structure of the growing plant. When animals and humans eat plants, the carbohydrates are digested, and glucose is made available for cells to metabolize as a fuel and energy source. As the glucose molecule becomes metabolized, it is taken apart piece by piece, and in that process – as electrons are transported along the respiratory 'conveyor belt' – energy is created and harvested.

These reactions occur because of glycolysis and the movement of glucose, protein, and fatty acid metabolites through Krebs' cycle and the electron transport chain - as that process breaks apart carbon and hydrogen bonds and captures the energy released via the transfer of electrons to ATP, and then to ADP, which is the 'storage battery' of the cell.

The transfer of this energy during this cellular respiration allows for a gradual release of energy from glucose to ATP to ADP and creates a controlled burning or oxidation of glucose (in contrast to a sudden release of energy). This ingenious mechanism allows for the harvest of this energy from its stored state and serves as an efficient way to capture and transfer energy held within the chemical bonds in food molecules, to the body - one electron at a time.

Because of these energy advantages, when it is available, glucose is the first fuel burned (even when there are abundant amounts of fat and protein present). There is an important point to make with regard to the practical application of this information.

With carbohydrate-centric diets, it remains difficult to convert to "fat burning" mode since carbs are utilized first. It also begs the concern for where fats that are consumed go, and how they are utilized if the predilection for fuel source favors available carbohydrates.

On a positive note, this means that carb-centric diets are both protein- and fat-sparing, allowing, or forcing the latter macronutrients to be used for other functions in the body, including the storage of fat for latter lean times.

Autophagy – Redox Driven Cellular Repair

Obviously, there are benefits to this, however there are also significant metabolic downsides.

In a carbohydrate-centric diet or lifestyle, fat is not readily utilized as energy because the energy equation favors glucose, and the energy dynamics shift less often and willingly to fat-burning mode for energy (without other factors entering in such as exercise or redox supplementation). In these situations, (especially with coexisting metabolic dysfunction and comorbidities), dietary fat and *de novo* fat (new production) is stored away for possible future use in liver and organ cells, and visceral fat storage depots – along with excess carbohydrates not needed for current energy requirements.

In states of starvation and fasting and glucose exhaustion, amino acids and fats are used for energy. Proteolysis and gluconeogenesis prepare amino acids, and fat oxidation prepares fats to enter Krebs cycle. However, in the presence of glucose and/or insulin, these processes are inhibited. With fats this is due to the effect that elevated insulin has in limiting the breakdown of triglycerides into independent fatty acids[184]. The point here is to highlight the main metabolic rule that as blood-glucose levels rise and insulin increases to move glucose into the cells, the use of fats as an energy source is inhibited. (This has interesting considerations for people with diabetes and metabolic disease!)

[As an aside, there are no doubt readers here who are acquainted with or will find many "credible" sources showing that a high carbohydrate diet is effective for weight loss. There are so many variables in this at the outset that it is difficult to know where to start. There is information in the Appendix on how to evaluate dietary advice that may be helpful. In summary, there are numerous points of definition related to what constitutes a 'high-carb' diet, as well as to what the end-point of such a diet is. If the purpose is weight loss, then a high-carb diet can work – if you eat very little calories and only from high quality 'healthy' carbohydrates. But the all-important follow up question should be – what kind of carbs? Or what is the likelihood of someone only eating 'healthy' carbs? If all carbs were only whole grain, fruits, vegetables, and "healthy" and there were no

Autophagy – Redox Driven Cellular Repair

refined carbs or processed foods, then it could fit within the rules of the cell for metabolic health. The right mix of healthy carb foods can supply protein, fat and complex carbs to meet many of the metabolic demands of healthy cells. However, today, that is very unlikely. The other all-important consideration relates to metabolic health. Seldom will weight-loss high-carb diets ever discuss metabolic health in any of its presentation. Weight loss as a measure of health is different from having genuine metabolic health! One can lose weight and still be metabolically unhealthy![185]

As we have reviewed previously, a cell cannot survive without energy and a source for producing it. Therefore, when glucose is absent, the cell is forced to switch fuel source to another energy source. The ability of the mitochondria to make the shift from glucose to fatty acids, is called *metabolic flexibility*. The success or degree of this ability is defined as *metabolic efficiency*.

Generally speaking there are three methods to achieve this shift in fuel sources. All three affect the state of glucose availability. These methods include:

- Fasting – elimination of food consumption
- Low-carb diet - restricted dietary carbohydrate consumption
- Exercise – 'spending' and using available glucose in the body

Whether carbohydrate (glucose) consumption is stopped through fasting, limited by restricted amounts of carbohydrates consumed, or is depleted through exercise-induced reductions in glucose, the net result is the same - lowered blood-glucose levels. When glucose and insulin levels fall it forces a change in fuel source, selection, and utilization. Since these methods are so tightly connected with the redox-related state of autophagy, we will review them in greater depth now.

Fasting and Autophagy

We spoke earlier about fasting and its effects in energy metabolism in the section on nutritional ketosis. Because the principles of ketosis and autophagy are so interconnected, this information here may seem redundant, but it presented through the lens of autophagy.

Autophagy – Redox Driven Cellular Repair

While <u>exogenous</u> redox supplements are a very effective method for shifting the metabolomic state from glucose metabolism to fatty acids, fasting is the most effective <u>endogenous</u> (natural) way to trigger a shift in the fuel source selected by the cell. The practice of repetitive intermittent fasting increases metabolic flexibility and efficiency and promotes the state of autophagy. Since the body must have an energy source to maintain cellular energy and function, eliminating food for protracted time periods forces cells to shift their fuel source from carbohydrates to fats. The degree of efficiency with which this occurs is a function of how well adapted, conditioned, practiced, or trained the body is to make this shift when the fasting state occurs.

From an immediate survival perspective, the body and its cells are not 'dumb.' They are well suited and conditioned to communicate and signal distress when carbohydrate (glucose) is diminished – especially if one is not conditioned to this reality. If one is not flexible or has not adapted or conditioned well to accomplish this, the body and brain will experience distress from the "sugar crash" (a carb withdrawal symptom), whereupon it triggers the hunger hormones to drive behavior that will 'rescue' the low glucose state with quick carbohydrate consumption.

As long as carbs are a regular and central part of one's lifestyle, "going without" through fasting will seldom be an enjoyable experience - as low levels of glucose produce agitation, tremors, clouded thinking, and feelings of distress, in tandem with this glucose roller coaster. Your unconditioned hormones want you to eat to fix this problem as it perceives it.

The persistent existence of the "fed" state eliminates and shortens any possibility that quality autophagy will occur. However, fasting and ketosis favor the conditions of mitochondrial flexibility and create the hormetic state that allows redox-sensitive transcription factors to initiate and maintain cellular renewal through autophagy.

Carbohydrate Restriction and Autophagy

Next to fasting in effectiveness in autophagy activation is the reduction of carbohydrate consumption to very low levels (generally considered to be about fifty grams per day), leaving fats and proteins as the two predominant

Autophagy – Redox Driven Cellular Repair

constituents of the diet. Within popular diet and science literature a distinction has been drawn between what is a "low carbohydrate" (LC) and a "very low carbohydrate" (VLC) diet. These diets are ketogenic and are often referred to as a 'keto diet,' due to their ability to induce nutritional ketosis.

The respective goals for low and very low carbohydrate diets in reference to the number of calories (not grams) consumed is 10-30% LC, and 5-10% VLC, respectively.

Many popular dietary guidelines call for a carbohydrate range between 45-65% of calories from carbohydrates. Again, from a cellular rules perspective, chronically elevated carb/glucose levels in this range would diminish quality autophagy, and less capable metabolic flexibility.

It is interesting, yet frustrating, that low-fat diets (the same thing as high-carb) have been strongly positioned as the solution to heart disease over the last three decades. This necessarily dictates that carbs be a dominant part of the daily diet – which leaves many questions for the common person as to how the rules of the cell reconcile this with the rules for metabolic flexibility and cellular health and redox stability.

The point is that cells always utilize glucose first if it is present, to drive its energy metabolism. If absent or low enough, the effect of fasting or carb restriction is essentially the same as it relates to energy metabolism and its effects on hormones and the redox state.

Because the metabolic shift happens due to the relative unavailability of free glucose, the primary objective is to *periodically* limit carbs in the diet and force the cell to shift to fats for energy. (Note the emphasis on 'periodically' – as flexibility implies the conditioned back-and-forth ketone cycling and movement in the ability to switch out fuel platforms in the cell).

Since limiting carb consumption brings near-equal benefits as fasting outright, it is often considered to be "fasting without fasting" – a metabolic shortcut of sorts to create the same beneficial metabolic effects.

Autophagy – Redox Driven Cellular Repair

Due to the effects of redox supplementation in providing a mild level of oxidation, the same outcome is seen with exogenous sourced agents to provide the equivalent effect on the metabolomic shift. From the cell's point of view, the limitation of dietary carbohydrates and/or the presence of redox supplementation is a key strategy to "training" the cell to use other fuel sources.

Recall that low glucose levels activate the hormone glucagon in an attempt to first find and liberate more stored glucose in the form of glycogen. Glucagon is the hormone that becomes active when glucose levels fall and breaks down glycogen. When glucagon levels rise in response to low glucose levels, it contributes to the activation of autophagy[186]. And then when carbohydrate consumption resumes again in the diet and glucose and insulin levels elevate, glucagon is suppressed – thus lowering the mild state of nutritional stress and stopping autophagy.

Whether the low glucose levels occur due to fasting or to a low-carb diet, the resulting lowered glucose and insulin levels along with a rising glucagon level, are correlated with the autophagic response. Thus, carbohydrate absence or restriction activates glucagon and helps initiate autophagy, while the presence of insulin inhibits autophagy.

It should be noted that carbohydrate restriction is not the same thing as caloric restriction. With caloric restriction, the calories consumed could still be majority carbohydrates above the threshold that denies ketosis. While avoiding energy excess is important by overconsuming food, restricting energy (food quantity) does not necessarily assure ketosis or comfortable flexibility – or metabolic health for that matter!

Due to the way hormones respond to macronutrient ratios and blood sugar concentrations, simply reducing total calories is not as strategically beneficial as managing the relative amounts of food types – especially those calories that come from carbohydrates specifically.

A related application of this knowledge is the manipulation of timing related to food consumption. One of the health miracles of restorative sleep is that autophagy generally happens during sleep – during periods of nightly

Autophagy – Redox Driven Cellular Repair

fasting. This explains why quality sleep is so essential. Fragmented sleep and obstructive sleep apnea dysregulates autophagy in the brain[187][188]. Throughout the various cycles of sleep, the brain is busy "taking out the trash" and cellular repair. This occurs because of redox-sensitive autophagy and is optimized when the rhythm of autophagy is not altered by sleep fragmentation[189]. Literally, sleep equals brain autophagy – or "garbage night." This is where the proverbial "Pac-man" moves through brain and all other cells of the body, gobbling up cellular debris and trash, and recycling and disposing of them in healthy fashion. By doing so, they restore cellular function and homeostatic redox balance. This is the essence of detoxification, rest and repair, and cellular renewal.

As a useful strategy, knowing that autophagy will only initiate with low glucose and insulin levels, and that this works best in a fasted state, we can take advantage of this each night by avoiding food intake 3 or 4 hours before bedtime. If the body is preoccupied metabolizing a late dinner, or bedtime or midnight snack, it reduces the amount of sleep time in a low glucose state wherein autophagy can begin to operate. Rather than spending precious sleep time digesting a meal and disposing of the glucose and elevated insulin that results from late-night eating and snacks, the brain and body can more easily initiate autophagy and use the precious sleep time to renew, repair, and replace, and improve metabolic cellular health.

As an even stronger strategy to lengthen time in autophagy, a morning "break-fast" of a low- or no-carbohydrate meal can extend the autophagic state through the daytime, adding more hours in cellular repair - before cycling out of autophagy and a 'keto' state.

Additionally, knowing the effect of synergistic redox phytochemicals and redox replenishment on metabolomic flexibility and function, layering a supplement strategy over the above can increase the effect further and longer and more profoundly, helping to fill in the gaps.

With regard to those with pre-existing metabolic health challenges (metabolic comorbidities) who may be less able to fast, a carb-restricted diet combined with specific redox enhancement may prove very beneficial. In these cases, physician advice and supervision is desirable due to the many

Autophagy – Redox Driven Cellular Repair

metabolic side-effects related to altering energy metabolism and glucose levels in the body.

Exercise and Autophagy.

Exercise is a third strategy for managing glucose levels and causing a shift in fuel source inside a cell. It is a non-diet mechanism for reducing glucose/glycogen levels in the body. During exercise, free glucose along with glycogen is metabolized first. As glucose levels are depleted through exercise, a metabolic shift occurs which favors fat burning to provide and maintain energy metabolism.

The effect of exercise on lowering blood sugar levels is easily sabotaged with consumption of carbohydrates in the form of energy or rehydration drinks, fitness bars, or anything that offsets the effect of exercise on glucose levels. This should give pause to athletes and those exercising who think their exercise offsets rehydration or "sports" drinks – or who even have a 'bad' diet. From a metabolic health perspective, you cannot outrun a bad diet with mismanaged energy metabolism.

The effects of exercise on muscle physiology is that it improves its capacity for using fat for energy. It also increases the muscle cell's ability to utilize glucose during insulin-stimulated conditions. This has profound impact on the ability of exercise in the prevention of insulin resistance and metabolic disease[190]. The opposite effect is seen in individuals who do not exercise or who are metabolically inflexible[191].

Physical exercise and the contraction of muscle fibers is an ATP-based biochemical phenomenon and requires the production of energy in mitochondria. In addition to producing cellular energy, this Krebs-based process creates reactive molecules (ROS) which function with a dual role – one which activates redox-sensitive healthy pathway genes, and the other in causing damage to proteins and cellular components.

Because of this, muscle cells require an efficient mechanism for dealing with folded, damaged, and toxic proteins, and the damaged organelles within the cell[192]. This is accomplished through autophagy mechanisms which clean out

Autophagy – Redox Driven Cellular Repair

the 'spent' and damaged molecules and use lysosomes to degrade and recycle this 'cellular garbage.'

This autophagic process occurs cyclically over time as a function of the dual effect from demands of energy metabolism and the presence of mild oxidative stress. In most tissues its effect is transient, lasting for a few hours. However, muscle cells exhibit an ongoing level of autophagy that may continue for days[193] following exercise, and especially through the rest and repair phase trailing exercise.

Combining or layering these strategies of intermittent fasting, patterns of carbohydrate restriction, and exercise (while protecting the liver from "added sugars" and processed foods), has shown to be an effective and powerful way to enhance cellular and overall health. Manipulating the types and timing of food consumed allows for an added level of control and management over cellular health and hormone regulation not obtainable in other ways. This is nature's method for shifting the body's metabolism into a fat-burning mode which results in natural weight loss - and in correcting fundamental metabolic dysfunction.

According to the "cell's rules," the body doesn't 'think' its way through these issues or conditions. (That is the readers job!) It merely responds to and acts based upon the existing physiologic state as dictated by the biochemistry, pH levels, oxygen levels, hormonal balance, stress factors, and the fuel sources that are consumed. Understanding these principles and how they function, allows for the judicious addition of lifestyle and supplementation measures that promote mitochondrial efficiency, and provide a gentle redox stimulus – all of which helps a cell to become increasingly flexible and metabolically healthy.

It is worth noting that experts in this field have yet to come to a clear consensus on the amount of time needed in a fasting or carb-restricted state, for autophagy benefits to begin. This brings up the question as to why?

At this point in time, the data is limited. However, this optimum autophagy parameter is likely a variable number from person to person - having more

Autophagy – Redox Driven Cellular Repair

to do with one's body physiology and diet, genetics, degree of cellular damage and state of overall metabolic health and flexibility (fat adaption) - than the clock. This is a function of hormesis and conditioning as well. This makes sense because each person's hormetic zone is different and is no doubt affected by many intrinsic and extraneous factors.

While some claim that as few as eight hours can induce autophagic flux, others claim it takes 16 to 18 hours - with some claiming two to four days – thus enabling the argument for a parallel ketogenic diet and periodic intermittent fasting to help maintain this state for prolonged periods of time. This also lends credence to the idea of ketone-cycling, so as to present varying degrees and timing of nutritional stress to the cells.

Additionally, the utilization of redox supplements in the form of redox signaling molecules and redox-based polyphenols and vitamins, can 'supercharge' this strategy to facilitate better metabolic flexibility and autophagy support.

Because of the related physiology, the same principles of time duration to activate autophagy apply to ketosis. Technically, ketosis can be quantified in units of millimolar (mM) content, and the generally accepted threshold for ketosis is ketone blood levels of 0.5mM. How quickly this threshold is reached will depend on carbohydrate intake and upon how much physical activity / exercise occurs.

The ketosis threshold can be reached with an overnight fast and can increase to between 1-2mM in two days and rise to 7-8mM with 5 days of intermittent fasting and carb restriction. For some people it may take a week or two of "keto dieting" to reach sustained ketone levels that are significant.

Ketogenesis and autophagy are related in that both are induced by the relative absence of glucose and glycogen and the increase of glucagon. Ketosis is the result of shifts in energy metabolism and flexibility, and autophagy is a stress-response phenomenon when the redox state is achieved which initiates cellular repair. This means there is an increased benefit for longer states of ketosis and autophagy. The point to not miss is

Autophagy – Redox Driven Cellular Repair

that for those well adapted and metabolically flexible, these transitions are much easier and quicker to cycle into and out of, than for those not well adapted to this level of metabolic health.

The time-benefit curve applies to both ketosis and autophagy – meaning that the more time in each state the more beneficial the effect - obviously up to a point. It is the cycling in and out of ketosis and autophagy that proves beneficial to the training of cellular metabolic flexibility, plasticity, and adaptability.

Additionally, cycling out of ketosis favors consumption of foods such as vegetables and foods that boost plant polyphenols, and which diversify the gut microbiome. (Obviously, supplementation with quality dietary supplements greatly helps in this regard as well.)

Contrary to some people's belief (as noted from the bias in the research that low-carb diets are necessarily assumed to have low vegetable content), fiber-rich plants provide a muting effect on glycemic levels despite their carb classification. Periodically consuming foods with higher carbohydrate amounts also allows for replenishing muscle glycogen storage after physical exercise or activity. Switching back and forth helps maintain the bodies' ability to 'flex' between the two extremes.

The health benefits from this are that skeletal muscle is healthier and more conditioned in people that can switch easily between glucose and fatty acids as their energy source[194]. This is because those who are metabolically flexible have more robust fat oxidation in muscle and increased stimulation of glucose oxidation when it occurs. Those who are inflexible or not fat-adapted have a blunted preference for fat oxidation in muscle and experience less stimulation of glucose oxidation. This is largely a function of insulin sensitivity. All of this occurs because being in ketosis decreases muscle glycolysis and plasma lactate concentrations and provides a cleaner burning fuel for Krebs cycle. This improves physical endurance by altering the fuels used for energy metabolism in the mitochondria[195], decreases lactate buildup, and improves post-exercise recovery.

Autophagy – Redox Driven Cellular Repair

This is the reason for better dynamic flexibility in aerobically fit lean individuals where there is a high reliance on fat oxidation during fasting conditions, as opposed to the greater reliance on glucose oxidation in metabolically inflexible individuals.

The concepts and practice of intermittent fasting and keto-friendly eating strategies allows the body to provide a consistent energy supply regardless of the environment or state of physical activity. This is the ultimate of stress adaptation and redox survivability.

Finding individual application requires experience, and a bit of applied science. Managing this energy metabolism and redox state is the essence of optimum metabolic flexibility and health. This assures that glucose levels can return to normal quickly after eating carbohydrates, and that in their absence fat is quickly used - without the uncomfortable effects of run-away hunger hormones.

Improved metabolic fiber-rich diets also respect the gut such that digested carbohydrates leaving the gut do not overload the blood stream with a wave of glucose. High fiber foods allow a metered release which helps control blood sugar levels - and in combination with the natural effects of metabolically healthy insulin action, this guards against spiking rises and falls in glucose levels.

With this understanding we are now ready to learn more about the relationships between autophagy, aging, and the redox connection.

Autophagy, Aging and The Redox Connection

Aging is characterized by epigenetic shifts, genomic instability, altered nutrient sensing ability, mitochondrial dysfunction, senescence and stem cell exhaustion, and mismanaged redox communication[196]. Each of these are inexorably associated with defects or deficiencies within the Redoxome related to excessive oxidation and inflammation, and the inability for cells to maintain homeostasis and to repair and replace themselves through cellular renewal mechanisms.

Autophagy – Redox Driven Cellular Repair

So far, we have presented in broad generalities the science of autophagy as an important part of cellular renewal and health. We will now discuss it in more detail and review the redox biochemistry and biology that makes it work.

The aging processes, associated as they are with low-grade chronic inflammation, is often referred to as "inflamm-aging." This affects all tissues of the body and presents as slow aching joints, altered metabolic function, and degeneration of brain cells which produce cognitive decline and dementia.

A major source of sustained inflammation during aging is the undigested and unprocessed cellular debris and damaged molecules that occurs during cellular function. The impairment of autophagy to renew, repair, replace, and restore (or any combination thereof), allows for accumulation and retention of damaged and folded proteins that have become distorted and have lost their electrical charges and functionality. Clearly, compromised autophagy is a hallmark of aging![197]

This happens when redox signaling and autophagy are impaired or negatively affected in any way. For true cellular repair and maintenance to occur, it requires the diligent and regular work of the cell's autophagy and custodial service.

Predictably, aging is closely related to impairments in, or lack of, autophagy. In particular, the age-associated dysfunction in autophagy means the cell is less able to clear molecules and sub-cellular elements including nucleic acids (DNA/RNA), proteins, lipids, and spent organelles. The mechanism for doing this is the process of cellular phagocytosis. Just as white blood cells capture and kill bacteria and virus (phagocytosis), cells also isolate and 'process' damaged particles and eliminate or recycle those components for reuse through lysosomes (autophagocytosis)[198]. This means that autophagy is the clearance mechanisms that utilize phagocytosis (autophagosomes and lysosomes)[199]. It is a very regulated process.

The accumulation of cellular debris contributes to the increase of oxidative stress within the cell., along with the effects of gut dysbiosis, cellular- and

Autophagy – Redox Driven Cellular Repair

immune-senescence[200]. It is this accumulated cell debris and spent immunoglobulin particles that occur during aging which trigger the innate immune system activation which leads to chronic low-level inflammation and glycosylation (browning)[201] – which further damages and changes proteins and cell structures.

This "browning" reaction endogenously, is similar in effect as that which happens with the Maillard reaction during food cooking; the high-heat degradation and cross-linking of proteins - which itself is now linked with pathophysiological conditions including diabetes, and kidney and heart disease[202].

With the 'cousin' reaction happening inside the body, the glycation of proteins, fats, and DNA is the process of attaching sugar molecules to proteins. This reaction is called the Amadori rearrangement reaction between glucose and proteins[203]. This can lead to irreversible chemical modification, 'browning,' and cross-linking of proteins inside cells and within tissues. Short-lived proteins such as hemoglobin, are glycated and can give a measure of the amount of glucose in the blood stream over time. The hemoglobin A1c test is reflective of and uses this index to diagnose and manage diabetes.

Other longer-lived proteins such as collagen can also glycate and become damaged. These irreversible cross-links in tissue proteins are known as *advanced glycation end products* (AGEs). These glycation reactions accumulate gradually but can be accelerated with increased blood sugar levels and oxidation conditions.

These damaged proteins tax the cell's ability to maintain stability and homeostasis and require a robust defense mechanism to both guard against undue oxidation, as well as to remove damaged proteins as expeditiously as possible. This is why the redox-controlled mechanisms for antioxidant defense and autophagy are so critical to health. The faster glycation and browning occurs, and the more cellular dysfunction present, the sooner disease and death happens.

Autophagy – Redox Driven Cellular Repair

This accumulating protein damage of glycated and folded proteins is a significant source of cellular debris which impacts cellular function and contributes to redox degradation within the cell. This produces long-term and high-levels of mismanaged oxidative stress leading to inflammation and disease.

In normal settings, inflammation subsides after the causative agent is removed or eliminated (i.e., bacteria, virus, trauma, etc.). This allows tissues to be rebuilt and restored. This is an essential aspect to the body's innate immune system – where inflammation in short stretches is actually an important element in guiding the healing processes.

However, with on-going chronic threats or with problems related to 'house-cleaning,' the cell's ability to "repair and replace" and to restore order in the body is compromised - which leads to disease and the common need for medical intervention.

Rather than utilizing interventions which focus on treating symptoms of disease or attempting to block the effects of inflamm-aging, the better route is to improve the cell's natural ability to clear the debris and restore redox stability to the body. Without this cellular house-cleaning functionality, the non-communicable metabolic diseases related to aging are increased. This is because the function of autophagy plays an important role in maintaining redox homeostasis within each cell[204], and helps prevent dangerous oxidation states.

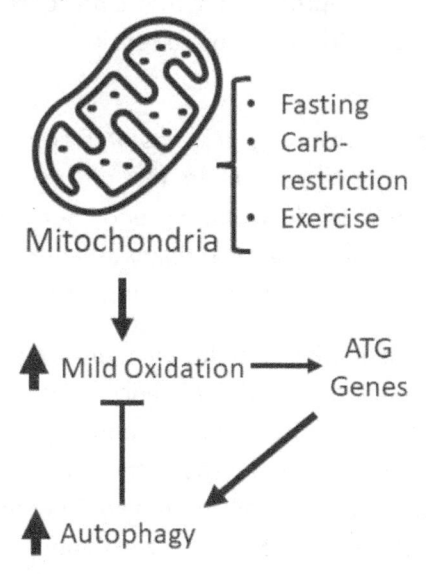

Autophagy is known to have a direct effect in upregulating the antioxidant pathways (Nrf2) as well as other metabolic pathways which effect homeostasis. Many of these pathways diminish oxidative

Autophagy – Redox Driven Cellular Repair

stress (through NADPH levels) and change glucose metabolism[205], adding increased abilities to maintain redox homeostasis within the cell.

Because ROS have a definite effect on cellular health and function, the redox basis for autophagy is interesting to consider. It is a paradox that cellular oxidation produces damage to cell structures and proteins, and that at mild or physiologic levels it activates signaling messengers and autophagy.

This happens especially so inside mitochondria. Oxidative damage is directly correlated with mitochondrial dysfunction and inefficiencies, which results in higher oxidation, reduction in energy production, and the accumulation of toxic by-products[206].

While we have discussed the dietary and macronutrient connections related to autophagy, there is yet one further level of control related to the mechanism of action which relates to cellular redox status.

We have established that a change in the redox status inside a cell is the molecular mechanism that induces autophagy. This happens due to the effect on redox-sensitive transcription factors that activate autophagy genes (e.g., ATG4), which in turn leads to the induction of the autophagic process. The redox state of a cell affects this process due to the presence of cysteine residues on the ATG4 protease molecules that are sensitive to mild oxidative states[207, 208].

Thus, the activation and inactivation of autophagy depends on a complex array of biochemical reactions that are responsive to the presence of oxidative stress within the cell, which is made worse by poor nutrition, cellular debris, etc. This response is the result of a cell's ability to detect the status of its environment using nutrient sensors and "redox switches."

Taken together, this means that a mild oxidative stimulus uniquely provides the ability to upregulate cellular renewal[209] and enhance metabolic flexibility. This reduces runaway oxidation and inflammation and maintains normal cell function. This baseline regulation of redox status gives an additional level of control over this important cellular renewal process, which can be manipulated with exercise, carbohydrate restriction, and fasting[210]). By varying – even willfully manipulating - the conditions of a cell

Autophagy – Redox Driven Cellular Repair

with nutritional lifestyle measures and redox activity, one can intentionally initiate the process of cellular renewal.

Cellular Death - Apoptosis

While we have been largely focusing on the "repair" aspect of the cellular health process, the other half of the "repair and replace" functionality is the feature of programmed cell death. This "replace" function is about the activation of apoptosis and mitosis – cell death followed by cell replacement.

There is an essential correlation that exists between the dual processes of autophagy and apoptosis. Redox signaling plays an important role in the crosstalk and the switching that occurs between the two. There are multiple proteins that control the redox-sensitive switches that participate in the induction of autophagy and/or apoptosis. These switches are also highly responsive to oxidative stress conditions in the cell[211].

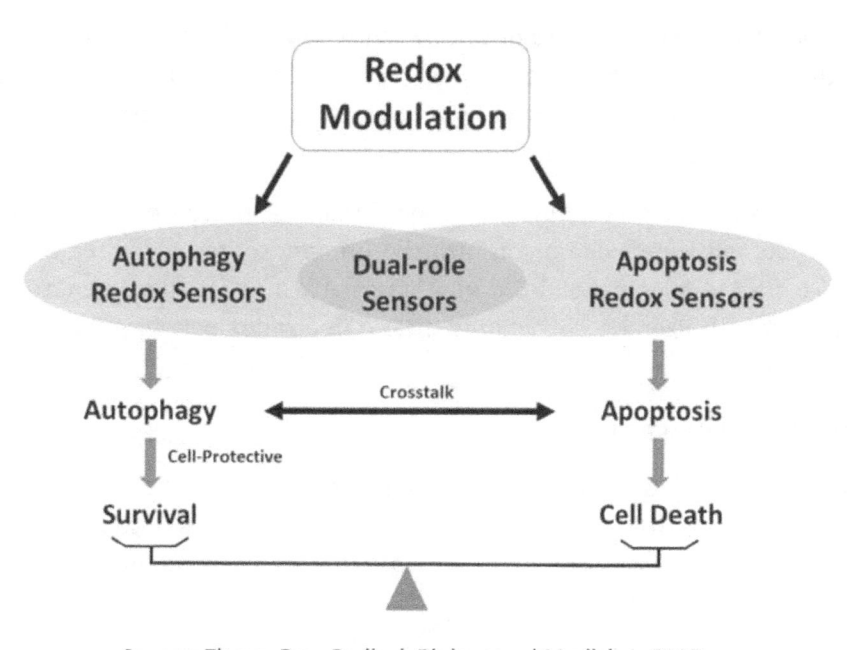

Source: Zhang. Free Radical Biology and Medicine, 2015.

Autophagy – Redox Driven Cellular Repair

Because both autophagy and apoptosis are regulated by redox sensors, and because it is a redox-sensitive mechanism that manages the crosstalk between them, there is a possibility for better management through dietary means.

The early theoretical models are now being aggressively researched and developed. They teach us that impaired autophagy leads to mitochondrial dysfunction and damaging levels of oxidation, which yields accelerated aging and disease. It is a positive feedback loop where more damage creates more damage.

The feedback loop runs the other way as well where mild oxidation creates a state of metabolic stability. Because increased autophagy improves mitochondrial function and redox function, it leads to homeostasis and cellular repair and lessens the forces pushing toward aging and disease. All of this functionality occurs on interconnecting pathways grounded within the Redoxome.

As such, these pathways are driven by redox-sensitive mechanisms tied to pathway genes which initiate cellular defense and autophagy processes. This is why the role of hormesis and stress adaptation response is so important in restoring cellular homeostasis[212].

From the available literature, it appears that the presence of hydrogen peroxide and superoxide anions are the primary source redox molecules which arise from mitochondria during states of fasting[213] and macronutrient management. Exercise also utilizes these same redox pathways to induce autophagy[214].

Summary of Autophagy

The triggers for activating autophagy are based on subtle increases in oxidation levels inside the cell. This occurs with exercise-induced oxidative stress, nutritional stress related to glucose metabolism, and through direct redox supplementation.

The blending of lifestyle (exercise and diet) with redox replenishment, work together to activate redox-sensitive switches which activate foundation-

Autophagy – Redox Driven Cellular Repair

level functions on the cell's 'motherboard,' to provide a metabolically sophisticated yet straight-forward method to activate cell defense and cellular renewal mechanisms.

Being mindful of how and why to be metabolically flexible and how to activate autophagy are the first steps in any real effort to purposefully manage one's health. The blending of these strategies and approaches creates a more complete "redox landscape" approach to overall health.

Applied Autophagy and the Redox Lifestyle

In further examining the redox connections with autophagy and metabolic health it will be helpful to understand the influences of lifestyle, both generally and metabolically. When viewed through this prism, the two principal lifestyle modes can be categorized as what we can call the "flexible" lifestyle and a "sedentary" lifestyle[215].

The flexible lifestyle could be better thought of as a "flexible redox lifestyle" - characterized as a "hunter-gatherer" type lifestyle in its core metabolic groundings. The metabolic rules of this lifestyle are consistent with the physiologic settings where those most responsive and capable have advantage and are better able to survive while foraging for food, where its availability is anything but assured.

We shall see that the "flexible" lifestyle characterized by a "foraging behavior," can also be accurately thought of as a "redox" lifestyle. This lifestyle and everything that supports it, promotes metabolic flexibility through efficient fatty acid oxidation, ketone creation and utilization, appropriate and optimal redox signaling – and enjoys many cell protective mechanisms such as autophagy and natural antibody production.

This is different from today where our "modern" age of agricultural abundance and food production and storage capabilities, make food available on demand. Modern "hunting and gathering" requires only a few steps into a kitchen pantry or a short drive to a grocery store or restaurant, to completely satisfy the food and energy needs of brain and body – on demand, with the excess stored away as fat for periods of famine and deficiency which never occur. This rewards an almost effortless sedentary

Autophagy – Redox Driven Cellular Repair

lifestyle that fills us with excess calories and sets the stage for today's diseases that arise from processed foods and 'quick energy.'

In describing the sedentary lifestyle, "sedentary" is not just about lack of physical activity (which certainly fits), it is more about "redox-sedentary" – as in not having activated redox pathways which otherwise drive the metabolic resourcefulness to assure better cellular health.

In a metabolically flexible redox lifestyle, there is an enhanced sensitivity to both natural and supplemented mild-oxidative stress, which is the driving mechanism that sets in motion the numerous redox-switches that fight premature aging. It artificially simulates and even mimics the true "hunter-gatherer" metabolic rules by depriving the body of energy sources as though still living in an era where the next meal was never guaranteed; eating in times of plenty to store energy, to be later utilized during periods of ketosis- and redox-driven metabolic functionality.

In contrast, in a sedentary lifestyle with high energy availability and a constant "fed" state, the combination of physical inactivity, high meal frequency, high added sugar and carbohydrate foods, and excess calories, overwhelm the body with excess fuel. The fuel excess beyond what the liver and muscles can use, is stored for a future 'famine.' As this occurs, redox

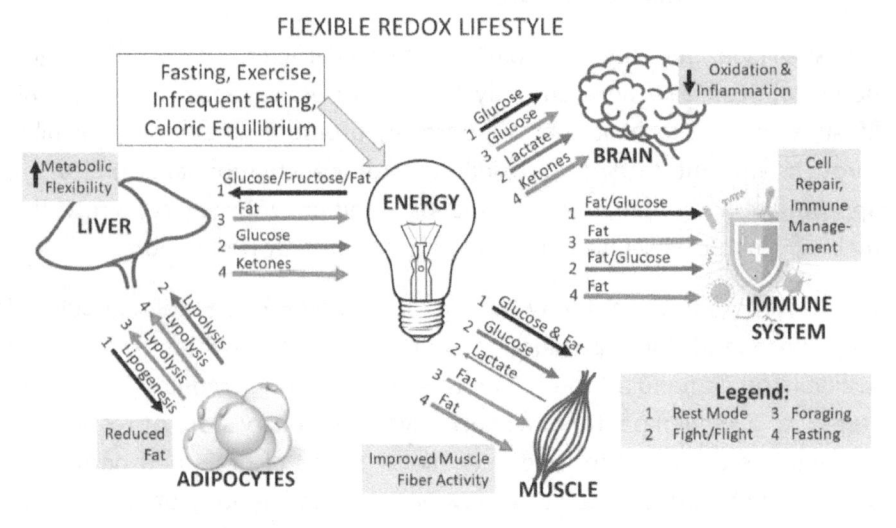

FLEXIBLE REDOX LIFESTYLE

Legend:
1. Rest Mode
2. Fight/Flight
3. Foraging
4. Fasting

Autophagy – Redox Driven Cellular Repair

mechanisms are seldom if ever activated or supported, which otherwise would provide for optimum cellular defense and cellular renewal.

Adding insult to this injury is the effect of processed and toxic foods such as processed fructose, which is largely metabolized in the liver and is converted into fats through a process of *de novo* lipogenesis – leading to increased visceral fat and 'fatty liver disease.' This accumulation further degrades metabolic health and erodes metabolic function.

In the metabolically inflexible and redox-inactive sedentary lifestyle, the ability for muscle cells to efficiently use glucose is degraded, as well as their ability to access and use fatty acids for energy. As a result, the immune system is easily challenged with high oxidation and chronic low-grade inflammation.

With the sedentary lifestyle, since there is little or no ketones being created in the liver, the brain's only energy source remains glucose. This means that when glucose levels decline and the body cannot "flex" to utilize fats and ketones, the brain quickly activates hunger hormones to drive carb consumption to restore glucose for the brain.

All of this is very different in a flexible redox supported lifestyle. Because of fasting, exercise, optimally timed eating, and the cycling of ketones, the

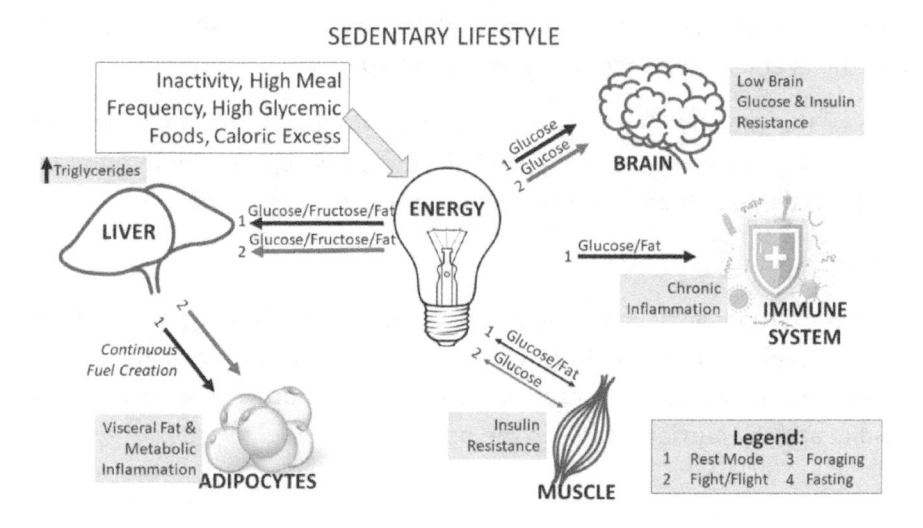

Autophagy – Redox Driven Cellular Repair

body's energy requirements are much more easily met without exaggerated hormone fluctuations. This is how the redox lifestyle supports and modulates hormone balance to support metabolic vitality and wellness.

The liver is the key organ in this scenario, which is why it is so important to "protect the liver" and keep it metabolically healthy with proper energy nutrition rationing and clean unprocessed foods to the extent possible. When it is protected and functioning in a healthy manner, and with a healthy non-inflamed gut, the liver remains flexible and responsive to dietary manipulation, nutritional supplements, and redox replenishment. It easily shifts and harvests fats from visceral storage depots and uses them for energy ("fat burning") thus lowering triglyceride levels in the body and resolving the myriad of presenting signs and symptoms related with metabolic disease and dysfunction (chronic disease).

Additionally benefits include an overall improvement in energy metabolism in muscles, enhanced immune system protection, improved inflammatory response, overall better cardiovascular health, and enhanced cellular repair and cell signaling. The brain and vital organs are especially blessed, helping the brain stay calm and energized and protected against the forces of neurodegeneration.

In short, when autophagy happens as it was designed to happen, the incidence and severity of chronic age-related diseases is positively affected, and the ever present forces of aging are tamed.

Due to the specific effects of autophagy on the brain and the important relationship between autophagy and diabetes, it is appropriate to finish up a discussion on autophagy exploring those connections further.

Autophagy and Diabetes

Because autophagy is highly dependent on the status of energy metabolism, special mention is made here of this condition. Those challenged with severe insulin resistance, metabolic diseases have added concerns relative to diet and the nutrient status in the body.

Autophagy – Redox Driven Cellular Repair

The strategy for the level of management related to a redox-supported lifestyle, can become problematic for those with blood sugar disorders, and/or liver disease or dysfunction. This is largely due to the rather intense and direct effects which energy metabolism has on metabolic function. This includes fuel/food type, its nature – whole vs. processed, refined vs. complex, plant nutrition, etc. All of this presents challenges for stable redox environments which promote cellular defensive and repair mechanisms.

To better understand the reasons metabolic disease is so impactful to health and the important role autophagy plays in diabetes, consider the following effects of impaired autophagy. In reviewing this list of effects, consider that diabetes carries with it several consequences or complications, each associated with the progressive and protracted elevation in blood sugar levels and inflammation in various tissues throughout the body. These complications affect the blood vessels, eyes, kidneys, pancreas, and nerve tissues, to name a few.

A quick look at the critical role of autophagy and autophagy dysregulation in blood sugar disorders reveals:

- Impairment of the autophagic pathway in pancreatic B cells results in the development of type 2 diabetes[216]. When these cells function abnormally glucose levels rise.
- Dysregulation increases heart failure, cardiomyopathy, atherosclerosis, heart attacks and strokes, and microvascular disease[217]. Enhancement of autophagic flux improves diabetic cardiomyopathy[218].
- Autophagy in pancreatic cells is a vital process to protect against the toxic effect of amyloid proteins that are toxic to B-cells, while lack of robust autophagy degrades pancreatic beta-cells ability to produce insulin[219].
- Impairment of autophagy in adipose tissue affects the size/mass and homeostasis of adipose cell[220].
- Insulin resistance in kidney cells suppresses autophagy and increases nephropathy. The functional role of autophagy in kidneys plays a pivotal role in renal protection during both normal aging and after kidney injuries (in animal models)[221].

Autophagy – Redox Driven Cellular Repair

- Autophagy has a protective role in high-glucose-induced neurotoxicity by clearing protein aggregates and damaged cell organelles and other cell structures. It also helps to protect nerve cells from loss of myelination and against metabolic energy crises[222]. Furthermore, autophagy is suppressed in neurons with high glucose levels, due to its effect on autophagosome synthesis[223].
- Impaired autophagy in the retina due to persistent elevated glucose levels compromises the ability to clear advanced glycation end products, oxidized proteins, and LDLs in the eye. Abnormal autophagy is a pathological feature of diabetic retinopathy as the balance between autophagy and apoptosis and cell damage is affected[224].

For those with insulin resistance and who may require supplemental insulin to reduce blood glucose levels, high sugar levels are often managed by increasing insulin artificially. Since insulin is something that shuts down autophagy, the additional insulin may counteract the effects of having lowered glucose levels, notwithstanding the desirable lower glucose levels.

Even while these insulin resistant situations are challenging to say the least, the objective remains to eat and live such that cells become more sensitive to the effects of insulin, which. This results in less need for supplemented insulin to manage blood sugar levels. This addresses the foundational metabolic health issues that create insulin resistance in the first place. This is accomplished by eliminating processed foods and oils, improving the quality of nutrients consumed, having a healthy mouth and gut microbiome, staying hydrated, increasing activity levels and exercise, and assuring that redox signaling pathways are optimally functioning.

The important point here is that blood sugar control is not the major objective; metabolic health is. This is a paradigm shift for most people (including some health professionals). Blood sugars can be managed with drugs and insulin (without affecting underlying metabolic health). When metabolic health and insulin sensitivity are successfully address with redox lifestyle strategies, the resulting blood sugar issues have a better chance of improving naturally, requiring less medical intervention. From the cell's

Autophagy – Redox Driven Cellular Repair

metabolic point of view, if additional insulin is required to override the inherent resistance, it may prove to be counter effective, as higher insulin levels limit autophagy.

In summary, autophagy is an important regulatory signaling pathway, and a vital cell protective and clearance mechanism in diseases affecting blood sugar control, as well as the numerous complications that arise from this condition[225].

Autophagy and the Brain

A healthy uninterrupted autophagic process is an essential part of the central nervous system's ability to deal with the consequences of oxidative stress in brain and nerve cells. This plays a major role in creating optimal CNS physiology and nerve cell survival. Autophagy dysregulation in the aging and diseased brain diminishes the function of microglia (the macrophage immune cell in the brain) in promoting repair and correcting poor brain cell function. Since nerve and brain tissues are already at a disadvantage in their ability to manage undue oxidative stress, the lack of, or interruption of, autophagy, adds insult to injury.

The accumulation of damaged proteins plays an important role in mitochondrial dysfunction. The proper function of microglia immune cells native to the brain is to assist in the cleanup that is essential in the brain to clear beta-amyloid and neurofibrillary tangles which encumber the brains of those with serious neurodegenerative disease. Whether the disruption of this microglial-mediated autophagy in the brain is causative, protective, or simply a side-consequence occurring during different stages of neurodegeneration, is not known for certain. However, what is certain is that autophagy there plays a key role[226].

This role includes but is not limited to phagocytosis of beta-amyloid deposits and the cleanup in the microenvironment around neurons[227]. In the brain, when autophagy is impaired, it leads to neuroinflammation and contributes to the development and progression of neurodegenerative disease[228]. This dysregulation of autophagy along with inflammatory mediators created in dysfunction, also substantially impacts cellular brain injury in all

Autophagy – Redox Driven Cellular Repair

neurodegenerative conditions, including in the aftermath of cerebrovascular accidents.

What is certain is that autophagy is a critical mechanism which impacts nerve and brain cells, heart cells, skin cells – literally all cells in the body. Because of this it is closely tied to the aging process.

Part 4 – Redox Functional Nutrition

Functional Nutrition in the Redox Lifestyle

The subject of nutrition today encompasses many beliefs, ideologies, and systems. It involves everything from what is trending, to which 'expert' says what, to trying to reconcile the constantly shifting base of nutrition science, and even the messaging used to market it all.

Because of its focus on cellular function the current branch of nutrition which most closely matches the Redox Lifestyle is called "functional nutrition." This is broadly defined as a personalized nutritional approach which supports optimal physiological cellular function where cells are nourished with foods that "best address the root causes of symptoms and disease"[229].

Functional nutrition holds that medical disorders can be food-related due to nutritional deficiencies, food allergies and sensitivities, and that each person needs a unique holistic dietary approach that considers one's lifestyle and backdrop of chronic disease problems. Because each person has a unique set of symptoms and diseases, functional nutrition generally holds that "one size does not fit all."

As has been emphasized throughout this book, the foundational nutritional concepts that should rule are those dictated by the cell related to optimum cellular redox function. This applies to the energy extraction side of nutrition, as well as to the quality of nutritive elements within food (cellular building materials, enzymes, and co-factors), or which are supplemented.

With the arrival of redox biology and the redox lifestyle, the definition of functional nutrition can now shift from "addressing the root causes of symptoms and disease," to become a focus which "addresses the root causes of cellular health."

There is in this a subtle difference in focus which is a step above the already enlightened functional nutritional ideals. It cares less about what is individualistic or unique to a person's situation (usually oriented around symptoms and disease and lifestyle), and more about engineering the

Functional Nutrition in the Redox Lifestyle

lifestyle that sustains proper health function. This aligns redox nutrition with the orientation that wellness is more than the absence of symptoms. This fully recognizes that all disease is the result of cellular dysfunction, and therefore that health is the result of healthy cellular function.

Rather than the primary focus being on which diets work best for specific diseases, the redox diet focuses on which foods and diets work best for cellular health processes (which is also what works best for nearly every disease!)

It matters that the primary focus is on what is best for cellular metabolic pathways first, and then secondarily on what is good for this or that common disease condition. In real life, because disease and metabolic dysfunction is such a prevalent part of each life, there is logical room for both considerations. For this reason, bio-individuality, and personalization via a 'functional approach' is still desirable, except with the nuanced recognition that it is about cellular rules and processes first, and secondly about dietary or herbal fixes which address specific disease and symptoms. This aligns diet and lifestyle in a more congruent way with the foundation rules that create health – followed with focused attention on disease and symptoms, as needed.

This is more about shifting the diet and eating plan to align with the principles of how cells are designed to function for health. It also establishes the hierarchal importance of foundational redox principles which are first and foremost the solid basis for everything happening within the Redoxome. The dietary strategy and overall lifestyle then are built upon this foundation – not the other way around. This is the essence of protecting the liver and feeding the gut; the essence of metabolic health and metabolic flexibility; the essence of cellular renewal and cellular defense. This is the redox way!

The variability from person to person with regard to each having different hormetic zones, along with each person's unique background of both disease and genetic influences, allows for individuality within their redox landscapes. Each person will discover their own "sweet spot" or hormetic

Functional Nutrition in the Redox Lifestyle

dosing which serves them best, which may change over time with improved redox functioning and improved overall health.

This new definition for the "best" diet can therefore be called the Redox Functional Diet. It is an important part of the overall Redox Lifestyle - acting as a pivotal pillar of health in the redox landscape. As a functional diet, the redox approach addresses the universal and foundational basis for cellular and metabolic health, which in turn allows the "Inner Doctor" to begin improving cellular function. As cells correct and heal themselves, symptoms and disease processes improve, requiring less medical intervention or outside "agents" aimed at forcing an effect upon receptor sites in drug-like action, to suppress a symptom.

Applied Redox Nutrition

Even though everyone wants the subject of food to be easy (to wit: processed and fast food) and yearns to have a detailed if not ready-made diet spelled out for them with exact instructions and methods for meal planning, shopping, cooking, and restaurant eating, the purpose here is not to provide that level of detail. This is about thinking independently and with knowledge to make informed decisions about what you put in your body and knowing how it affects your cells.

Redox "dieting" is manipulating your cellular state on purpose with food and supplements, while factoring in your unique health and genetic makeup. Knowing the principles of redox biology and how the Redoxome work, will provide broad guidance that will assist in dialing in the right foods and eating practices, in parallel with other redox enhancing strategies. This is the redox nutrition aspect of the redox lifestyle.

This is an important shift in thinking because the truth is that "diets" do not work! They come and go along with the motivation and circumstances and mood of the moment. The proof for this is in the fact that every "diet" you or anyone has ever "done," didn't last long! Otherwise, you and they would still be on it! That is because it is and forever will be a "diet," and not a "lifestyle."

Functional Nutrition in the Redox Lifestyle

Almost always "diets" are utilized as a high-burst short-term project to kickstart a resolution to be better. That is good – but it seldom lasts for anyone. Often the focus is on what cannot be eaten and less on what you should eat - or how it should be eaten.

Diets require great discipline because they are usually about deprivation – and if in the face of this deprivation the hunger hormones are not appeased, the diet is usually short lived.

Most diets do not have as their primary focus true metabolic health. Most of them are marketed for weight loss. The fact of the matter is that you can "diet" and even lose weight, and not be metabolically healthy. Even with successful weight loss in the short term, cells remain metabolically unhappy and wrapped 'around the axle' of hungry hormones and unbalanced metabolic function.

A "redox diet" focuses first on metabolic health, recognizing that the weight and hunger issues cannot be solved with any meaningful result without good metabolic stability.

A redox nutrition lifestyle is more than doing a "diet." It's more than being a carnivore or a vegan or eating high-carb or low-carb diet, or low-fat or high-fat. It is more than Mediterranean, keto, Weight Watchers, or South Beach, or even using meal replacement to meet an objective.

In truth, a "redox diet" or lifestyle runs on principle (the cell's rules, rule!). It is dialed-in to be unique for each person's metabolic situation, genetic background, and medical situation. It can embrace and utilize all of the foregoing approaches – in time and substance – but it never loses focus on the basic rules of how cells metabolize food for energy, or how that process affects redox-sensitive cellular health processes throughout the body.

Because of this, there is inherent flexibility amidst this strategy, provided it does not violate general rules related to food processing, environmental toxicity, added sugars, etc. As well this 'flexibility' must consider and include prebiotic fiber status, plant nutrition and phytochemical content, a wise mix of macronutrient fuel sources, respect for nutritional ketosis and hormesis

Functional Nutrition in the Redox Lifestyle

principles, and the manipulation of food consumption in a way that supports cellular health mechanisms.

So what is it that works?

Lifestyle works! That is the only thing that does work! It isn't a flash-in-the-pan effort to drop pounds, or fit into skinny jeans, or to even improve blood sugars and cholesterol levels. All of this happens as a byproduct of a redox lifestyle done right. And - as a generalization, if it isn't working, then it's not being done right!

This is why knowing the principles and the natural laws are so important. This will sustain and move you through the pitfalls of habit and non-support from those surrounding you. Making informed decisions based on principles will outlast any and all "diets" you will encounter or be tempted to "do." This is the power of correct principles, for with those you can govern yourself!

For example, drawing upon the principles presented here in Healthy Matters, understanding that cells shift from predominant glucose burning to fat burning when glucose and insulin levels are low, will inform your choices in meal planning and snacking and fasting. Knowing that purposeful planned ketosis cycling enables fat adaptation and metabolic flexibility, also helps with these decisions and motivations. Understanding autophagy and being clear on your intended metabolic health outcomes, provides motivation regarding late night snacks. Knowing the risks that go with processed, refined, sugar-added foods leads to better decisions for all food and beverage choices. Knowing that you are not locked into only one way of eating provides freedom and flexibility (except with regard for the rule about processed and high-sugar foods!).

When approaching lifestyle with the rules of redox under the belt (literally), then satiety, satisfaction, flexibility, variation, and so much more can be navigated - because they are grounded on the rules of how cells work.

In all of this, the functional and operational groundings within the Redox Lifestyle are oriented around the rules of the cell. These relate to both how energy is extracted from fuel and energy sources (i.e., food), as well as to

Functional Nutrition in the Redox Lifestyle

what is done with this energy over time in the body, and how all this impacts the cells and metabolic pathways in the process.

The reader is referred to earlier chapters to review the principles of redox energy metabolism and the principles of hormesis, nutritional ketosis, metabolic flexibility, and of redox-driven autophagy. These principles matter because energy metabolism is an essential part of the nutrition equation. These relate to the consumption and timing of eating of, macronutrients in the diet.

In addition to the relative mixture and amounts and timing of macronutrients in the diet (food as fuel), is the important role of micronutrients and their role in metabolic pathways and processes. This includes their role as energy co-factors and synergistic redox agents to promote redox functions and biological reactions throughout the body. As such, they affect both the redox biology and the redox energy equations - especially as it relates to hormesis-driven and redox-sensitive mechanisms.

Micronutrients provide antioxidant defenses and are instrumental in cellular protection and tissue repair. These are also grounded on the principles inherent in the Redoxome landscape and all up and down the redox backbone. As such they are crucial in maintaining a healthy biological system. Physiologic doses of supplemented antioxidants are useful in maintaining redox homeostasis[230]. This effect occurs directly via their action as metabolic cofactors and redox antioxidants, and indirectly through hormetic influence on the Redoxome.

Nutrition and Hormesis - Review

Our attention will next focus on micronutrients and their specific relationship within the Redoxome. Before beginning a more detailed review of plant phytochemicals, herbs, and vitamins, it will help to emphasize the important redox principle of hormesis. The reader may want to refer back to the earlier discussion about nutrition and hormesis and autophagy. Briefly stated, this principle is that dose matters. Too much and too little are not healthy, but the dose within the hormetic zone is where the optimal benefit occurs.

Functional Nutrition in the Redox Lifestyle

This hormetic dose is a "therapeutic dose." This may be something entirely different from the "recommended dietary allowance" (RDA) dose which is defined as the minimal dose set to prevent diseases of deficiency. The RDA is oriented around diseases of deficiency, not the 'therapeutic' dose that activates optimal cellular and metabolic function.

Admittedly, this is a controversial topic because vitamins and nutrition are not intended to be "therapeutic." With this context we are not implying or stating that vitamins are "cures" or "therapy" for disease. We are saying that they are part of the equation for awakening the Inner Doctor so that the cell can heal itself. Within this context the intent is to speak of the optimal hormetic dose that maximizes the redox effect within a cell.

Obviously, this is not usually a measurable metric and can vary between individuals depending on their state of redox deficiency and organic load of health problems, but the principle is nonetheless a true principle which applies to every person.

Hormesis teaches us that too little vitamin dosing is just as detrimental as mega-dosing because both are outside the hormetic range. While it seems intuitive that too few vitamins can lead to poor cellular health, the other side of the hormetic dose range is less well understood by many people, including health enthusiasts. Excess vitamins and polyphenols and minerals can be toxic, cause interactions with prescription medications, and have other untoward effects in physiology. High amounts of isolated compounds can be toxic due to their prooxidative effects at high concentrations[231].

Excess vitamins and antioxidants suppress the necessary mild states of oxidation required to activate cellular defenses and for optimal cellular functioning[232]. By artificially subduing the mild oxidative environment within the cell needed to activate the stress-adaptive cellular defenses, high nutrient doses can deprive the cell of its natural restorative abilities.

At physiologic levels, mild oxidation plays an important role in redox signaling, pathway gene expression, regulation of antioxidant defense mechanisms and cellular repair (autophagy), and a decrease in inflammation and cytokine levels.

Functional Nutrition in the Redox Lifestyle

Antioxidants at high levels disrupt the redox balance and degrade the ability for cellular function, leading to cellular dysfunction. The harmful effects include increased oxidation, glycation of proteins and DNA, and increased inflammation and cytokine production[233][234].

These concerns highlight the importance of being judicious and selective in the blends, and concentrations utilized when supplementing with micronutrients. "If a little is good, a lot is better" is not a good rule to live by when it comes to nutrition.

Bioavailability

A final important point to make about nutritional dosing has to do with bioavailability, absorption, and the pleiotropic effect of micronutrients (i.e., one producing many redundant effects).

The number of micronutrients which enter the mouth may not necessarily be the amount that actually enters the blood stream. Impairments in gut health, gut dysbiosis, varying levels of digestive chemicals and other hormones can impact the absorption of dietary nutrients - as well as the

Hormesis and Vitamin Dosage

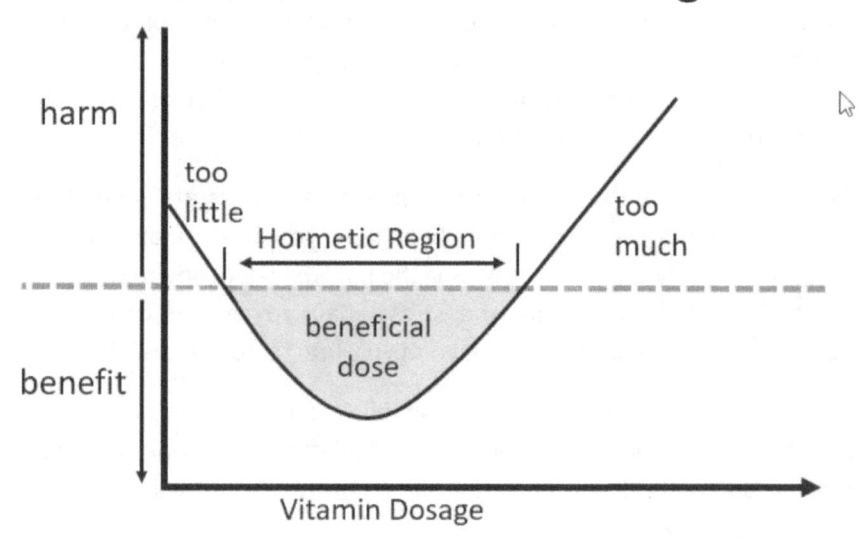

Functional Nutrition in the Redox Lifestyle

creation of vitamins and neurotransmitters from within the digestive tract from healthy bacteria.

A healthy gut may mean that lower doses of vitamins are necessary, and that those which are eaten are used with better efficiency. As enhanced redox signaling awakens the "Inner Doctor," there is often less need for "more" in both quantity and variety. The pleiotropic effects of herbs and polyphenols create cross-over benefit, meaning that fewer varieties are necessary due to the redundancy and overlap in benefit which varying herbs have. For example, many herbs have similar effects upon redox functionality.

Redox Micronutrients and Phytochemicals

Phenolics are among the most active substances from natural plant sources. They exert a variety of health-promoting properties that are cytoprotective, antimicrobial, anti-aging, anti-inflammatory, antiallergenic, antimutagenic, vasodilatory, anxiolytic and antidepressant, and neuroprotective and cognitive enhancing[235]. Those acquainted with the redox biology associated with each of these processes will quickly recognize the close and interdependent interaction with redox signaling and their place within the Redoxome.

Polyphenols, vitamins, and micronutrients are abundant in nature and throughout the plant world. Over thousands of years these have been broadly available in native diets and have been used both as herbal remedies (with drug-like effect) and as stress-adaptive adaptogens which help stabilize and normalize physiological processes and cellular functions. They are found in "common" foods, as well as more exotic foods and spices which source from unique locations around the world. Due to better understandings of their benefits and how they help stabilize cellular health, the practice of nutritional supplementation has taken on new life.

However, not all supplements are created equal. While the role of micronutrient supplementation is now well accepted, (except by those who still believe the standard diet is sufficient), there remains a wide variability from one supplement product to the next, which relates to how they are

Functional Nutrition in the Redox Lifestyle

sourced, prepared, and delivered to the human experience. Many are synthetic and unnatural, and others are mishandled in ways that diminish their nutritional quality and redox interactivity. The better supplements always adhere to the highest standards, are from whole foods, are blended and combined to support the synergism that exists across the redox landscape.

When used with proper knowledge of how they impact energy metabolism and the multitude of reactions within the Redoxome, they provide a balanced effect on redox biology. This means they promote both homeostasis as well as the mild-oxidative stimulus which activates redox-sensitive defense mechanisms in the cell.

There are several natural compounds with special ability to impact cellular health and energy throughout the body, brain, and mind. They accomplish this because of the effect they have on cellular defense and antioxidation pathways, and by optimizing cellular energy production in Krebs cycle and the electron transport chain in the mitochondria. Many of their effects on energy are indirect because they are co-factors and secondary messengers in the redox pathways related with neuro-chemicals, hormones, digestion, inflammation, fatigue, sleep, cognition, and mood to name a few.

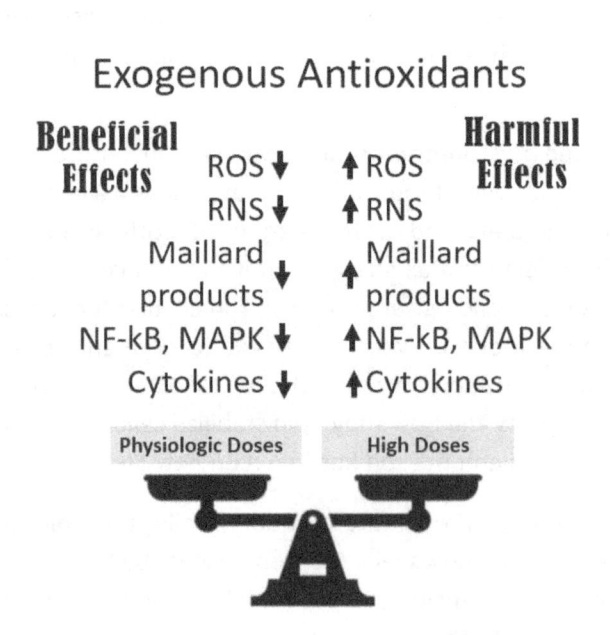

Exogenous Antioxidants

Beneficial Effects	Harmful Effects
ROS ↓	↑ ROS
RNS ↓	↑ RNS
Maillard products ↓	↑ Maillard products
NF-kB, MAPK ↓	↑ NF-kB, MAPK
Cytokines ↓	↑ Cytokines
Physiologic Doses	High Doses

Functional Nutrition in the Redox Lifestyle

The following representative list of nutritive compounds in this next section is far from all-inclusive. However, it presents a number of well-researched redox-based micronutrients which have profound abilities to enhance cellular energy and support vital metabolic pathways, boost cognitive and neurological health and well-being, and enrich psychological balance. When these micronutrients are strategically blended and used together in proper amounts, and when complimented with an appropriate redox lifestyle and redox supplementation, they provide an optimally synergistic approach to improved energy and function in both mind and body.

As this list is presented and reviewed, pay attention to the redox-specific actions which each one is involved in. Because each of these nutrients participate in numerous redox interactions, you may come away impressed with the integral role they play inside the Redoxome as they work together in special ways to support redox health. Furthermore, you may well note the cross-over and synergism between them. Each biological agent has multiple effects within the body and the redox landscape, many of which overlap in repeated manners – all a part of the synergistic overlay that exists within the marvelous Redoxome as designed. This is nature's way of conserving biological survival and in assuring that basic redox functions are supported horizontally across the redox landscape and vertically up and down the redox spine.

Your knowledge of the redox biology connections related to energy metabolism, transcription factors, redox-sensitive switches, pathway genes, autophagy, etc., will be helpful in understanding the powerful interplay these micronutrients have with core redox biology and cellular energy processes.

Functional Nutrition in the Redox Lifestyle

Functional Redox Nutrition - Supplementation

Functional Redox Nutrition - Supplementation

Acetyl-L-Carnitine

Acetyl-L-carnitine (ALC) is made from the amino acid L-carnitine in the brain, liver and kidneys, and is found in all cells of the body. Both forms are utilized by the body to facilitate the metabolism of fat into energy. This is accomplished by its break down into carnitine, which is used to transport long-chain fatty acids across the mitochondria membrane, where they are metabolized (beta-oxidation) to create Acetyl-CoA, which then enters Krebs cycle to produce energy. Carnitine's role in fatty acid metabolism also affects other fuels that are metabolized, including glucose metabolism.

Both of the acetyl and carnitine segments have neurobiological properties. Carnitine participates in the metabolism of fatty acids, and the acetyl segment is used to maintain acetyl-CoA levels to support mitochondrial and Krebs-based energy production. As such it modulates brain energy, neurotrophic factors, neurohormones, neuron synapse shape and function[236].

ALC enhances acetylcholine production, which is a chief neurotransmitter of the nervous system, and is important for muscle control, autonomic body functions, and in learning, memory, and attention. It stimulates production of proteins and membrane phospholipids and stabilizes membrane fluidity by regulation of sphingomyelin levels, which is important to prevent nerve degeneration.

Neuroprotection by ALC when supplemented above physiologic levels has been demonstrated in animal models and is associated with decreases in brain lactate levels and increases in ATP. The markers of oxidative stress are reduced in both brain tissue and cerebrospinal fluid, which inhibits excitotoxicity in settings of acute injury as well as chronic neurodegenerative disorders[237], thus preventing cell dysfunction and death.

ALC reacts with the Keap1 repressor protein (which ordinarily keeps Nrf2 transcription factor inactive) in a way to liberate Nrf2 and induce the cellular antioxidant defense response. It also causes expression of the Heme-oxygenase-1 genes which are associated with cellular defense responses.

Functional Redox Nutrition - Supplementation

ALC also upregulates heat-shock proteins (HSPs) which play a protective role in guarding against damage from damaged proteins, and in maintaining the proper ratio between oxidized and reduced forms of glutathione[238].

Supplemented ALC can correct immunological functions and improve energy metabolism, as well as restore age-related mitochondrial defects. ALC has the ability to influence expression on many gene pathways, notably those which control antioxidant capacity, cellular defenses, restoring and stabilizing mitochondrial activity.

Carnitine improves insulin resistance by promoting mitochondrial function and improved regulation of autophagy[239]. It is also used to improve cognitive thinking and memory and mood, and to reduce neuropathic pain.

ALC supplements increase the enzyme (acetyltransferase) which converts choline to the neurotransmitter acetylcholine[240], which is important for memory, mood, muscle control and other brain functions. Supplemental choline administration is also helpful as it speeds up the creation and release of acetylcholine.

Choline is a source of methyl groups that are utilized in the methylation cycles involving methionine and homocysteine and in the one-carbon chemistry reactions[241]. Choline is necessary for the body to synthesize phosphatidylcholine and sphingomyelin, two important phospholipids within cell membranes and are required for structural integrity.

Improved mitochondrial efficiency, along with its effects on neuroprotection, aging, and energy metabolism, and its ability to protect and balance the cellular redox state, makes ALC an important player in cellular health.

Alpinia Galanga

Alpinia galanga is a plant in the ginger family (Zingiberaceae) native to Southern Asia. It bears an underground root system or rhizome which is used as both as a medicinal herb and culinary herb. Traditionally, and in Chinese medicine it has been used for upper respiratory conditions, general discomfort, and stomach and GI distress.

Functional Redox Nutrition - Supplementation

Galanga's phytochemical makeup is rich in flavonoids and polyphenols which give them effective anti-inflammatory, antioxidant, antiviral, antiallergic, and gastroprotective properties. As a class these herbs are most commonly used for anti-inflammatory purposes. Galangal has shown to decrease cell senescence in normal fibroblast cells which highlight its promising anti-aging effect[242]. Due to these anti-inflammatory properties, it has shown to reduce both inflammation and discomfort and to boost the immune system. It also has exhibited cardioprotective effects in animal testing[243].

Alpinia galanga is a natural energy enhancer and central nervous system stimulant[244]. When used in conjunction with caffeine, it impedes the 'caffeine crash' with sustained attention and alertness[245]. It's primary effects in the body are to improve mental alertness and focus, the support of cognitive function and brain processing[246], and to synergistically amplify the nootropic effect of companion ingredients (i.e., agents that improve cognitive and executive function, memory, creativity, and motivation in healthy people).

Ashwagandha root extract

Ashwagandha (*Withania somnifera*) is a traditional Indian Ayurvedic medicine. The root of this plant smells like horse (*"ashwa"*) which is the derivation of the name, as consuming it gave the recipient the 'power of a horse.' This traditional herb is said to promote a youthful state of physical and mental health and happiness.

It is an adaptogen which means it helps the body better handle stress and anxiety due to its ability to manage various mediators of stress, including heat shock proteins, cortisol, and stress-activated kinases[247]. In this effect, it compares well with Panex ginseng in its adaptogenic properties, which is why it is sometimes known as Indian Ginseng.

The chemical constituents of ashwagandha include alkaloids, steroidal lactones, and saponins. These compounds are anti-stress agents and have immunomodulatory actions.

Functional Redox Nutrition - Supplementation

It has GABA-mimetic effects in helping support neuron development and repair. Ashwagandha appears to slow and stop cellular damage to brain cells and neurons and to prevent synaptic loss, making this supportive in the care of neurodegenerative diseases across the neurological spectrum, and in supporting cognitive function[248].

Stress, anxiety, and poor sleep are pervasive and are linked to many disease processes. Ashwagandha is often used to reduce stress, improve sleep, and enhance general wellbeing and to provide an extra measure of stress resistance through tis anxiolytic effects[249].

B Vitamins

Vitamin B is a family of water-soluble B vitamins which include:

- B1 thiamine
- B2 riboflavin
- B3 niacin
- B5 pantothenic acid
- B6 pyridoxine
- B9 folate
- B12 cobalamin

The family of B vitamins are intimately and widely involved at all levels of redox activity and cellular function. The family of B vitamins are essential in the NAD- and FAD-dependent reactions that are part of the energy metabolism pathways of glycolysis and Krebs cycle[250]. Through their activity in the folic acid cycle and methionine cycle and transsulfuration pathways they participate in redox-related reactions that involve DNA metabolism and repair, cell signaling events, and the antioxidant defense mechanisms. Therefore, they regulate cellular homeostasis and ROS balance. Their combined effects are particularly important in brain function, energy production, DNA / RNA synthesis and repair, methylation reactions, and the formation of numerous neurotransmitters, signaling molecules, and proteins[251].

The various roles of these micronutrients in energy metabolism include:[252] [253].

Functional Redox Nutrition - Supplementation

- Thiamine B1: Thiamin is a component of the coenzyme thiamin pyrophosphate which helps in the breakdown of glucose via glycolysis and helps convert glucose to energy. It also helps in the metabolism of amino acids which prevents fatigue and sustains endurance training[254]. Thiamin participates in the synthesis of RNA and DNA, and various proteins and neurotransmitters, helping to maintain cognition and mental alertness. Thiamin facilitates the completion of Krebs cycle reactions by supporting oxidative carboxylation, and the release of CO2. It is also required for normal muscle function.

- Riboflavin B2: Riboflavin is a cofactor in the electron transport chain and helps extract energy from glucose, fatty acids, and amino acids. It is an antioxidant and a part of the antioxidant enzyme glutathione peroxidase.

- Niacin B3: Niacin is a cofactor in the Krebs-based electron transport chain. It helps release energy from glucose and fatty acids. It plays a key

Energy Metabolism & B Vitamins

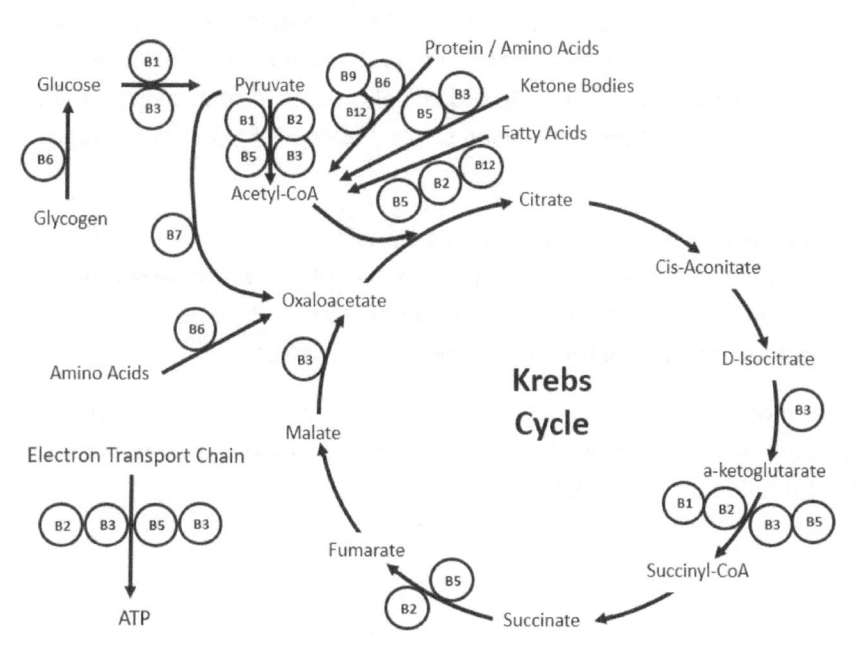

Functional Redox Nutrition - Supplementation

role in the electron carrier redox couples NAD+/NADH & NADP+/NADPH, which is a central role in redox reactions in cells.

- Pantothenic acid B5: Pantothenic acid is a component of coenzyme A, which is a necessary part of the acetyl CoA step within Krebs cycle. This is critical in the energy metabolism of carbohydrates, fats, and proteins.

- Pyridoxine B6: Pyridoxine is a coenzyme for more than one hundred enzymes involved in the metabolism of amino acids. It is necessary for transamination – the conversion of one amino acid into another. This means that without pyridoxine, all amino acids would become essential and need to be dietary sourced. It assists in the metabolism of energy of carbohydrates. It helps in the delivery of oxygen in the body because it helps create hemoglobin. It is a cofactor in the creation of neurotransmitters and helps sustain nerve cell function. It lowers blood levels of homocysteine, converting it to cysteine which can then be transformed into glutathione and metallothionine.

- Folate B9: Folate is involved with DNA creation and the health of red blood cells. It is also helps reduce homocysteine levels in the blood. Healthy folate levels protect nerve cell health and is especially important in early growth and development in fetal development to prevent neural tube defects in utero. Folate also helps with amino-acid metabolism

- Cobalamin B12: Cobalamin helps transform folate into its active form within the folic acid cycle, and to enable folate to form DNA, create red blood cells, and to metabolize homocysteine. It helps maintain nerve cells by protecting the myelin covering of nerves.

Taken together, the complex of B vitamins are mandatory in the processes that extract energy from foods, and control many of the nerve and brain health functions that create clear thinking and mental energy.

Functional Redox Nutrition - Supplementation

Vitamin B3 – Niacin

Niacin or Vitamin B3 – also called nicotinic acid or nicotinamide - is one of eight B vitamins. Its name comes from the word **NI**cotinic **AC**id vitam**IN,** so as to not confuse people that it has anything to do with nicotine. B3 plays an important role in energy metabolism due to its role in converting carbohydrates into glucose, metabolizing fats and proteins, and in keeping the nervous system working properly. Its multiple effects across a landscape of metabolic action qualifies it as a pleiotropic agent affecting many cellular functions.

Niacin is found in many foods such as meat, fish, milk, eggs, and green vegetables. It is required for the proper function and metabolism of food and to maintain health in cells. As such, B3 is a vitamin that is necessary in many cellular redox reactions including being a key player in mitochondrial energy production.

Niacin serves important roles throughout the cell and metabolic environment. One of the critical points of interaction is within the energy creation pathways and their interactions with the electron carrier redox couples.

The NAD+/NADH and NADP+/NADPH redox couples are responsible for moving electrons in the production of cellular energy. Their role in glycolysis and within Krebs and the electron transport chain is that of being a shuttle to carry electrons through the series of reactions that harvest ATP. These redox couples are necessary for glycolysis and the biosynthesis of nucleotides and amino acids, and for providing electrons for oxidative phosphorylation and ATP production within the electron transport mechanism.

Maintaining steady levels of these redox couples ensure normal metabolic function and redox homeostasis, along with the regulation of many signaling pathways related to cellular and energy metabolism[255]. Elevated NAD+ levels affect energy metabolism and increase ATP production by activating proteins in the mitochondrial respiratory chain – and niacin is an integral part of making this happen.

Functional Redox Nutrition - Supplementation

In human cells NAD+ is created from four precursors which include tryptophan, nicotinic acid, nicotinamide, and nicotinamide riboside. Intracellular NAD+ levels can be increased by supplementing with these NAD+ precursors. Redox-based lifestyle measures favors increasing NAD+ levels naturally through exercise, nutritional ketosis, and mitochondrial redox activation. The evidence suggests that supplemented niacin is an effective booster of NAD+[256].

Deficiency of NAD+ plays a major role in the aging process because it limits energy production, nuclear repair, and decreases cellular signaling[257]. Like many other things in life, NAD+ levels decline with age. And deficient synthesis of NAD+ is associated with accelerated aging. When cells lose energy and experience dysfunction it leads to various metabolic and age-related conditions.

There is also a strong relationship with the activation of sirtuin proteins through the NAD+ activity, which are deeply involved in regulating cellular metabolism and in supporting the family of NAD-dependent enzymes which directly affect gene expression.

Niacin aids in dealing with inflammation. It inhibits oxidative stress and redox-sensitive inflammatory genes (NF-kB) and is associated with decreased endothelial cell oxidation and reduced LDL oxidation and cytokine production – all key events in the formation of oxidized plaque in the walls of blood vessels. These anti-atherosclerotic and vascular anti-inflammatory properties operate independent of its effects on the regulation of lipids[258]. These anti-inflammatory properties are also involved in the decrease seen in beta-amyloid toxicity in neurodegenerative diseases[259], an obvious factor in brain cell health, alertness, and cognitive function.

The antioxidant properties of niacin are due to its effect on the glutathione antioxidant redox cycle. NADPH is an important coenzyme in the functioning of glutathione reductase which converts oxidized glutathione (GSSG) to its reduced form (GSH) allowing it to be used over and over within the body. GSH in turn is a co-substrate for glutathione peroxidase (GPx) which is an antioxidant and important part of the regulatory antioxidant defense system[260]. This guards against oxidation and lipid peroxidation of cell membranes and other cellular proteins and fats. The anti-inflammatory effect of niacin involves the activation of the heme-oxidase protein (HO-1) which activates nuclear translocation of Nrf2 and the activation of signaling pathways that generate antioxidant production within the cell[261].

Vitamin B5

Pantothenic acid, or pantothenate, participates in the synthesis of acetylcholine, an important neurotransmitter involved in focus, memory, learning, and improved brain synapse function and prevention of nerve damage. It is critical for converting food into energy, and in balancing blood sugar, controlling cholesterol levels, managing blood pressure, and in nerve cell repair and maintenance. It plays an important role in the synthesis and metabolism of proteins.

Because of its role in the mitochondria in producing energy, it is a significant contributor to mental energy, mental clarity and alertness, and in memory and mood. The energy vitamin B5 helps produce is the energy that fires neurotransmitters in the brain and carries nerve signals throughout the body. As part of Coenzyme-A (CoA), it participates in the creation of central nervous system neurotransmitters such as acetylcholine, epinephrine, and serotonin. Because of this role, it is often referred to as a significant anti-stress vitamin.

Pantothenic acid is an obligate precursor to Coenzyme-A. CoA is a cofactor in many pathways that affect protein, fat and carbohydrate metabolism, neurotransmitter synthesis, hemoglobin synthesis, and phase II detox acetylation where toxins are converted to less harmful and easier to excrete molecules.

The upstream 'sister' of Acetyl-CoA is essential for synthesis of myelin proteins which sheath and protect nerve cells, and pantothenate B5 localizes to myelin-protected nerves and white-matter brain structures[262].

CoA participates in cholesterol synthesis and its downstream metabolites, steroids, vitamin D, and bile acids which aid digestion of fats. CoA is also

Functional Redox Nutrition - Supplementation

needed to transport long chain fatty acids into mitochondria for energy conversion.

Vitamins B6

The significance of the broad reaching impact of B vitamins as a class, are no better illustrated than in its involvement in the various metabolic pathways within the body. Collectively, B vitamins merit this significance because of their roles as co-enzymes in a wide array of enzymatic reactions within the cell – especially the metabolic pathways related to the so-called "one-carbon chemistry" reactions (also called methylation cycle), and the transsulfuration pathway.

In these metabolic one-carbon pathways a single carbon atom is[263]:

1. <u>Transferred</u> to tetrahydrofolate (THF) to form methylene-THF (used in the synthesis of thymidine which is incorporated into DNA)

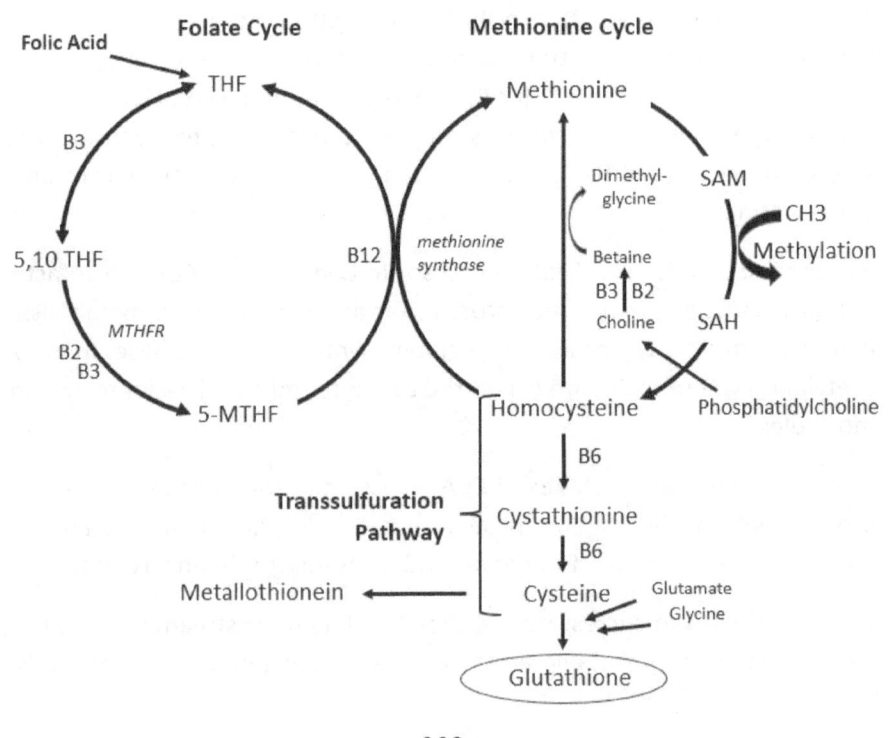

Functional Redox Nutrition - Supplementation

2. <u>Oxidized</u> to formyl-THF (used in the synthesis of purine, the building blocks of RNA and DNA)
3. <u>Reduced</u> to methyl-THF (which is used to convert homocysteine to methionine, which then becomes a source of methyl groups for DNA, RNA, hormones, neurotransmitters, membrane lipids, proteins, and epi-genomic histone modification / "gene silencers").

Vitamins B6, 9, and 12 are obligate cofactors in these metabolic pathways and are responsible for their optimal functioning. They are integrally involved in homocysteine metabolism and glutathione synthesis.

Translated, what this means is that carbon atoms (within the methyl group CH_3) are moved or rearranged within metabolic cycles and pathways. Any reaction in these pathway cycles or "circles" which do not work or function well for whatever reason, impedes the progress of the reaction throughout. This is a metabolic defect or blockade. Enzymes and cofactors are necessary to catalyze and facilitate these reactions. That is the role of B vitamins in these pathways. At any point along their respective paths and cycles, perturbations or dysfunction can stop or slow down the process, causing disease and distress to occur.

It is from the latter metabolic step (# 3 listed above, involving homocysteine), that homocysteine can be converted to cysteine (using the enzyme cystathionine synthase and the co-enzyme B6) - which then is converted into the sulfur-rich proteins metallothionine and glutathione. The latter is as an important redox pathway set in motion by redox signaling molecules.

These two proteins play important roles in cellular stability by providing antioxidant support. They are also both participate in detoxification of metals and toxic organic compounds, by making toxins water-soluble and capable of being excreted through the kidneys and bowel.

Metallothionine is especially effective in reducing metals (i.e., zinc, cadmium, copper, mercury, iron, and bismuth)[264], and in protecting against oxidative stress from the dangerous hydroxyl radical (which comes from the

Functional Redox Nutrition - Supplementation

iron Fenton-type reactions), which causes free-radical damage to cellular membranes[265].

This redox path involving homocysteine-to-cysteine-to-glutathione, plays a crucial role in the biological role of these detoxifiers and antioxidants. When toxins accumulate in cells, these molecules associated with the transsulfuration pathway are intimately involved in their detoxification.

Vitamin B6 (pyridoxine) and its derivatives are co-factors to nearly one hundred different reactions and pathways in the body. It is involved throughout the folic acid cycle, methionine/methylation cycle, and transsulfuration pathway. As mentioned previously, it is in the transsulfuration pathway where they play a central role in the redox reactions that involve glutathione synthesis[266] - where homocysteine is converted to cysteine and then to glutathione.

The formation of glutathione requires the amino acid cysteine. Glutathione is a thiol- or Sulphur-rich amino acid that combines with glutamate and glycine to form glutathione. Glutathione is not absorbed well in gut and has a difficulty crossing cell membranes to enter cells. Therefore, the constituent amino acids must enter the cell where glutathione is synthesized *in* situ inside the cell - with cysteine either coming from dietary sources or converted from homocysteine from within.

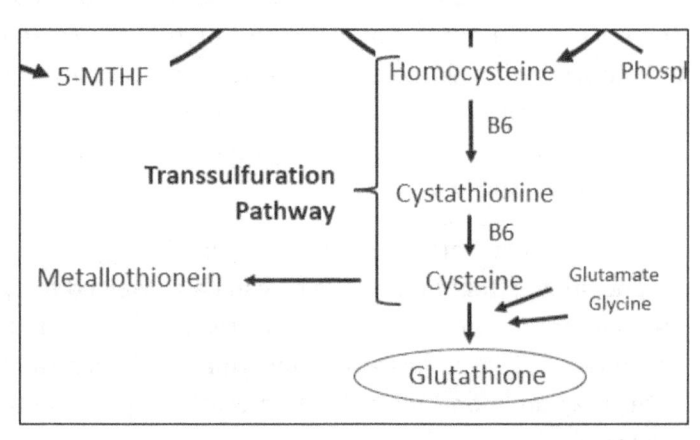

This breakdown of homocysteine to cysteine is dependent on B6. Approximately 50% of the required cysteine comes from dietary sources, with the remainder coming from this B6-dependent conversion of homocysteine to cysteine.

Functional Redox Nutrition - Supplementation

Thus, there are three rate-limitations in the synthesis of glutathione; the first being the amount of cysteine present; secondly the presence of vitamin B6 present; and third the amount of gene expression which induces its production (i.e., redox signaling and Nrf2 activity).

Vitamin B12

Vitamin B12 is a family of cobalt containing compounds that are a part of many reactions in the body, specifically the manufacture of red blood cells which affects oxygen transport throughout the body. It has an important role in energy metabolism and is often promoted as an energy enhancer and an athletic performance an endurance booster. It is essential for DNA synthesis and hemoglobin synthesis which is responsible for carrying oxygen to the cells of the body. Low B12 produces feelings of fatigue and tiredness, and in impaired muscle capacity and muscle performance.

B12 assists in the metabolizing of glucose, fats, and proteins because it is a key enzyme in the production of succinyl-CoA, one of the steps in Krebs cycle and which is associated with the metabolism of fatty acids and ketogenic amino acids[267].

Vitamin B12 is helpful in dealing with stress and feelings of overwhelm. This is because it is helpful in reducing cortisol release from the adrenal glands and improved regulation of the autonomic nervous system[268].

Vitamin B12 deficiency is associated with

- autonomic sympathetic and parasympathetic nervous system problems[269]
- autonomic dysfunction and defective sympathetic activation[270]
- accumulation of homocysteine, a risk factor for cognitive dysfunction[271]
- impairment of DNA synthesis
- faster cognitive decline and risk of neurodegenerative disease[272]
- increased breakdown of the myelin sheath covering nerves[273]
- increased depression[274]
- cognitive decline and dementia[275]

- decreased hemoglobin and oxygen carrying capacity of red blood cells[276].

In order for B12 to be absorbed, the stomach, pancreas and small intestine must be functioning properly. Stomach cells secrete a protein called *intrinsic factor* that is necessary for Vitamin B absorption in the small intestine[277]. Deficiencies in intrinsic factor happen with autoimmune disease and inflammation in the stomach. Malabsorption is more common in the elderly and those with gut dysbiosis and GI diseases.

GABA

Gama-aminobutyric acid is an amino acid which acts as a neurotransmitter chemical made in brain and nerve cells. It is also found in some foods (cruciferous vegetables, beans, peas, tomatoes, spinach, mushrooms, sprouts). In the brain and spinal cord, it is the primary inhibitory neurotransmitter because it blocks and diminishes nerve signals. Its primary role is in reducing neuronal excitability throughout the central nervous systems[278].

Disorders in GABA signaling participate in many neurologic and mental health disorders. In addition to inhibiting neuronal firing and unwanted motor signals, it helps calm heightened respiratory rate. In the spinal cord it helps to manage activated proprioceptive nerve signaling which facilitate smooth movements and better integration of sensory information[279]. This makes them highly relevant for neuroprotection, and in dealing with neurodegenerative disease and cognitive functions.

It plays an essential role in promoting sleep[280] and calm, easing anxiety and stress, aids with relaxation, and protects the brain. Within the nervous system, GABA modulates the transmission of signals between neurons and promotes nerve development. It's pharmaceutical-like effects on tissues and organs of the body are varied and include improved blood pressure and blood sugar management, antioxidant and anti-inflammatory effects, and improvements in liver, kidney, and intestinal health[281].

GABA provides neuroprotective effects that prevent nerve cell injury, and respond to damage from toxins, oxidation, inflammation, and ischemic or stroke injury. It suppresses neurodegeneration, improves memory, and increases cognitive function.

GABA is also able to be produced within the intestinal tract (the so-called enteric nervous system - ENS) by strains of *Lactobacillus* and *Bifidobacterium* bacteria. GABA and its receptors are widely distributed through the ENS[282], and the effects of GABA in the gut are transmitted to the brain through the vagus nerve – part of the so-called gut-brain connection.

The role of redox agents in the nervous system is well illustrated by how redox molecules can regulate inhibitory neurotransmission mediated by GABA receptors in the nervous system.

Various redox signaling molecules can modulate both the phasic and tonic responses that are controlled by GABA receptors in nerve synapses. Redox molecules can induce potentiating or inhibiting actions on GABA receptors, which is a homeostatic mechanism used by neurons to regulate the function of GABA receptors[283]. Excessive motor activity such as with dystonia and spasticity are believed to be a deficiency in GABA signaling[284].

The brain is particularly vulnerable to oxidative damage due to its requirements for high oxygen utilization. The effects of this produce oxidative insult which translates to increased aging and neurodegenerative disorders.

Antioxidant defense mechanisms and cellular renewal (autophagy) processes which remove damaged proteins have neuromodulatory redox effects in brain cells. Glutathione's role is to exert a protective antioxidant defense against this oxidative stress, and to aid in the regulation of synapses and neuronal plasticity.

GABA receptors are thus the target for the actions of these redox signaling agents. Thus the redox-dependent involvement of GABA and its receptors provide a foundational physiologic mechanism for modulating brain and nerve cell inhibition[285] - and is a prototype for the same mechanisms throughout the central and peripheral nervous system.

Functional Redox Nutrition - Supplementation

Garden Sage and Spanish Sage

Garden sage or *Salvia officinalis* is an aromatic herb of the mint family and is a culinary herb used as food flavoring and in poultry stuffing and in pork sausages. Spanish sage *salvia lavandulifolia* is a small woody herb native to western Europe. Both garden and Spanish sage are beneficial for improving memory, executive function, mood, and cognition[286][287]. They enjoy excellent antioxidant and anti-inflammatory properties that help them in protecting against the progressive decline seen with neurodegeneration.

Sage leaf contains a variety of phenolic acids, flavonoids, terpenoids, and polysaccharides. These compounds include tannic acid, oleic acid, ursolic acid, carnosol, rosmarinic acid, sage coumarin, sagerinic acid, yunnaneic acids, carnosic acid, fumaric acid, alpha-pinene, 1,8-cineole, chlorogenic acid, caffeic acid, flavones, luteolin, apigenin, hispidulin, kaempferol, quercetin, camphor, arbinogalactans, and pectin.

Sage is also high in vitamin K and minerals like magnesium, zinc, and copper. Vitamins A, C, E, B3 niacin, and nicotinamide are also found in small amounts. It has high antioxidant activity which protects cells against oxidative free radical damage.

Sage enjoys a reputation for being brain-enhancing with *in vitro* and animal studies confirming that the active compounds in sage may enhance cognitive activity and protect against neurodegenerative disease[288].

These multiple compounds work together to give Salvia its many pharmacodynamic effects on the brain. This rich array of phytochemicals influences many physiological pathways with improvements in:

- cholinergic activity effects
- neurotrophic effects
- antioxidant effects
- anti-inflammatory effects
- anti-depressive and anxiolytic effects
- beta-amyloid peptide reduction
- cellular redox balance effects.

Functional Redox Nutrition - Supplementation

Improved cholinergic signaling activity with the neurotransmitter acetylcholine plays an important role in cognitive function and behavior, including attention, orientation, learning, memory, and motivation. Disruptions in this signaling lead to multiple neurodegenerative disorders[289]. Sage inhibits human acetylcholinesterase[290], the enzyme that breaks down acetylcholine neurotransmitter, thus protecting and improving neurotransmitter function.

Sage is noted for its neurotrophic support of brain cells, cognitive and nerve cell protection and neurologic health. Neurotrophins are important regulators of nerve cell survival, neural development, and function, and in neural plasticity[291]. They provide a well-recognized protective mechanism against stressful insults in the brain where they defend neurons against injury and disease[292].

Brain derived neurotrophic factor (BDNF) is a neurotrophin which plays a significant role in brain cell survival, and in encouraging growth and differentiation of neurons and brain cell synapses[293]. As such it and many of the other neurotrophins support the survival of neurons and brain cells, promote synaptic junctions, and are essential for learning and long-term memory storage. Of interest is the fact that the BDNF signaling pathway is associated with the Early Growth Response gene[294] (EGR) and is one of many activated through redox signaling. The mild to moderate levels of oxidation in the spinal cord stimulate BDNF expression through redox-sensitive transcription[295].

The mechanism of redox-sensitive transcription, which follows physiologic levels of oxidation stimulus, activates transcription and pathway genes to induce the production of BDNF in mRNA in brain cells[296,297], and is the same mechanism of action preserved and conserved through nature to affect the activation of all cellular defense processes.

Antioxidant effects of sage help reduce oxidative stress which is implicated in many neurological and mental health disorders. Sage also has been shown to reduce the production of reactive oxygen species by inhibiting oxidases (which help transfer electrons between molecules), thus improving mitochondrial efficiency and reducing the production of superoxide and thus reducing oxidative stress. It is also associated with the increase of the cellular antioxidant response with increased levels of catalase, superoxide dismutase, glutathione, and glutathione peroxidase[298]. By inhibiting lipid peroxidation and with enhanced antioxidant defense it can be helpful in protecting against metabolic dysfunction and disease.

Anti-inflammatory effects for sage are significantly robust. *In vitro* and animal studies demonstrate that sage exhibits anti-inflammatory effects[299]. It was found that several markers and pathways are influenced by sage, including COX-2, hypoxia-inducible factor1 (HIF1), NF-*k*B, and several cytokines that are a product of the activation of inflammation genes. Sage has shown to blunt gene expression for many of the inflammation-related genes including prostaglandin, cyclooxygenase-2, nitric oxide synthase, cytokines/interleukins, and chemokines.

Antidepressant and anxiolytic effects of sage are extensive. The variety of anxiety and depressive disorders are all marked with stress and diminished effects on cognitive and mental performance. Interventions and preventions to these conditions always have as a component of care, a strong focus on the positive effects on cognitive performance. The anti-stress effects of sage are more pronounced than with oils (chamomile, rosemary, lavender) and occur due to its ability to increase dopamine activity[300]. Some action is also derived from the activity of flavones on benzodiazepine receptors[301]. Sage's phenolic acids also exert antidepressant and anxiolytic-like activity in animal models[302].

Human studies have shown significant cognitive-enhancing effects of sage. Positive cognitive effects (memory, attention, word recall, memory speed) and mood-enhancing (alertness, calmness) effects have been observed. These studies lend support for the cognitive and mood-enhancing ability of sage, at least in short-term studies[303].

Beta-amyloid peptide reduction in brain neurons is a topic of growing interest. People with mild to moderate neurodegeneration suffer from gradually diminishing cognitive function due to the effects of oxidation, lipid peroxidation, DNA fragmentation, and the accumulation of beta-amyloid peptides. Collectively these deleterious processes produce neurotoxicity and decreased cellular function leading to neurodegenerative disease. Because present therapeutic approaches are often limited to dealing with symptoms, many investigators are turning to phytochemical compounds and blends which can offer neuroprotection.

Sage has shown the ability in cell cultures to protect against induced neurotoxicity[304]. Sage possess considerable antioxidant capacity and neuroprotective properties against experimental beta-amyloid induced cell death. These two combined properties lean favorably toward sage's ability to combat neurodegenerative disorders[305].

Cellular redox balance and regulation of redox-sensitive mechanisms is a central player in the ability of sage to participate in cellular health processes. The ability of sage to protect cells against oxidative injury by enhancing cellular function and cellular renewal processes, to inhibit ROS production and to decrease lipid peroxidation, and to increase endogenous antioxidant levels (glutathione, catalase, superoxide dismutase, glutathione peroxidase, and heme oxidase 1), qualifies sage as a significant regulator of cellular redox balance in brain cells[306].

Guarana

Guarana is a plant that is native to the Amazon basin. It is also known as *Paullinia cupana*. It is a climbing plant prized for its fruit and has been used for centuries for its therapeutic properties[307]. Over the years the seeds of this fruit have been used as a key ingredient in energy drinks and other formulations that are alleged to boost one's libido (aphrodisiac) due to a vascular relaxing effect on the microvasculature networks throughout the body.

It contains an assortment of antioxidants, along with many bioactive compounds including methylxanthines such as caffeine, theobromine, and catechins, as well as tannins, saponins, epicatechins, and proanthocyanidins[308,309].

The cellular effects of guarana include a decrease in cell mortality, cell membrane oxidation, DNA damage and rapid cell division[310], cellular oxidation, and an increase in superoxide dismutase (SOD) via Nrf2 activation[311]. These strong antioxidant properties contribute to its anti-aging[312] properties and is often included in skin and hair care products. Additionally, guarana has an antioxidant effect on nitric oxide metabolism, mainly when nitric oxide levels are overly elevated (which if left elevated increases production of the oxidant peroxynitrite).

It has been linked with reductions in obesity and metabolic syndrome[313]. This is likely due to the chelating effect on redox-active transition-metal ions, and the *in vivo* effects to downregulate redox active transcriptional factors that produce pro-oxidant enzymes, and by activating antioxidant enzymes[314]. The cyto-protective effects of guarana is also believed to be helpful with age-related eye disorders and retinal damage as it has shown to decrease *in vitro* oxidative damage in retinal cells[315].

Behavioral effects of guarana are dose-related and improve mood and cognitive function throughout the day, with better effects occurring using lower doses rather than higher doses[316]. The combined effect of Panax ginseng and guarana demonstrated enhanced memory performance, which evidenced the psychoactive effects of guarana and confirmed the same properties of ginseng[317].

Guarana has shown interesting antibacterial properties which may justify some ethnopharmacological use (traditional medicinal use of plants), such as against digestive tract bacterial pathogens. It's antioxidant activity could also explain the ethnopharmacological application against vascular disease[318]. Further studies have shown that guarana is associated with lower prevalence of cardiovascular metabolic diseases and positively influences lipid metabolism and reduced LDL oxidation[319].

L-Theanine

L-Theanine is an amino acid derived from green tea and mushroom (edible bay boletes). Because of its effect on improved cognition and mood, it is available as a supplement and is now an ingredient in functional energy drinks.

L-Theanine is active within the redox landscape by sustaining the pools of Krebs cycle intermediates that are crucial for cellular energy creation and

Functional Redox Nutrition - Supplementation

biosynthesis processes throughout the mitochondria[320]. Additionally, it reduces aging by inhibiting the formation of advanced glycation end products (AGEs) generally[321], and beta-amyloid deposits in the brain[322][323], and by stabilizing oxidative stress and inflammation[324][325] through inactivation of kinase and NF-kB pathways. Taken together these redox-related functions have the effect to attenuate cognitive dysfunction and neurotoxicity from oxidation and beta-amyloid deposits.

L-Theanine's ability to reduce advanced glycation formation and its effect on improved regulation of the sirtuin family of proteins and the expression of brain-derived neurotrophic factor (BDNF) signaling pathways, has been noted in the literature[326]. This is noteworthy because it was found to mitigate brain damage by inhibiting AGEs/RAGE signaling pathways and by upregulating sirtuins and BDNF, qualifying it as a "functional food" to prevent neurological disease.

L-theanine helps maintain healthy levels of gamma aminobutyric acid (GABA), dopamine, and serotonin – each important neurotransmitters which impact happiness and coping abilities in everyday life. It also enhances alpha wave activity in the brain. It's anti-fatigue effects arise from increase in dopamine and liver glycogen levels, and the reduced 5-HT and serum urea levels[327]. The potential for promoting and supporting mental health, countering stress-related problems, improving attention and memory, and overall cognitive impairments are noteworthy[328][329][330].

L-Theanine's ability to prevent neuronal loss, mitochondrial failure, and also improve neurotransmitters function, occurs because of its antioxidant, anti-inflammatory, and its neuromodulatory properties[331]. L-Theanine has been shown to decrease memory loss associated with beta-amyloid accumulation, as well as to reduce nerve cell death, diminish lipid peroxidation and protein damage, and to increase glutathione levels in the cell[332].

The role of L-Theanine's biochemical cousins help explain its role in the body. L-Theanine is derived from glutamine, the latter being one of the basic twenty amino acids. Glutamine also converts into two neurotransmitters, GABA and glutamate, which each share the same cell receptor site.

Functional Redox Nutrition - Supplementation

Glutamate is an excitatory neurotransmitter which activates or excites this receptor and is associated with memory and learning. Gaba calms the receptor. Excess stimulation is responsible for a state termed "excitotoxicity." GABA on the other hand has the opposite effect where it silences this effect and produces calm.

Because theanine is structurally similar to both glutamate and GABA it binds to glutamate/GABA receptors throughout the nervous system. L-Theanine has a dual effect on this receptor because it is generally calming like GABA, but it can also function as the receptor agonist (stimulant) similar to glutamate. As such it protects against neurotoxicity produced by both excess dopamine[333] and excess glutamate[334] – thus inducing alpha wave brain activity and alleviating anxiety[335].

The physiological effects of L-Theanine include[336]:

- Neuroprotection
- Hypotensive activity
- Blood sugar regulation
- Anti-fatigue
- Anti-neoplastic cell effect
- Mood modulation
- Antioxidant activity
- Improved immunity
- Lessened liver damage from alcohol
- Cardioprotective effects
- Improved cognition and memory
- Reduced menstrual discomfort
- Sleep maintenance

Functional Redox Nutrition - Supplementation

L-Tyrosine

L-tyrosine plays an important role in the central nervous system and in supporting the thyroid and adrenal glands. It helps the body produce important brain neurotransmitters, including dopamine, and the catecholamines epinephrine and norepinephrine which participate in stress response and management. Because L-tyrosine promotes the body's production of brain chemicals and thyroid hormones it is able to support healthy stress management and helps maintain healthy adrenal gland function. L-tyrosine serves as a precursor for the thyroid stimulating hormone thyroxine[337] and for the skin pigment melanin. L-tyrosine also stimulates growth hormone release[338]. Among the effects reported are the ability to prevent declines in cognitive functions in response to acute physical stress, and in affecting mood and sleep.

Because it improves the rate of neurotransmitter production, it helps relive the physical symptoms of stress and mood swings. People with chronic stress may be less able to convert phenylalanine to tyrosine, which makes supplementation with L-tyrosine desirable. This makes L-tyrosine a 'conditional' essential amino acid because under normal conditions the body is able to synthesize it from phenylalanine. However, when it is depleted, as can happen during stress, L-tyrosine increases the production of neurotransmitters. This has been the basis for studying the effect of tyrosine on the human stress response phenomenon[339].

Due to its phenolic structure and make up, tyrosine is a powerful antioxidant, neutralizing oxidative molecules and free radicals, and inhibiting peroxidation of lipids. This soundly qualifies it as a redox-supportive micronutrient.

Nicotinamide Mononucleotide

Nicotinamide mononucleotide (NMN) is a powerful precursor to NAD+. It is rapidly absorbed and quickly results in elevated NAD+ levels. This is especially important since NAD+ is one of the more abundant molecules in the body and is a critical component within the mitochondrial energy production pathways. NAD+ triggers cellular repair and enhances cellular survival[340]. Because it participates in these redox energy pathways, it slows aging and upregulates cellular repair.

NAD+ is used by sirtuins to repair damaged DNA. Sirtuins are known as the "guardian of genes" and requires NAD+ to become activated. Sirtuins help regulate the expression and activity of antioxidant enzymes through its effect on the Nrf1/Keap1 redox switch, and via the alteration of the NAD+/NADH redox couple (which carries electrons in energy metabolism). They play an important role in redox homeostasis through their feedback mechanisms.

Sirtuins initially gained their popularity due to the connections with health benefits seen with calorie restriction (ketosis-induced antioxidant production). They have been connected with increased longevity due to its histone modification effect in epigenetics, and its effect to oppose gene shortening and to enhance telomer maintenance[341].

Aging significantly reduces the body's ability to convert NMN to NAD+, with NAD+ levels decreasing by half at middle-age[342]. This parallels the reduction in redox signaling and declining mitochondrial function and collagen production, which are also associated with normal aging[343]. Long-term supplementation with NMN helps alleviate physiological decline in aging animals. In fact, in animal models, older animals enjoyed increased responsiveness to NMN when compared to younger animals. With NMN and NAD+ supplementation there was also significant improvement in weight problems, energy metabolism, physical activity, insulin sensitivity, eye health, cognitive function, reduced oxidation, and improved gene expression[344].

Because of NMNs effect in improving NAD+ levels, the association with energy production is well established due to its effect in the mitochondria. NMN supplementation increases acetyl-CoA levels in Krebs cycle as well as NAD+ levels which enhance sirtuin activity, thereby increasing mitochondrial energy metabolism in the brain. While it is unclear exactly how NMN improves depression (in animal models), there is strong evidence that NMN can improve depression through improved mitochondrial function by enhancing NAD+ and sirtuin activity[345]. Targeting the mitochondria with NMN and NAD+ in this fashion to improve mitochondrial dysfunction, makes this an important element in dealing with depression[346].

Interestingly, the threads that weave these interrelated processes together are all managed through the effects of redox-sensitive redox signaling.

Panax Ginseng

Panax ginseng (Pg) is a plant native to Far East China, Korea, and Siberia. There are many forms of ginseng and Panax ginseng, or 'Korean ginseng' is perhaps the most commonly used and researched. There are many active phytochemicals in Panax Ginseng, and the most important are ginsenosides, also called panaxosides. These are triterpene saponins.

The beneficial effects from Pg include anti-inflammatory and antioxidant actions, and the suppression of uncontrolled cell division. Its mental and psychological benefits include improvement in memory and mental alertness, and cognitive function, along with improvements in dealing with neurodegenerative diseases.

Research on the main active component ginsenoside, has shown an effect on the hypothalamus-pituitary-adrenal axis (HPA) and the immune system[347]. This may account for the observed and documented effects for these polyphenol compounds. Animal research has documented enhanced immune function by way of improved white blood cell activity (phagocytosis), and higher levels of interferon. They also enhance vasodilation, increased resistance to stress, and hypoglycemic blood sugar control[348].

Other investigators are drawing attention to the hormetic redox effect and use of Pg in nutraceuticals, functional foods, and cosmetics, where ginsenosides induced the transcription of stress-response genes and increased heat shock proteins in skin cells[349], suggesting the broader utilization of physical, nutritional, and mental hormetins.

These stress-adaptive responses are activated through hormesis-driven activation of the redox state within the cell. Individual ginseng constituents commonly induce this redox-sensitive response (hormesis) which is known to produce effects of clinical relevance. To date, the principal focus has been with regard to its effect on neurodegenerative processes and enhancing nerve cell repair and in reducing discomfort[350].

As with almost all polyphenol plant constituents, the hormesis-driven dose response with ginseng is prototypical of all classes of plant chemicals – firmly grounding their effects within the structure of the redox landscape and Redoxome.

Phosphatidylserine

Phosphatidylserine (PS) is a key component in cell membranes. It is a negatively charged phospholipid containing both fatty acids and amino acids. It plays an important role in cell cycle signaling, especially as it relates to autophagy and apoptosis. Phospholipids are necessary to protect and provide structure for cells. It is required for healthy nerve cell membranes and the myelin covering which protects brain cells[351] and is part of the inter-cellular signaling mechanisms[352]. Thus, it is an important building block for cell membranes which directly affects cellular function. Supplemented PS is absorbed well and easily crosses the blood-brain barrier and safely lowers, halts, and even reverses biochemical alterations and structural detonation in nerve cells[353].

The effect on human cognitive function is profound. "It supports human cognitive functions, including the formation of short-term memory, the consolidation of long-term memory, the ability to create new memories, the ability to retrieve memories, the ability to learn and recall information, the ability to focus attention and concentrate, the ability to reason and solve problems, language skills, and the ability to communicate. It also supports locomotor functions, especially rapid reactions and reflexes"[354].

PS safely slows, halts, and reverses biochemical alterations and cellular damage in nerve cells. Because of this, it assists with human cognition functions, both short and long-term memory, attention focus and mental concentration, reasoning and language skills, and communication[355].

Taken together, PS plays an important role in improving memory, alertness, and mood. It improves learning ability and mental focus. It helps with

Functional Redox Nutrition - Supplementation

neuroprotection and brain recovery and to offset the effects associated with age-related cognitive decline.

Red Orange Complex®

Red Orange Complex – ROC, (*Citrus sinensis*) is an extract obtained from crimson oranges grown in volcanic soil in Italy near Mt. Etna. These red oranges varieties (Moro, Tarocco, and Sanguinello) have a bright orange peel with red hues, from which their name is derived.

The active compounds of ROC are anthocyanins, hydroxycinnamic acid, flavanones (hesperidin, narirutin), and ascorbic acid. The properties and effects of each of these on their own and as they synergistically combine, yield significant health benefits.

Anthocyanins are water-soluble phenols called flavonoids that are colored pigments in glycosylated forms. They yield the colors red, purple and blue to various fruits, berries, and vegetables.

Anthocyanins as a class are redox-active molecules and can work as a mitochondrial electron-carrier. Their neuroprotection capabilities involve cellular redox state, and the modulation of mitochondria function. They have rich antioxidant activity and exhibit affinity for mitochondrial membranes and exert reversible redox behavior within the range of mitochondrial redox chain potentials. It is able to counter the effects of toxicity within the mitochondrial complex 1 [356].

Hydroxycinnamic acids are a group of aromatic phenolic acids or phenylpropanoids which are derivatives of cinnamic acid. They are a class of phytochemical often used in 'cosmeceuticals' for their ability to protect against sun damage and hyperpigmentation in skin. They have antioxidant, anti-collagenase, anti-inflammatory, antimicrobial and anti-tyrosinase activities, as well as they provide protection against sun damage.

This phenolic acid has potent antioxidant and anti-inflammatory properties and have health benefits with a broad range of metabolic disease conditions, including obesity, blood sugar disorders, and neurodegeneration[357]. The neuroprotective role of phenolic acids such as hydroxycinnamic acid is significant. They improve depression, neuroinflammation, glutamate-induced toxicity in brain cells, seizure, memory impairment, and several other brain related disorders and conditions[358]. They are noted for their effect in protecting brain cells and the effect they have on behavior and quality of life. Because of their positive effect in neurons and glial cells, and due to their efficient gut and brain absorption, phenolic acids such as hydroxycinnamic acids show promise when used in combination with supportive ingredients.

The **flavanones** hesperidin and narirutin are polyphenols or plant phytochemicals specific to citrus fruits, where they are generally found in high amounts. Hesperidin is a flavanone that is isolated from the rinds or peels of some citrus fruits. They have been found effective in various mental health conditions including neurological disorders, psychiatric disorders, and cardiovascular diseases, in large measure due to the anti-inflammatory, anti-lipid peroxidative and antioxidant, lipid-lowering, and insulin-sensitizing properties[359]. It has shown to be effective in improving endothelial function and reducing inflammatory markers in patients with metabolic syndrome[360].

Hesperidin helps support memory, brain synapse formation within the central nervous system, and it promotes neurogenesis and neuronal synapse formation, survival, and activity within the brain[361]. Narirutin is also found in citrus and has high beta-amyloid inhibitory activity, strong antioxidant activity, and along with other citrus flavonoids, it can modulate blood platelet function and help inhibit clot formation as a reversible process[362].

Flavonoids provide significant cytoprotective effect against oxidative stress, aiding normal redox homeostasis in cells and protecting against oxidative injury in cells, through the cellular antioxidant pathways. Glutathione levels are increased by phenolic and flavonoid compounds[363], inducing the phase 2 enzyme system driven by activation of the Nrf2 transcription factor.

These flavanones demonstrate neuroprotective properties and have positive effect upon blood-brain barrier function/integrity, which together helps explain the mechanistic actions by which these neurological effects are obtained[364].

Flavonoid supplementation has shown improvement in cognitive performance, lessened depression, and anxiety. These findings have remained consistent across several disease models which seems to validate the effects are due to modulation of fundamental processes.

The redox activity associated with ROC supplementation improves cellular antioxidant levels. The likely mechanism for this finding is its interaction with redox signaling pathways which activate the Nrf2 transcription factor, which in turn mediates the activity of the DNA-based gene expression on the nuclear antioxidant response element for glutathione and superoxide dismutase formation. The overall antioxidant effect for ROC is likely due to this as well as its direct scavenging ability as a reducing agent[365].

Using animal models, citrus peels improved longevity, motor movement, memory, antioxidant status, and improvements in enzyme systems. The most likely mechanisms involved the actions of flavonoids on neuronal signaling[366,367].

Rhodiola rosea

Rhodiola rosea (R. rosea) is a stress reducing adaptogen containing many active compounds, the two most potent being rosavin and salidroside. It enhances natural resistance of the body to stress, fatigue, and depression. Today, R. rosea is promoted to increase energy, stamina, strength, and mental capacity, improve athletic performance, resist the effects of stress, and help manage depression, anxiety, cognitive decline and memory problems, and other symptoms.

The anti-stress properties have been linked with the hypothalamic-pituitary-adrenal (HPA) axis, and key stress mediators such as heat shock proteins, nitric oxide, kinase inhibitors, and cortisol, among others[368]. Animal models have shown reduction in pituitary ACTH activity, the hormone responsible for activating stress hormones from the adrenal gland.

Functional Redox Nutrition - Supplementation

R. rosea's effect as an antidepressant in humans is due to the interactions with those mediators which are involved with neuroendocrine and immune and neurotransmitter systems. It is through these molecular networks that the general claim for its beneficial effects on mood are anchored[369]. R. rosea influences the release of stress hormones and enhances energy metabolism as demonstrated in animal models and offers a safe way to address symptoms of stress and stress-related complications[370].

The significant antioxidant effects are due to the phenolic-based molecules ability to scavenge reactive oxygen molecules, as well as its ability to activate Nrf2 to produce cellular antioxidants. The active compound salidroside inhibits kinase phosphorylation and NF-kB activity, while activating Nrf2 antioxidant signaling[371].

The principal mechanisms which R. rosea utilizes for its multi-targeted effects include, the mTOR pathway where salidroside activates the mTOR pathway to protect and repair neurons, blood vessels and muscles, whereas in dysplastic cells it inhibits mTOR to reduce their growth. R. rosea helps with DNA repair and diminishes mutations in DNA. It is able to enhance cellular adaptation for hypoxic conditions such as high-altitude living. It has a stimulating effect on immunity, improving T cells and immunoglobulins, and it has anti-inflammatory activity by blocking the NF-kB signaling pathway[372,373].

Saffron extract

Saffron (*Crocus Sativus*) is a plant used to make saffron spice, food coloring, and medicine. Its active compounds have been used traditionally for a wide range of disorders including vascular disease, gastrointestinal disorders, menstrual problems, and learning and memory impairments. It is also claimed to have an effect to alter mood, inhibit or kill dysplastic cells, and decrease inflammation. It has been used traditionally for its effect as a sedative, and its antidepressant properties[374,375]. Because of its mood-improving effect it enhances satiety and aids in appetite control and weight loss[376].

Functional Redox Nutrition - Supplementation

The bioactive compounds are apocarotenoids (which give it its red color), terpenoids, flavonoids, phenolic acids, and phytosterols. These collectively are responsible for the wide range of therapeutic effects, especially in the nervous system because of their ability to cross the blood-brain barrier. Multiple trials support its neuroprotective, anxiolytic, antidepressant, and learning and memory-enhancing effects. Its ability to moderate depression is due to the increase in glutamate and dopamine levels in the brain[377].

Due to the phytochemical and phenolic nature of these active compounds, it has an antioxidant effect and can maintain the redox status of cells and can protect against progressive oxidative damage. This contributes to its brain and heart-protective effect[378]. These obvious redox connections are manifest, as crocus helps preserve the glutathione redox system[379].

Zinc Citrate

Zinc is an essential mineral and plays an important role in cellular metabolism and in metabolic pathways. It is part of the catalytic activity of approximately 100 enzymes involved in immune function, protein synthesis, wound healing, DNA and RNA synthesis, and in cell division[380]. Daily dietary or supplementation sources are necessary since it is not stored within the body.

The list of psychiatric and neurodegenerative disorders that involve deficient zinc levels is steadily growing. "Brain fog" as it is commonly called, results when brain cells are not properly communicating with each other. Zinc assists with communication among and between brain cells. This communication is centered in the axonal and synaptic transmissions between nerve cells in both excitatory and inhibitory amino acid receptors[381].

Zinc is necessary for nucleic acid metabolism and brain tubulin growth and phosphorylation[382]. Zinc is concentrated in nerve synapses and is therefore involved in the stability of the nerve synapse and as a natural neuromodulator. It plays a key role in synaptic plasticity and is believed to play a vital role in learning and memory[383].

Functional Redox Nutrition - Supplementation

Zinc plays an important role with viral immunity. Due to its positive double charge, a transporter is required to move it across the cell membrane. These transporters for zinc are called zinc ionophores. Certain flavonoids and polyphenols (quercetin and resveratrol) function as ionophore transport carriers[384].

The decreased presence of zinc in neurodegenerative disorders has led some to suggest that beta-amyloid deposits are in part causing cognitive impairment because they may be trapping zinc in the synapse, leading to its lack of function in brain cells[385]. Whether this is the exact mechanism or not, research has shown decreased levels of zinc in people with neurodegenerative diseases. The same associations are drawn with the relationship with mental health disorders that reflect stress, anxiety, depression, and more extreme psychiatric disorders[386].

Taken together, studies have shown that zinc deficiency is surprisingly prevalent in people with mental health and neurodegenerative disorders[387]. Zinc deficiency affects nerve generation and repair, increased brain cell death, increases memory and learning deficits, and is a risk factor for neurodegenerative disorders[388]. Zinc deficiency is also critical for growth, development, and maintenance of immune function and is associated with approximately ten percent of the human proteome and hundreds of key enzymes and transcription factors. It plays an essential role in antiviral immunity[389].

Conclusion & Quick-Start Recommendations

Conclusion & Quick-Start Recommendations

Pulling together a working plan for how to be healthy is or should be the order of the day for anyone seeking a better life. The old adage of "if you don't have your health, you have nothing" is best appreciated by those who have lost their health and spend their fortune and their years trying to find it again.

Still, in a world filled with conflicting and conflicted voices and agendas, it remains difficult to judge without understanding the ground rules for what makes the human body tick. To that end, this expose about Healthy Matters, grounded on the redox science of Redox Matters, presents relevant information to enable that better judgment.

With elevated understandings comes better choice. The enticement offered from food and media establishment, and even from our own mismanaged hormones and cellular processes, are powerful forces to be reasoned with and tamed. With ignorance and misinformation, our cellular and health fates are almost sealed - doomed to be forever managed through medical intervention, as marvelous as it may be.

For those who want it differently, there is hope and a path forward, regardless of where they are on the pathway of life. It is never too late to provide support and recourse to cells that have languished from years of neglect and abuse. 'Now' is always a good time to begin prevention in all its forms.

With the "rules of the cell" in mind, sorting through and applying the right "diets" and lifestyle adjustments should come easier and with a higher level of motivation and willpower. Succumbing to and remaining captive to the power of hunger hormones, weight challenges, dull thinking, hurting mobility, and premature aging just doesn't have to happen. At least not in the 'ordinary' manner – and not without a good redox-oriented fight!

The solution is not in finding the right diet or exercise plan. The answer is in finding the right lifestyle! The redox lifestyle should be an everyday thing – not just something you resort to "fix" something that isn't working well. The idea of "going on a diet" or starting an exercise regimen, should be

Conclusion & Quick-Start Recommendations

something that is a common practice in how you fuel and treat the body. Every day. If there is such a thing as a New Year's resolution – this, is it! Except it should be a "New Lifestyle" resolution!

This lifestyle is more than the managed control of symptoms. Real health, true health, is more than the absence of disease. It is a properly functioning metabolism that enjoys metabolic health. This includes the process of energy creation in the cell, and the proper metabolic functioning of redox pathways. These are the "rules" that govern health, wellness, and anti-aging. There are no other rules!

A redox lifestyle is one that incorporates all the good points of anything that promotes true metabolic health **and** are anchored on the foundation of the Redoxome. This "and" is an important conjunction!

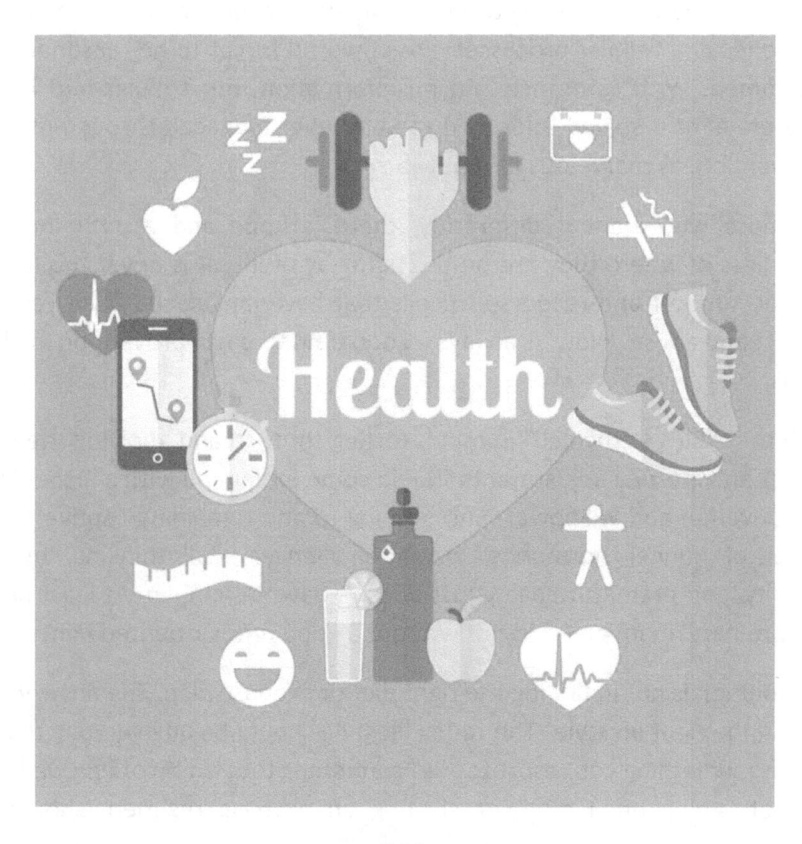

Conclusion & Quick-Start Recommendations

Now that we know these ground rules, we have increased power to change our lives. However, it doesn't promise to solve everything overnight or to eliminate medications over a weekend. These problems were developed slowly over decades of ignorance, misdirection, abusive eating, and failing redox support. Like an onion, they are layered, and it will take time to reset and retrain the metabolic pathways and redox functions.

Fixing this lifestyle and making better choices will, however, begin to make changes in how your redox landscape functions. Begin with the low-hanging fruit. Start with eliminating processed foods and oils, replacing them with better food selections that obey the rules. Eliminate (or seriously cut back at least) carbonated and sweetened beverages and replace with clean pure water. Choose whole fiber-rich foods. Begin to move your body – today. A simple walk will do for starters, some pushups or jumping jacks or burpees will help – and cost nothing. Brush your teeth better and get adequate sleep and fix or support the airway if sleep apnea is happening. Change your stress by talking things out, meditation, prayer, physical activity, and serving others.

The rules that govern your redox landscape allow redox supplementation to work in harmony with proper nutrition and physical activity. It will increase mitochondrial efficiency and promote higher levels of redox signaling and healthy gene expression and metabolic health. Therefore, jump start the redox platform with quality supplements, and begin or increase redox supplementation. The latter holds great power to immediately create that important hormetic redox stimulus which activates pathway genes and is a powerful redox force-multiplier.

All of these solutions are in harmony with the redox landscape and are how cells are designed to function, repair, and renew. They fit and work together bio compatibly and with synergism. When they are working, health is the reward. They are grounded in the rules of the Redoxome.

Conclusion & Quick-Start Recommendations

That is why the discovery of redox signaling molecules and the way they impact the Redoxome, is the most important discovery in health in our lifetime. It operates at the deepest levels of the cell to manage energy metabolism and direct all the business of the cell – precisely at the interface between energy and matter. It is the most exciting new arena and category of health.

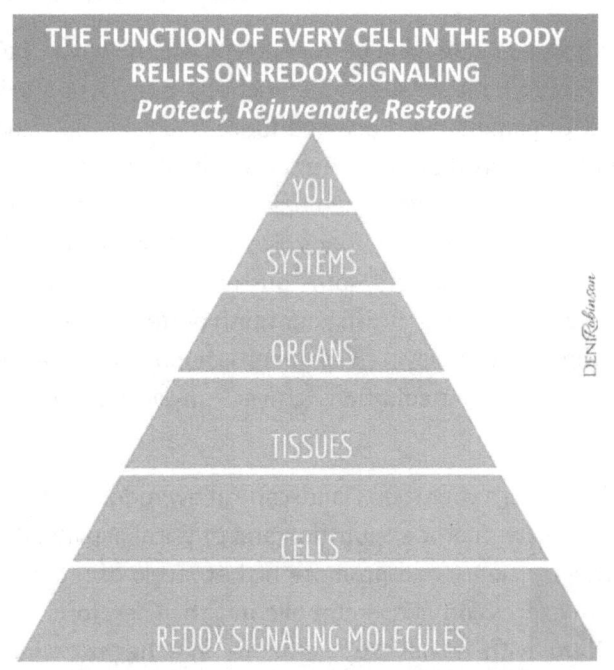

THE FUNCTION OF EVERY CELL IN THE BODY RELIES ON REDOX SIGNALING
Protect, Rejuvenate, Restore

- YOU
- SYSTEMS
- ORGANS
- TISSUES
- CELLS
- REDOX SIGNALING MOLECULES

The grand secret to health, the *modus operandi* and biological mechanism-of-action for how the body stays strong and healthy - even how it senses, detects, interprets, and responds to stress – is based in this redox landscape.

The rules which govern the thousands of interactions in the cell are so profound and foundational that they govern all cellular function. This includes mitochondrial energy metabolism and cellular 'housekeeping' – all of which remain obedient to the rules of redox biology, hormesis, and redox-sensitive gene activation.

While prevention has long been heralded as the answer to long lives with less medical intervention, the science about how cells really work to activate their own defense and repair has been absent – until now. The trial-and-

Conclusion & Quick-Start Recommendations

error methods of the past had very incomplete cellular science grounding because they simply did not have the complete picture of the Redoxome. This explains why yesteryear's explanations for good health through nutrition sounded empty and void of logic.

This information can now be used to your benefit as it informs your daily decisions. This will change how you move, eat, relax, sleep, and care for your liver, mouths, and gut. These rules rule because they are what drive nature's designed health defenses and cellular renewal processes. They keep us healthy and responsive to a changing and challenging world around us.

However, it happens, the goal is to improve redox signaling and to activate cellular processes within the Redoxome which utilize the principles of metabolic flexibility, nutritional ketosis, hormesis, and autophagy - to improve cellular health and function.

Healthy Matters!

Conclusion & Quick-Start Recommendations

Anti-Nutrients

APPENDEX

Anti-Nutrients

A list and description of anti-nutrients include:

Phytic acid

Phytates are inositols containing phosphate groups and are common in the seed of many grains and legumes. They can reach concentrations of 10% in dry matter. They assist in blocking bacterial enzymes from digesting or damaging food while the seeds are in dormancy and awaiting germination, which occurs when they are planted or soaked in water. Their antinutritional effects are related to their ability to chelate or bind to minerals and proteins[390]. As a storage form of phosphate, they are used by the seed during germination. In the human gut phytates complex with calcium, magnesium, copper, iron, and zinc, which inhibits their absorption.

Enzyme inhibitor

Trypsin and amylase inhibitors resist enzyme degradation of proteins and carbohydrates. These often inhibit digestion and places additional stress on the pancreas.

Tannins[391]

Proanthocyanidins or catechins (including tannin acid) is one of the more abundant secondary plant metabolites in the human diet. Condensed tannins include various forms of catechin (EC, EGC, & EGCG). They form strong bonds with proteins and carbohydrates which increases their plant-defense, and gives them antioxidant, anticarcinogenic, detoxification, and health protective properties. Because they can inhibit absorption of dietary minerals (copper, zinc, and iron) they are classified as an 'anti-nutritional'.

Lectins[392,393]

Plant lectins are proteins which bind to carbohydrates and are widely distributed in the plant world. While insignificant amounts exist in fruits and vegetables, legumes and grains contain higher amounts and have drawn the

Anti-Nutrients

most attention there for their 'anti-nutrient' effect. They are resistant to enzymatic digestion in humans and are stable in acidic conditions – a feature that protects lectin-containing plants in nature. Because of their affinity for glycoproteins, they bind to glycan receptors located on cells in the intestinal tract. Due to their strong long-lasting bonds, they are theorized to play a role in autoimmune and inflammatory conditions. They interfere with absorption of minerals (calcium, iron, phosphorus, and zinc), and affect the diversity of intestinal bacteria. These effects cause Lectins to be classified as 'anti-nutritional.' However, they do have beneficial effect in small amounts by providing antioxidant support and by slowing down the digestion and absorption of carbohydrates. The use of non-toxic low amounts have shown useful in stimulating cell growth in the gut and in defending against cellular dysplasia[394]. There are also many studies showing the health benefits from lectin-containing foods (legumes, whole grains, nuts), strongly suggesting the hormetic effects[395] from properly managed and prepared foods with lectin significantly outweigh the potential harm of lectins in these foods. Lectins derived from legumes have considerably more impact than those from grains, but in all cases can be removed from and denatured in foods, by soaking, cooking, and fermentation.

Saponins

Saponins resist microbial infection in plants and have moderate toxicity in human diets in higher concentrations. They disrupt epithelial function, damage red blood cells, and can create digestive issues, inhibit enzymes and thyroid function. Chemically saponins are a steroid or triterpene and as such can interact with lipid molecules in red blood cell membranes leading to their breakdown. They are difficult to remove by soaking or cooking. Nonetheless, saponins contain high antioxidant activity, and in low hormetic doses have shown to activate adaptive response-related signaling pathways to produce cell-protective responses in animal models, whereas high doses produced the opposite hormetic effect[396].

Phenols

Anti-Nutrients

Phenolic and polyphenolic compounds are secondary metabolites widely seen in plants and act as antioxidants and detoxifiers of pro-oxidant metals. They prevent oxidation and DNA damage.

Alpha-galactosides

Otherwise known as "flatulence factors," this galactosides[397] functions as a prebiotic in the food industry and is changed during processing. They are involved during plant and seed development and are beneficial to beneficial gut bacteria (bifidobacterial and lactobacilli) in the human colon. When unaltered through soaking ahead of cooking, they produce a measure of gastrointestinal distress and flatulence as bacteria work harder to digest starches.

Gluten

Gluten is a lectin – one of many in grains. It is often difficult to digest[398] and can cause digestive disorders and allergies in sensitive people. Because it is a lectin it has toxic properties for intestinal cells[399].

Artificial Sugar

Artificial Sugar

Not all sugars are created equal. And that is certainly true of carbohydrates on the simple-to-complex continuum. Other forms of sugar are also worthy of understanding better, owing to their ubiquity and popularity among both consumers and food manufacturers. Artificial sweeteners have occupied a sizeable place in our food marketplace and the lexicon of both the food marketing world and that of ('wannabe') wellness advocates.

Recognizing the inherent dangers in sugar and believing (or wanting to believe) that all would be well if we could use substitutes for sugar and not 'real sugar,' our food industry and society at large began the plunge toward 'anything-but-sugar.' These substitutes include a broad array of artificial sweeteners that have images bigger than life and have been propped up by massive Big Food marketing budgets and product development that appeals to the narrative that "diet this" and "diet that" is somehow healthier than regular sugar. (It's not! But that shouldn't give free license to consume sugar! That misses the point!)

Reducing "sugar" content and substituting artificial sweeteners, shifted the metabolic insult from being that of excessive energy metabolism, to cell toxicity.

Although it was and remains a false dichotomy or argument in the first place and even a 'red herring' distraction from the genuine issues, the notion that artificial sweeteners are somehow safe and harmless is anything but the truth. While there may be less sugar involved that in turn impacts rising blood sugar levels less, the use of artificial sweeteners to maintain sweetness and palatability of food, is anything but healthy. However, it remains a major component of foods and beverages oriented around a "low-calorie" dietary philosophy – believing that most of our health and obesity problems are due to consuming too many calories.

This leads to the packaging of foods and the marketing of ideas that the reason why people are overweight or unhealthy is because they consume too many calories. This runs parallel and strong within the fitness movement

Artificial Sugar

which suggests that more exercise helps burn off excess calories and that one can out-exercise a bad diet and an unhealthy cell.

The extension of this argument is that substituting sugars and reducing calories means not having to burn off as many at the gym. This is the faulty "energy in – energy out" philosophy which cannot address what is really happening in the Redoxome. However, it is very difficult to do combat with powerful forces that have educated multiple generations that "diet" anything is good. It has become very polarizing.

A popular artificial sweetener, aspartame, sits front and center in the great sugar debate. At 4 calories per gram, it is equal to regular sugar, but it is about two hundred times sweeter than sugar. Therefore, the allure is that less is used or needed to obtain the same degree of sweetness in foods or beverages – using a fraction of the calories. While our purposes will not include a detailed analysis of aspartame, and notwithstanding the fact that very early science declared it as safe[400], there are many studies and reports that document and explain its hazards to the brain and the body[401][402] due to its cellular and metabolic toxicity (poison).

While many people have been 'educated' to believe and think that diet sodas are healthier, the evidence says just the opposite. In fact, consumption of sugar-sweetened and artificially sweetened beverages are associated with increased risk of mortality – meaning premature death[403]. Research has shown that it disturbs amino acid metabolism, protein structure and metabolism, integrity of DNA, nerve functions, endocrine hormone balances, and changes in neurotransmitters and stress-hormones (catecholamines)[404]. It disrupts oxidant/antioxidant balance, increases oxidative stress, damages cell membranes, and deregulates cellular function leading to systemic inflammation[405]

Biological Redox Switch

Biological Redox Switch

The body has amazing mechanisms in place to regulate its biology and processes. One that has come to light in recent years is the principle of redox sensitive mechanisms that detect and interpret biological status, and which initiate adaptive responses within cellular functions. These mechanisms are often described as "redox switches[406]."

Notwithstanding that the principles of redox biology are "older than dirt" (literally), it has only been in the last decade that research has identified and explained the pivotal role which redox signaling plays in health and disease. This explains why many health professionals and the public at large are just now learning about the importance of redox signaling and how to improve health and slow down premature aging by enhancing and protecting the level of signaling function in the body.

Most biological redox switches rely on oxidation of sulfur molecules (thiol groups), especially related to cysteine molecules, or 'residues.' The research that has emerged over the last several years has changed our understanding of how cells and biological systems detect and respond to changing conditions in their environment and their biochemical status.

Cellular redox signaling affects the entire cellular redox environment and is the mechanism of action for the multitude of redox-sensitive switches that identify and turn on and off pathway genes that control how our DNA operates.

From a health perspective, cellular dysfunction (and disease) happens when this signaling becomes altered or diminished – a natural consequence of disease and aging. By improving the ability of redox switches to function properly, it is now possible to counterbalance oxidative stress, inflammation, and to guarantee cellular survival in oxidative conditions.

This is the essence of properly functioning health processes (i.e., hormesis, autophagy, and all redox-sensitive mechanisms) which rely on amplified redox signaling and which provide the required mild-oxidative stimulus to maintain and manage a redox-sensitive environment inside the cell. When this becomes diminished with time, aging, and disease, it is necessary to re-

Biological Redox Switch

focus on lifestyle measures and supplementation to restore and stabilize the redox environment. To date, drugs are unable to make this happen because metabolic disease at its most foundational level is not "drugable." The Redoxome, however, is "foodable" and "redox-able" and is very responsive to the manipulation of energy metabolism and the development of metabolic health.

Brain Health and Function

Brain Health and Function

Brain cells are at very high risk for excessive ROS generation and oxidative damage. This is because of their high requirements for oxygen consumption and energy creation. About 20% of total body oxygen consumption and about 25% of all glucose are utilized by brain neurons to maintain brain and cerebral functions[407]. Their vulnerability arises from the large number of redox-active metals, promotion of ROS formation, the higher levels of poly-unsaturated fatty acids (PUFA – which are more sensitive to oxidation), and from less-than-robust levels of antioxidant enzymes such as glutathione and superoxide dismutase[408].

The reduced activity of enzymatic antioxidants glutathione, superoxide dismutase and catalase, and the reduced total antioxidant potential within plasma (i.e., the amount of all antioxidants in the blood), which exists in neurodegenerative brain conditions, helps explain the compromised oxidative stress defense mechanisms known to exist in neurodegenerative disorders. In other words, brain cells are disadvantaged in their ability to mount stress-defense mechanisms and to compensate for oxidative damage that occurs therefrom[409]. Combining the increased levels of oxidation occurring in affected brain cells, and the compromised ability to mount an intra-cellular defense in brain cells and in tandem with decreased antioxidant defense in peripheral tissues, helps explain the early causes of age-related neurodegeneration in affected brains. Furthermore, the progressive deterioration over time is known to be associated with this interplay between oxidative stress, amyloid deposition, and the continuation of inadequately defended inflammation.

Knowing this, lifestyles and strategies that can target this oxidant / antioxidant imbalance and to restore more optimal brain repair and metabolic function, become highly desirable. These strategies, to be congruent with the metabolic and defense pathways of the cell, must of necessity follow the rules of a Redox Lifestyle.

Fats

The beginnings of the movement against fat began in the mid-1900s when studies seemed to show a correlation between high-fat diets and high-cholesterol levels, suggesting that low-fat diets might help reduce cholesterol levels that were correlated with the rising incidence of heart disease and heart attacks. By the 1960s the low-fat approach became the predominant medical and nutrition ideology, promoted by the medical establishment, federal government, and food industry. Even though there was no clear evidence that it actually prevented heart disease or was the independent variable responsible for heart disease and weight gain, it nonetheless became the ruling dogma. Only recently has this prevailing wisdom begun to be challenged - with evidence of an emerging paradigm shift occurring that reflects recent science about fats.

An excellent review of the history of the low-fat ideology was published in 2008, titled "How the Ideology of Low Fat Conquered America[410]. Softening attitudes and recommendations are coming in as better science is emerging which doesn't lump all fat together in the same box. There are good fats and bad fats. All fats exist in nature, and when they are adulterated and processed, they take on completely new properties that are almost always bad in their effect on cellular health.

There is new thinking on fats and how they relate to metabolism, cell cycle, and redox functioning[411]. New research is emerging giving a fresh look at saturated fats and re-analyzing old data in the context of modern-day understandings of metabolic health. They are acknowledging that the last forty years of low-fats have been a "failed experiment, and that the type of fat matters and that healthy fats are necessary and beneficial for health[412].

However, the presence of any suggestion of "high-fat" diet, or even *not* following a low-fat diet strategy, remains entrenched in our society at large, and is almost anathema in the modern world of contemporary medical and nutrition ideology. This has ruffled the feathers of many leading 'authorities' in health, wellness, nutrition, and healthcare, as the ever-present dogma and orthodoxy is in open display villainizing anything high-fat. The ongoing narrative from all of The Bigs, is still squarely in the low-fat camp, which has

Fats

institutionalized processed oils as the mainstay for "health" as they suppose it to be.

Processed seed oils have gained significant popularity and enjoy widespread use given the food industries promotion of them based on questionable science data which early on linked animal and saturated fats with increases in LDL cholesterol (facts that are now being "modified" and updated in current literature). Nonetheless, processed oils have become the mainstay both at home and for commercial food preparation due to their cheap(er) costs and handling characteristics.

The most common fat in our "modern" diet is linoleic acid. This polyunsaturated fatty acid (PUFA) is easily transformed into a number of oxidized metabolites which are linked to a variety of chronic disease conditions such as cardiovascular disease, neurodegenerative disease, liver disease, and even chronic pain. Humans lack the ability to synthesize this fat in their bodies, so any accumulation or presence of this fat must be sourced through food. Cultured cells have shown that exposure with linoleic and linolenic acids increase oxidation in fibroblasts[413] creating a pro-oxidant state. Research has shown that lowering or eliminating linoleic fat in the diet significantly reduces the synthesis and accumulation of oxidized linoleic derivatives in the body[414].

Because these PUFAs are processed oils they enter the bloodstream quickly similar to high glycemic carbohydrates – the ultimate definition of a "fast food!" Processed oils are empty of nutrition, meaning they have no micronutrients and contain zero fiber. They add calories with no nutritional value and in fact drive overeating behavior[415].

Even worse, foods fried in processed oils create carcinogenic and mutagenic aldehydes[416]. Adding insult to injury, these oils experience multiple repeated heating to high temperatures which further degrades the oil itself as well as the oil fumes that are given off – all of which contributes to increased risk for cancer and lung disorders[417].

Tracking information from the late 1800s, daily vegetable oil consumption in the US has risen from zero to 80 grams/day, where 86% of added fats are

Fats

from vegetable oil[418]. Because vegetable oils are "seed oils," they are known as: polyunsaturated vegetable oils, PUFA, edible oils, Om-6 oils, and 'plant oils.' They consist of soybean, corn, canola, cottonseed, rapeseed, grapeseed, sunflower, safflower, and rice bran oils. These oils collectively are the primary sources of Omega-6 Linoleic Acid (LA). (Omega-6 exists in very low levels in saturated fat sources such as coconut oil, butter, palm oil, and lard).

The effect of excess Omega-6 (LA), in combination with a westernized diet and nutrient deficiencies, is highly problematic for metabolic health. The lipid peroxidation cascades which are initiated therefrom affect mitochondrial membrane integrity (cardiolipin – the inner membrane) and create mitochondrial dysfunction by affecting the electron transport chain. This results in a complex array of metabolic problems including reduced fatty acid beta-oxidation, glycolysis reliance, DNA mutations in mitochondria and cellular nucleus, cell death, neurodegeneration, and insulin resistance and fatty liver development.

Because these processes are pro-oxidative, pro-inflammatory, toxic, and nutrient deficient, it leads to metabolic disease. Furthermore, lipid peroxidation from Omega-6 PUFAs (LA) also is cytotoxic, genotoxic, mutagenic, carcinogenic, atherogenic, thrombogenic, and obesogenic.

The takeaway from this emerging information is that it is better to eliminate processed seed oils of every kind, and to utilize natural oils such as olive, avocado, coconut, butter, and lard – in moderation – and always with principles of a metabolic redox lifestyle in play.

Gradually the pendulum is beginning to shift, but not quickly enough for real metabolic health.

Ketosis and Exercise

Ketosis and Exercise

Exercise demands and uses increased amounts fuel to power the increased need for energy during increased physical activity. As such, it is another physiological condition that benefits from metabolic flexibility to better match fuel availability with energy demand.

As we have learned, the first fuel burned is the available glucose, which comes from freely circulating glucose and that which is stored in the form of glycogen. As glucose is utilized and insulin levels drop and glucagon hormones rise, a metabolic shift occurs in the cell to sourcing fatty acids as the next fuel source. As this happens, triglycerides are broken down from adipose storage sites, to provide these free fatty acids.

Hormones play an important role across the landscape of energy signaling. AMP kinase (AMPK) is an enzyme that senses need for energy. It can be pharmacologically activated which simulates the gene activation similar to that seen with exercise. Activation of related metabolic genes have been found to enhance running endurance in mice by 44%[419], showing that exogenous agents have the ability to upregulate gene expression to enhance metabolic adaptation and increase endurance without exercise. This has led to the conclusion that combining exogenous agents which affect fuel preference in the mitochondria potentiates the effect of exercise, at least in mice.

Exercise is healthy precisely because of its effect on mitochondrial efficiency (i.e., the creation of redox molecules), and its effect on decreasing glucose and insulin concentrations, which "flexes" or shifts the cell fuel choice from oxidizing sugars to oxidizing and burning fats.

Exercise training promotes conditioned changes in the epigenome, transcriptome, and proteome of skeletal muscle, all of which increases metabolic flexibility and the cellular autophagic repair which happens following the induced stress from exercise[420].

The noted benefits of a ketosis-induced shift to fat burning, has prompted some to advocate using exogenous ketone supplements to "artificially" manipulate a ketone-like effect and to force a cell to utilize fat as the

Ketosis and Exercise

primary energy source. The use of ketone salts to obtain a state of nutritional ketosis without limiting carbohydrate intake, has met with mixed results. Nonetheless, it proposes an interesting strategy to increase post-exercise glycogen replenishment (glycogen sparing), decreased protein breakdown for energy production, and possibly to modulate metabolic action and signaling messengers[421].

Metabolomics Study – The Supercharging of Krebs

Metabolomics Study – The Supercharging of Krebs

[The following section was published in Redox Matters and is provided here for convenience to show the effect of a novel nutrition ketosis-induction agent which facilitates the metabolically-flexible shift from glucose to fatty acid metabolism in Krebs cycle, independent of food and macronutrient consumption. Note that this information is a critical 'jumping-off point' which massively impacts the new redox science, of how the redox-sensitive state in a cell can be manipulated through replenishment to mimic the effects of fasting, low-carb eating, and exercise while in a 'fed' state. This highlights the principles and supports the observations that a mild hormetic oxidative stimulus within a cell has the power to activate heathy pathway genes, which in turn manage the cellular 'business' of all-things health! This is a critical launch point in understanding the Redoxome and in establishing a healthy redox lifestyle.]

The physiology of Krebs cycle is central to redox metabolism and is of special interest to researchers in the field of metabolomics. Researchers have intently studied the molecules involved in these reactions, their precursors, metabolic rates, by-products, enzymatic activity, and how they cross react with other metabolic pathways. From this they are able to draw conclusions about cellular and molecular biology, metabolism, exercise physiology, and the related effects on diseases and treatments.

Metabolomics is a rapidly emerging field of science employing technology to analyze various cell functions including gene expression, transcription factors and mRNA translation, and cellular metabolites. The established so-called 'omics approaches to this science include genomics, transcriptomics, proteomics, and metabolomics. Each level helps researchers understand cellular biology and how the body responds to both genetic and environmental distress[422].

Metabolites are the 'spoken language' that is the phenotypic and functional display that becomes the physiologic state of an organism[423]. Because metabolites are closely linked to phenotype (gene expression), and give

Metabolomics Study – The Supercharging of Krebs

researchers something straightforward to measure and evaluate, they help us understand how to bridge the gap between genetic programming and genetic expression. Understanding the physiologic shifts that occur with different variables in the redox biology spectrum, leads to new insights in how to manipulate and better manage the physiology related to energy production and the creation of helpful redox signaling.

With our better understanding of the layered responsive states of cellular physiology, an additional "ome" can be added to this picture – one that represents the foundational role that redox biology plays in human physiology. That layer is the *Redoxome*[424].

Admittedly this is a new addition to the field of metabolomic science, albeit the existence and influence of redox biology is as old as cells. The sovereign facts are that nothing expresses, displays, exhibits, or functions (phenotype) without there being 'upstream,' or foundational signaling and direction. Redox signaling as seen through the Redoxome, is the force of nature or *vi naturae* which makes it so.

One of the impressive studies to date for the effect in nature of redox biology, is the redox metabolomics research conducted at the North Carolina Research Institute[425], a collaborative entity involving many university and linked research centers[426]. This investigation was conducted by a research team at the Appalachian State University's Human Performance Laboratory, renowned for its rigorous research into the effects of supplementation on exercise and exertion physiology.

While not identified as such or so named (i.e., "Redoxome") in this specific redox metabolomics study, the focus of this metabolomics study was to measure the effect of influencing the Redoxome on the human system, as measured in the throughput of easily measurable metabolites and metabolomic outputs, as the redox biology was altered.

The study design[427] was of 20 highly fit cyclists randomized into two groups of ten. They were double blinded as to which group received verified redox molecules and which received a control of normal saline suspension (i.e., without bioactive redox molecules).

Metabolomics Study – The Supercharging of Krebs

The objective of the study was to measure the effect of supplemented redox signaling molecules on the Krebs cycle metabolites and to observe any shift in their response or effectiveness due to supplementation. Shifts in these intermediary metabolites would indicate positive or negative effects on human physiology related to inflammation, oxidative stress, and physiologic stress.

In the test phase, the respective samples were consumed for seven days. At the end of this time each group participated in a 75-km cycling trial. Blood was drawn immediately before the trial, immediately after, and one hour after. After a three-week period of time allowing for washout where neither group used redox or placebo, a crossover switch of the research groups took place where again in a double-blinded design the original redox group now drank the placebo, and the original placebo group used redox molecules for seven days. Again, at the end of this second seven-day rest while consuming their respective test samples as before, both groups did the same 75-km cycling trial and blood was drawn as before.

The researchers anticipated that there would be some difference in metabolite shift between the redox and the placebo group following each exercise trial respectively, since most supplements normally generate a degree of shift when exercise is combined with supplements.

However, what was discovered was that the redox group in each part of the trial experienced a significant shift in metabolites prior to exercise – that is, before the exercise portion of the trial even took place. Furthermore, it was found that 43 metabolites shifted, representing about 40% of the total. (As a point of reference, generally in other unrelated trials most supplements studied in similar fashion show shifts in only 10 or 20 metabolites).

Again, the surprising and unexpected results were that these shifts took place before exercise was started, rather than after the exercise. It was not the combination of exercise and redox supplementation that was unique (which is the normal and expected outcome), it was that the shift preceded exercise. These findings proved that redox signaling molecules produce a major shift in metabolites independent of exercise.

Metabolomics Study – The Supercharging of Krebs

Stepping aside to examine the related physiology of these findings introduces a few questions and an expanded discussion about exercise physiology and matters of redox fuel usage in the mitochondria.

- What are Krebs metabolites or Krebs intermediates and what does their shifting and changed expression, mean?
- What causes triglycerides to breakdown and undergo hydrolysis or lipolysis which increases blood levels of free fatty acids?
- How does redox signaling affect the creation of lipase enzymes that create free fatty acids?
- What is the relationship of redox signaling on the presence and effect of catecholamines to stimulate the lipolysis pathway which liberates free fatty acids?

Metabolism is the biochemical processes that occur within a cell that are necessary to maintain life and control cell function. Metabolites are small intermediate, or end-product molecules used in these processes. They are useful in the regulation of the lymphatic system, stem cell function, immune modulation, thermogenesis, and in controlling out-of-control cell division[428]. Lipolytic products resulting from the process of lipolysis (the breakdown of fats/lipids) is increasingly recognized in participating in many cellular signaling processes, including redox signaling and control of oxidation[429].

The physiology of Krebs cycle and how it creates energy and redox molecules is at the center of this science. Recall that mitochondria convert

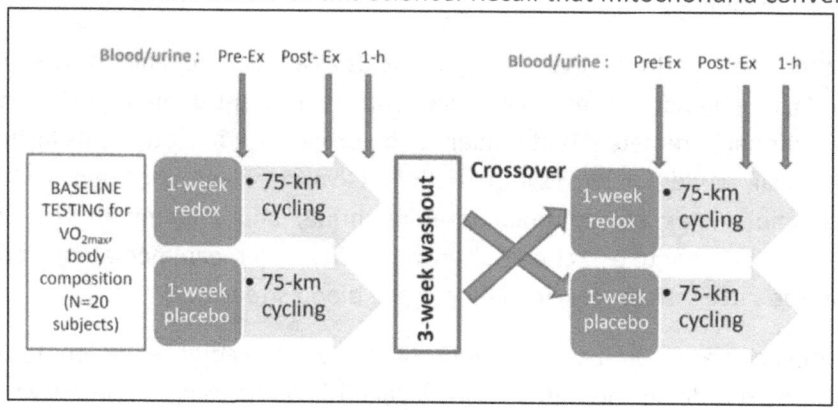

Appalachian State Human Performance Laboratory - Study Design

Metabolomics Study – The Supercharging of Krebs

food and oxygen to generate energy. This food or fuel source is provided via two paths representing carbohydrates and fats, with the 'final' fuel of each path being acetyl-CoA, which then enters Krebs cycle.

Sugars enter this mitochondria-based cycle through the glycolysis breakdown of glucose to create pyruvate, which in turn is converted into acetyl-CoA. Fats are broken down into free fatty acids (lipolysis) which then enter the mitochondria, and then through a reaction called beta-oxidation are converted to acetyl-CoA.

Both of these routes provide the required acetyl-CoA molecule which then enters the electron transport chain's oxidative phosphorylation reactions (oxidation and reduction), which generates ATP energy – along with the necessary ROS by-products useful in redox signaling.

Just as burning wood creates a certain amount of energy which can be measured, so also using food as fuel in the cell creates energy which can be measured. A gram of glucose produces four kilocalories (kcal) of energy and a gram of fatty acids release nine kcal of energy. That means fat has over two times the amount of stored energy as compared to glucose.

However, more critical to this system is the role each plays in providing this energy. The relative mix of glucose or fatty acids as a fuel and energy source is complex physiology. In the glycolysis pathway, glucose and stored glucagon are the fuel source, and lactate is produced as a side product of this reaction.

In the other pathway, the use of fatty acids as a fuel is dependent on states of fasting, gender, disease presence, and the present demand for energy. Additional parameters that influence the preference for fatty acids include physical conditioning, sympathetic activation, and hormones (the catecholamines epinephrine, norepinephrine, and dopamine), the diet consumed prior to exercise or physical activity, and the immediate quantity of free fatty acids freely circulating in the blood stream.

Fatty acids are stored as triglycerides within visceral adipose fat depots and are broken down through a process called lipolysis using lipase enzymes. This lipolysis is largely controlled by the endocrine system. When the need

Metabolomics Study – The Supercharging of Krebs

for energy increases, a cascade of hormone-mediated reactions result in the activation of lipase which hydrolyzes triglycerides to free fatty acids. These FFAs enter the circulation and find their way to other cells where they can be utilized as a fuel source.

At rest, the sympathetic nervous system is calm, and catecholamine (epinephrine) blood levels are low. With an increase of exercise, stress or sympathetic activity, blood levels of epinephrine rise which stimulates lipolysis and elevates serum levels of FFAs.

Both basal metabolic and sympathetic stimulated lipolysis is higher in visceral and mid-body adipose depots than subcutaneous fat. Notwithstanding that visceral adipose is more insulin resistant it is more sensitive to hormone stimulation and modulation.

The effect of this lipolysis is an increased release of free fatty acids into the blood stream. Whether the fatty acids elevation comes from lipolysis or from reduced ability to clear high fats in the blood stream following eating, the net effect is the same – elevated serum levels of FFA. This elevation makes more FFAs available as a fuel source in Krebs cycle.

There is an interesting crosstalk relationship between the glycolysis and lipolysis pathways. The formation of lactate from the glycolysis path, inhibits lipolysis[430]. However, increases in circulating FFA levels decrease the oxidation of pyruvate, the primary molecule of the glycolysis path, apparently helping to explain the shift in fuel source as fatty acids are liberated and more are made available to heart and skeletal muscles[431]. This shift from glycolysis to fatty acid oxidation decreases lactate levels in the cell.

On a negative note, an oversupply of FFAs in the absence of a demand for using the energy generated, creates an adaptive increase in beta oxidation which leads to incomplete oxidation of fatty acids, which in turn increases oxidation and redox pressure within the cell to increase the production of reactive oxygen species and oxidative stress, insulin resistance and cell damage[432]. This would seem to suggest that improvements in physical activity (which would increase the demand for energy generation) would

Metabolomics Study – The Supercharging of Krebs

pair well with any strategy that increases fatty acid release, whether pharmaceutical based or lifestyle/supplement based.

As noted previously, lipolysis requires the activity of lipase (i.e., adipose triglyceride lipase – ATGL). This plays an important role in the release of fatty acids from intracellular adipose and which activates peroxisome receptors[433], which in turn create peroxisomal redox signaling that regulates both lipolysis and reactive oxygen species. This introduces another redox-sensitive control mechanism to help balance oxidative stress within the cell.

Making practical application of this information to everyday life yields interesting assumptions and conclusions. Connecting this string of exercise and metabolic physiology together, shows the absolute complexity and redox sensitive responsiveness the body exhibits. Alterations anywhere along these multiple paths can exert deleterious effects, whereas enhancements yield a state of health and vigor unavailable any other way.

In skeletal muscle the uptake of glucose increases during exercise up to about sixty to ninety minutes, then gradually shifts to free fatty acids as their concentrations in the blood increase and mitochondria burn more fatty acids and less glucose[434]. With increasing duration of exercise, glucose utilization in muscle declines - creating an increased dependency on FFAs for energy metabolism. Therefore, after prolonged exercise FFA uptake increases and FFAs become the predominant fuel being used.

This means that as a general rule in normal situations (i.e., minus the introduction of redox signaling supplementation) during prolonged exercise, triglycerides are converted into free fatty acids and released into the circulation providing the primary fuel for working muscles. These principles of exercise physiology led to reduction in triglyceride levels (adipose tissue mass) and improved metabolism, insulin signaling, and overall health through its effect on mitochondrial function[435].

Returning now to the specific Redox Metabolomic Study it was found that when signaling molecules are supplemented there is a shift in Krebs cycle metabolites. This shift increased the quantity of FFAs in blood and led to the preferential oxidation of FFAs over glucose/pyruvate. This leads to

Metabolomics Study – The Supercharging of Krebs

reduction of lactate accumulations and the concept of glucose/glycogen sparing metabolism – a feature very appealing to athletes and others experiencing exercise or exertion fatigue. Also found was a corresponding elevation in glycerol levels, which is an evidence marker of extensive triglyceride metabolism (hydrolysis).

These metabolomic shifts are significant. The brain, muscles, and body tissues need a steady and predictable fuel with which to make energy. Except for heart muscle cells (cardiomyocytes) the first fuel generally used is glucose/glycogen through the glycolysis pathway. Then, when reduced or depleted, the body shifts to fatty acids that are stored in adipose cells and made available during this process.

These laboratory findings suggest and confirm that redox supplementation elevates serum FFA levels ahead of exercise demand and can become the preferred fuel even during rest.

The finding that redox supplementation can shift Krebs cycle in the mitochondria of all cells (except brain neurons) to prefer energy-dense fatty acids first, is important. This is highly impactful in cellular physiology because it manipulates the very core or foundation level of cellular function, energy production, and many downstream benefits including lipolytic fat-signaling. This suggests and explains that enhancing redox biology is nature's method for reducing adipose and triglyceride levels.

In some fashion yet to be understood completely, redox signaling replenishment facilitates these significant metabolomic shifts. In recognizing the various co-factors that play together in these pathways, the future research will be eagerly anticipated to elucidate and sort out the precise mechanisms-of-action whereby enhanced redox signaling facilitates these outcomes.

In summary the findings of this study reveal:

- Fatty acid levels increased in the blood prior to exercise.
- Increased fatty acid oxidation and mobilization prior to and during exercise. For the placebo group this occurred later.

Metabolomics Study – The Supercharging of Krebs

- Extensive adipose breakdown (triglyceride hydrolysis) and increased free fatty acids.
- Higher blood levels of free fatty acids linked to sparing of amino acid breakdown and increased Krebs cycle intermediates, post-exercise.
- Muscle glycogen sparing due to less inhibition of fatty acid oxidation.
- Redox supplementation produced higher levels of ascorbic acid (antioxidant) and lowered fructose levels.
- Less lactic acid / lactic acidosis (lactate).
- Reduced triglyceride levels.

The grounding thesis for this science (and this book) is that it is the Redoxome that has foundational influence over how DNA, proteins, and metabolites express and are utilized in the body – for better or for worse. This study on metabolomics further establishes that enhancing the 'Redoxome' – the basic foundational redox biology of the human body – can have profound effects on human health.

Nutrition Philosophy and Science

Nutrition Philosophy and Science

In Part One of this book, we presented various nutritional philosophies and schools of dietary advice. There are so many different nutritional philosophies and ideologies in the medical science, pop culture, wellness, and nutrition science space, that it is mind boggling!

Each dietary strategy has its advocates and critics. The common person has to wonder, if there is a difference between them, does it really matter? If it does, then what is the difference between them? If it truly is about health, then what is the best dietary strategy for creating and maintaining wellness?

In addition to a similar list presented in Part One, the following list is another sampling of an internet search for "nutritional philosophies." This extenuation of the discussion will show the width, depth, shallowness, differences, and sometimes erring concepts and advice that is readily present on the internet. Consider this analysis as an 'informed opinion' piece by the author with some incisive commentary from his analysis of the source materials and studies. The objective here is to be argumentative for that sake alone, but to demonstrate the wide variability of scientific evidence and available advice - all of which is highly determined by the interests of the vested parties and ideologies represented.

The point is that with a better understanding of the nature of a redox lifestyle and diet, the following morsels of advice can be accurately evaluated and adjudicated as to their merits or lack thereof. To that end, as this section is read, compare the recommendations and 'findings' with a reserved and enlightened yet critical "redox" mind.

As you read, remember that this is a sampling of leading recommendations from popular and 'authoritative' sources, and consider if this is all you had to go on, how deficient it would be.

Five key factors that make a healthful diet[436]:

- An adequate diet
- A balanced diet
- Calorie control

Nutrition Philosophy and Science

- Moderation
- Variety

Five key principles of nutrition[437]:

- Water is your friend
- Ban Processed foods
- Less is more
- Eat a well-balanced breakfast
- Add fruit or veggies to your meals

Three principles of good health[438]:

- Understand food
- Listen to your body
- Understand health as a whole

Ten principles of nutrition[439]:

- Avoid added sugar
- Avoid processed foods
- Eat only when hungry
- Drink water, tea, and coffee
- Eat veggies at every meal
- Eat real food
- Prepare food yourself
- Know difference between good and bad fats
- Choose your fuel based on your objectives
- Eat mindfully

USDA MyPlate[440]:

- Eat fruit at breakfast; focus on whole fruit
- Eat a variety of vegetables
- Make half of grains whole grains (includes whole grain puffs and flakes / cold cereal)
- Vary protein
- Beverages – less added sugar, saturated fat, and sodium
- Eat low-fat and fat-free dairy, including soy

Dietary Guidelines for Americans[441]:

Nutrition Philosophy and Science

- Discourages supplementation; recommends that nutrient needs be met from eating a variety of foods and beverages, except during pregnancy or with certain medical conditions.

United Nations Food and Agriculture Organization[442]

- Healthy eating pattern includes:
    - Variety of vegetables
    - Fruits, especially whole fruits
    - Grains, at least half are whole grains
    - Eat fat-free or low-fat
    - Variety of protein
    - Oils
- Healthy eating pattern limits:
    - Saturated fats and trans fats
    - Added sugars and sodium
    - Alcohol in moderation

Physicians Committee – Dietary Guidelines Recommendations[443]:

- Eat plant-based diets
- Eliminate low-carb diets
- Eliminate dairy
- Eliminate processed meat
- Eliminate saturated fat
- Do not include a low carbohydrate eating pattern or recommend limiting consumption of carbohydrates

Granted that all of this advice and the sources where it originates from, is well-intended and contains many dietary truths. However, taken together this sampling of mainstream advice contains many contradictions, inconsistencies, and incomplete overviews of what is claimed to be good nutrition – <u>especially as viewed through the lens of metabolic health and a redox lifestyle</u>.

Nevertheless, this cross-section of real-world nutritional guidance evidences the commonly available advice available to consumers and to health and nutrition specialists across the marketplace. While some may dive deeper into the subtext, most will lightly hover over it and take their

Nutrition Philosophy and Science

advice from the headlines and boldest print or infographics. Few think to question it deeper and to read the fine print, or even between the lines, to search out the truths, half-truths, misinformation, and disinformation. Even fewer will research the vesting interests which sponsor the representative ideologies behind the scenes.

Providing further analysis, note that within the last set of recommendations (Physicians Committee), this esteemed committee categorically advocates against low-carb diets, claiming that they are linked to consuming too few fruits, vegetables, grains, and legumes. Several studies are cited in their source materials, linking low carbs with death from diabetes, stroke, and heart disease. They also assert that low-carb diets which are high in animal protein and fat are linked to type 2 diabetes, insulin resistance, weight gain, atrial fibrillation, and heart disease. However, the studies cited within their sources to validate the claims against low-carb diets, make the case for "high fat" (the same as low-carb) using "high-protein," not "high-fat." There is a significant difference between a "low-carb high-protein" diet, and a "low-carb high-fat" diet. It is disingenuous to call out a "high fat" diet when protein (not fat) was the focus of the study which constituted the "low-carb" study design, and thereafter the "low-carb" scorn.

Specifically, the diabetes connection cites a study[444] that identifies low-carb diets (that are connected with disease) as being low-carb and high animal protein (actually red meat and processed meats) – yet the study conclusions identified "low-carb" as to imply "high fat" when it was truthfully a "low carb – high protein" diet that was evaluated. This is also different from a 'ketogenic diet ("low-carb and low-to-moderate protein and high fat") which is metabolically energy- friendly.

(If that is confusing, just realize that it is critical in study design that the conclusions are consistent with the variables actually studied and assumptions are not 'reached' to include what cannot be concluded. That is significant in this and many other similar studies which attempt to justify high-carbohydrate diets, processed oils, and more, as being healthy – especially when there was little investigation into the innerworkings of

Nutrition Philosophy and Science

cellular function or redox-related functionality. We may be inclined to give them a minor pass since the Redoxome is a more recent scientific discovery.)

Furthermore, it was noted that this did not affect women, but it did men – yet the conclusion broad-brushed the recommendation to imply the same effect for everyone across the board.

They also cite evidence that low-carb diets lead to higher risk for early death. They conclude that fiber-rich carbohydrates should provide most of the calories in a healthy diet and be the main fuel for brain and muscle (which by the way wholly omits the positive effects that ketone bodies from fat metabolism, have on brain cells). They also state that three-fourths of the daily calories source should come from carbohydrates in the form of fruits, vegetables, grains, and legumes – "which help prevent and reverse the risk of heart disease, type 2 diabetes, and obesity" – leaving unchallenged the assumption that a low-carb diet cannot by definition include fiber-rich vegetables and fruits that will also accomplish the same end points (protect the liver and feed the gut).

Another linked study, given as an authoritative source and published by the European Society of Cardiology[445], discusses the controversial nature of low-carb diets while acknowledging controversial results in previous studies. While discussing the links between low-carb diets and all-cause death, they likewise perpetuate the same confusion that defines all low-carb diets as being associated with increased death and disease – without any discussion of the important metabolic variables that dictate energy metabolism, or even acknowledging that there is no absolute equivalency between low-carb diets and low fruits/vegetable consumption. These broad-brush misunderstandings ignore the true connection of dietary source/type with metabolic disease, as well as that low-carb diets are not advocated or wise for 24/7/365 execution (one must cycle in and out of ketosis to be better adapted), as well as that low-carb diets can very well include rich amounts of phytochemicals, fiber, and healthy fat – at the same time.

The point is that half-truths and incomplete study design assumptions lead to less than accurate findings. The categorical conclusions that low-carb

Nutrition Philosophy and Science

diets lead to higher all-cause mortality, leaves out many vital pieces of information.

The ubiquitous problems in research and nutrition guidance are that there is obfuscation in what constitutes a "carbohydrate." There is also little if any consideration for the effect which different types of carbs have on the gut, liver cells, and mitochondria (or if they include fiber-rich or fiber-poor sources and types). To say that carbohydrate metabolism is the main fuel for brain and muscles[446] is only half the truth, because it clearly is not the best fuel, nor does it come at the cleanest healthiest benefit for peak cellular function. Other problems are that they assume a steady-state diet and that there is no benefit from cycling in and out of ketosis, ignoring the mounting data showing the benefit from fasting, ketosis, and autophagy.

The point is that not all carbs are created equal, yet the majority of studies and expert opinion seems to lump them all together. (Similar argument for all-things "fat.") Again, the implications drawn are that those eating low-carb diets are not getting adequate fruits and vegetables (assumes that a "low-carb" diet doesn't include complex phytochemical-based vegetables and fruits), and that those who do eat high carb diets, are.

They hold to these standards even while acknowledging that low-carb diets have great effect for weight loss, lowered blood pressure and improved blood glucose control[447]. Nonetheless, they insist that long-term low-carb continuance (implying it is 24/7/365) results in increased all-cause mortality from cancer, hypertension, diabetes, and cancer[448], completely overlooking the wisdom of "flexibility" between energy sources (ketosis cycling).

In the study previously cited[449], it should be noted that the results of the study are drawn out over 20 years in a prospective study design, done with periodic multi-year check-ins and assessments asking participants to declare their typical eating patterns. There are obvious (to me) questions that arise about a study designed to examine eating habits and practices of a fixed population group over a twenty-year time period (prospective). Factors of metabolic function and nutritional ketosis involve not just food, but eating practices such as fasting, liver cell health, gut health and function, added sugar and the amount of processed and fast foods in the diets – perhaps

Nutrition Philosophy and Science

different with each person – and again, over twenty years of variability, and collecting data in a rather subjective survey form. Notwithstanding these study weaknesses, great and impactful conclusions and recommendations are proffered from the information.

Continuing ... the notable and questionable correlations in the study paired the low-carb diet with having high levels of animal protein (again, not fat consumption), specifically "red and processed meat," and acknowledged that the "reduced intake of fiber and fruits and increased intake of animal protein, cholesterol, and saturated fat with these diets may play a role. Differences in minerals, vitamins, and phytochemicals might also be involved," they report. There was no indication given that attention was given to the metabolic nutrition factors that impact redox and cellular health (admittedly and to be fair minded, to the latter point perhaps when this study was performed this information was absent in the science landscape, or at least less known in the literature).

As an example of one of the assumptions, the question should be asked: is it possible to have a low-carb diet that contains no refined carbohydrates, and still has high amounts of phytochemicals, minerals, and vitamins, and is fiber-rich? These variables are not discussed or calculated within this, or the bulk of studies referred to which address the pros and cons of low-carb diets. Yet they are categorically lumped together without differentiating the important differences of carbohydrate type, the impact of refined carbohydrates and processed oils, and low-fat energy metabolism on the metabolic energy demands of cells, and their combined effect on redox status – to say nothing of the time-impact of eating as it relates to energy metabolism and glucose/insulin levels and ketosis and metabolic flexibility.

These 'authoritative' and often (out)dated studies are utilized over and over as proof that low carb 'anything' is dangerous. Yet while discussing the very metabolic diseases they rail against, they overlook or at least diminish cell-based laws related to redox cellular function and energy metabolism, let alone make little or no mention of the impact of processed foods, oils, and sugared beverages. They give poor attention or credit to the effect of food type, source, quality, and timing of eating – and how all that relates to redox-sensitive antioxidant protection and cellular repair mechanisms. Additionally, they disregard how excess carbs (which are seldom if ever quantified) contribute to triglyceride storage, liver health and gut dysbiosis, or the role of the liver in *de novo* lipogenesis from liver toxins such as fructose.

What is often missing in these discussions is the impact of refined carbohydrates. This is about what is done TO the food, not necessarily what type it is. Without this vital additional information and understanding and without consideration of these many variables, the conclusions are suspect at best. Following a blanket recommendation for carbohydrate-centric diets (assuming that means there are more vegetables eaten, if even then...), leaves a multitude of metabolic and redox related variables out of the picture.

Another witness to the shortsightedness in the language of these standards, and often ill-informed recommendations, is the standard advice to "let half of carbs be whole-grain." This is good advice if 100% of one's diet are refined processed grains! Eating half that amount would obviously be better than all of it being refined.

Saying that "half" should be "whole," leaves open the permission to let refined processed grains constitute the other half of one's carbohydrate consumption. And even then, it ignores the effect of the remaining refined "half" upon energy metabolism, and altogether omits the impact of the timing of consumption and the "rules" which dictate when, how, or if fats are oxidized in the energy equation. Additionally, it overlooks the effects of, or the percentage of calories obtained from this piece of the 'carbohydrate pie.' Seldom in any of the authoritative guidelines is any consideration given to the multitude of nuances with low-carb diets as it relates to processed and refined grains. And completely missing in most studies and recommendations is the impact of processed seed oils on cellular function.

Rather than "half," why not say "all?" That's what the science would dictate. People will naturally compromise from that mark downward, but if the starting goal is 50%, it feeds the permission to have at least half the carbohydrates as refined – no better than eating pop-tarts as the breakfast entre!

Granted, that at the epidemiological and public health level, many of these advisory standards are a considerable improvement for some people. But it would be refreshing if that were acknowledged and factored into the research designs and conclusions. Even that would elevate the quality of these studies by acknowledging the limitations of the research and openly declaring the assumptions upon with their conclusions are actually based. Even better would be to repeat these nutrition trials with the cellular rules of metabolic health and redox signaling firmly in place.

The point of this drawn-out commentary is to emphasize the lack of focus on metabolic rules and mechanisms. The focus is on symptoms of metabolic disease (which can evolve to be diseases themselves) but which are managed with medical intervention. Beginning with faulty or partially faulty assumptions along with dated science, often leads to conclusions that are not congruent, are often self-serving, and cater unwisely to interest groups. Perhaps current redox-oriented science of the next research era may help undo the entrenched conclusions and recommendations that have been chiseled into the granite rock of "Mount Nutrition."

To conclude, the point is that the 'polished' advice (admittedly for 'general' consumption) too-often offers ill-informed and usually ignorant arguments as they relate to the true effect which various foods have on cellular metabolic function. There are many types, combinations, ratios, consumption timing consideration, and cooking methods that make up and affect the quality and effect of food as it plays on the redox landscape. As such, many of the presenting arguments and guidelines are shallow and even 'red herring distractions' which simply confuse and create philosophical silos that do not serve individual redox health.

Processed Food

Processed Food

Processed foods are scientifically engineered to be irresistible and easy to consume large quantities. If you can't "eat just one" then they are doing their job!

The "stimuli stacking" formula for creating super appetizing food is to make it calorie dense, strongly flavored, convenient, quick-to-hit-the-taste-buds, and easy-to-eat and irresistibly overconsume. The more of these traits that can be stacked into a food, the better! Junk food is designed to make us respond with compulsiveness.

Given that processing food in today's modern era is a certain necessity in order for supply chains to be full, and vast populations to be fed (since they are not living on the farm any longer), let's take a deeper look.

There are a variety of processing methods and food science ingredients that are added to extend its shelf life, improve its color, make it more resistant to oxidation and rancidity, enhance its taste, make it easier to eat, and so much more. Here are some examples:

Extrusion is the process of milling grains and processing them into a watery slurry. This is then passed with high heat and pressure through a machine called an extruder. This transforms whole grains into an air-filled mash which can be formed into a variety of uniform shapes and made into cereals, crackers, and baked into crispy nuggets or flakes and combined with other crunchy 'foods.' Along the way many chemicals are added which affect its consistency, taste, texture, color, stability, and handling characteristics.

Through the extrusion process, it changes texture, affects digestibility, and destroys many nutrients and enzymes that were in the original source food. Starch composition is changed, and natural fiber is removed. Fats and proteins are also damaged and denatured. All of this affects the nutritional value so much that vitamins and minerals and fiber are needed to be added to "enrich" the product.

Emulsifiers are used to improve the feel of the food when chewed. They smooth and thicken and are responsible for creating a rich smooth feel

Processed Food

when in the mouth. While natural emulsifiers like egg yolk can be used, the food industry often uses chemicals such as Polysorbate-80, sodium phosphate, and carboxymethylcellulose.

Flavor enhancers are widely used. These artificial agents intensify taste without adding "real food" value such as fruits, vegetables, or spices. These include monosodium glutamate (MSG) which is a potent neurotoxin affecting the brain (hippocampus) which activates neurodegenerative pathways[450]. MSG gives a special aroma to processed food, and is linked with obesity, metabolic disorders, neurotoxicity, and reproductive problems. They release glutamic metabolites which act on glutamate receptors and disrupt neurons and have been implicated in behavioral – at even the lowest of doses. Because it increases palatability of food, it disrupts energy balance and disturbs the leptin-mediated hypothalamus signaling cascade. However, none of this fits the narrative of the public media supporting Big Food, as is witnessed with examples of "fact checks" from USA Today which defend its use[451].

Coloring agents are used to increase food appeal. Agents such as Yellow #5 (tartrazine) and Red #40 (allura red) are added for the look of food and add zero nutritional quality. They do, however, provide a toxic effect on the liver causing hepatic cell damage by increasing lipid peroxidation and decreasing antioxidant enzyme activity[452] such as superoxide dismutase, catalase, glutathione, and elevation of alkaline phosphatase (ALP) which is a liver enzyme associated with liver damage and bone disorders.

Oil hydrogenation renders fats more stable by adding hydrogen atoms, so they are less vulnerable to the effects of oxidation. This increases shelf life without changing taste or texture and other properties of the food.

Processed food manufactures "trick" us into eating more because of the pervasive Big Media marketing efforts to "educate" us that processed foods are "healthy." They come packaged with buzz words such as *organic, vegan,* and *gluten-free*. Chips and cereals prepared with avocado oil, which are baked not fried, that contain flaxseeds, or which contain real vegetables, or have real fruit in them. Their marketing appeals to self-care about your

Processed Food

deserve level or needing time away with a good food and friend, or a healthy soda beverage – "you deserve a break today."

In fact, the slick marketing took on a new pale when Coca-Cola partnered with the National Heart, Lung, and Blood Institute and other snack makers to join "The Heart Truth Campaign"[453], extolling the virtues of Coca-Cola products as heart healthy[454].

The *#ShowYourHeart* hashtag handle will lead you to this marketing campaign war which was waged not in the interests of heart health, but on the minds of a population wanting to justify their use of a beverage with zero nutritional value – notwithstanding the "diet" branding. In fact, diet beverages sweetened with artificial sweeteners, are worse than regular sweetened beverages in their effect on heart attacks and strokes, blood pressure and visceral obesity. They also have a 36% higher risk of metabolic disease and a 67% greater risk for developing diabetes[455]. Those believing that "diet" is where it is at, should ponder that!

We also eat more because of packaging and the serving of big portions plays a trick on our mind that we are getting better value. Waste not, want not! Buy more for less. Endless refills. All-you-can-eat. Fries with that hamburger. This creates confusion about the value of food, and its appeal to satiety and food security. However, this value conundrum poses a "health tax" as more unsuspecting people eat low-nutrient, over-processed, and energy-dense "foods" – purposefully designed to cause us to eat more of it and carry more of it around on us for years to come.

The "eat-more" strategies are also boosted with more varieties and flavors – meaning the more of each there are, the more we can't stop! The sweetness of sugar, fat's smooth texture, and the stimulating effect of salt combined with flavor enhancers, blend to create a non-stop selection of candies, chips, pastries, frozen confections, and almost every item in the frozen food, chips and crackers, and bakery sections of the grocery store. Their stacked-stimuli effect creates hyper-palatable food that is simply and overwhelmingly seductive.

Processed Food

One might mistake or dismiss the irony of Big Food's marketing campaign if it wasn't such a catastrophic move on the health of a willfully ignorant public. Notwithstanding the superficial and seemingly justifiable position of needing processed food to provide for a growing population, the direction processed food is going from a metabolic health perspective, is not good.

Redox Detoxification

Redox Detoxification

Redox biology and cellular detoxification are inexorably related. The word "toxicity" generally refers to the effect an outside or exogenous substance has on the body. The degree of toxicity is determined by the relative damage done to an organism. Cytotoxicity specifically refers to the effects of toxicity on cell function and metabolic pathways.

In a broader and more fundamental sense, cell toxicity refers to dysfunction at the cellular level. This does not necessarily require an outside agent to induce toxicity, as any dysfunction within a cell and its functional processes can result in a state where oxidation and inflammation are elevated. This dysfunction allows metabolic "toxins" as well as outside elements (such as metals, xenobiotics, etc.) to accumulate. This occurs as the detoxification pathways which are related to metabolic pathways (such as the folic acid cycle, methionine cycle, and transsulfuration cycle) become impaired in their ability to methylate and properly detoxify cells of toxic agents that are not present in a state of health.

Absent overt poisoning via outside sources, inefficient elimination at the cellular level and the organ level (i.e., liver and kidney function) allow for gradual accumulation of harmful agents and conditions in the body. Inefficiency or inability to remove toxicity and toxic conditions and processes places greater stress on cells.

In popular use are many methods and means aimed at detoxifying and removing from cells and the body general, toxic agents, and situations. Generally, these are seen in the form of herbal remedies, often combined with strategies that assist elimination through improved bowel function, fasting, nutritional supplements, sauna, liver cleanses, etc.

All remedies, strategies, tonics, and 'treatments' per se, have as the intended result to improve cell function and to thereby cleanse or detoxify cells, and to efficiently remove them from the body via sweat, urine, and fecal elimination. Often during these healing processes and procedures - as cleansing and detoxification proceed and as the body works to awaken detox pathways and eliminate waste products that have accumulated over

Redox Detoxification

time - the 'awakened' cellular processes begin to detox faster than the body can properly manage.

The common pathways that enable detoxification, and by definition which create toxification through their dysfunction, are intricately related to the redox signaling mechanisms that control pathway genes, which in turn activate antioxidant and anti-inflammatory pathways. Any degree of inefficiency in these pathways – directly or at their 'headwaters' – will decrease the cell's ability to efficiently detoxify and eliminate cellular waste and environmental toxins. Likewise, any and all methods that improve cellular homeostasis and enable detoxification, are redox controlled pathways.

Thus, improving the redox state is axiomatic and central to detoxification. Indeed, detox happens if/when redox pathways are normalized and functional.

Glutathione and metallothionine are both sulfur-rich proteins synthesized from cysteine in the transsulfuration pathway and play an especially important role in detoxification. These Sulphur moieties convey increased detoxification ability to them within the body.

The Nrf2 antioxidant gene pathway is responsible for initiating the production of these molecules Glutathione and these other cysteine conjugates, play important roles in detoxification and in protecting against toxicity and disease[456].

While properly not speaking to every person's situation, some errantly assume that because they feel worse through the detox process (regardless of how the detox comes about or is engaged), that their chosen detox strategy is making them "sicker." However, these reactions are signs that the detox process is working in a positive way to help the cells and the body cleanse itself of impurities, toxins, metals, and foreign agents. As cellular function improves and normalcy returns, these reactions naturally begin to dissipate.

This healing process is a basic part of redox biology. It is a sign that cells are beginning to regain function and efficiency. By "taking out the garbage"

Redox Detoxification

through the various elimination channels, the body is resetting itself. Proper hydration during this period of time is important, as this is the fluid medium that helps to efficiently remove toxins (that are made water soluble in the liver), and that have been processed and mobilized and targeted for elimination.

Those with genetically based metabolic pathway disorders (such as MTHFR), or who have gut dysbiosis, may find more difficulty through these detoxification steps. Specific protocols have been developed for hyper-challenged individuals to help them with "work-arounds" and cellular assistance during these processes and are best guided by knowledgeable health providers to assist in removal of heavy metals and in supporting overall detoxification and gut health. Others may require an added dose of patience and perseverance while the body works its way into and through the detox process.

It is also reasonable to titrate the detoxification process. Chronic illness and a toxic state do not happen quickly; neither does detoxification. Slowing down or adjusting the detox challenge by reducing the intensity of the chosen strategy, or by increasing the time variable, or by persisting longer, may be helpful through the detox process. Adjunctively supporting the cells through allied strategies such as hydration, supplementation, improved sleep, stress reduction, lymphatic massage, and proper nutrition, are always wise.

To the point of gastrointestinal health, part of the detoxification process revolves around the processes of altered guy dysbiosis. As the balance of the gut microflora shift from unhealthy organisms to health-dominated, a certain degree of GI upset may be experienced, which may also translate into overall wellbeing or lack thereof.

The end result is to reset cellular function through improvements in redox controlled detoxification pathways, ultimately to create a better cellular state that does not accumulate toxins and responds as designed to environmental and metabolic stressors. Working With Physicians and Healthcare Providers

Redox Detoxification

In 'traditional healthcare' the paradigm or worldview largely revolves around making a diagnosis and finding a medication or procedure that matches with the diagnosis. Accordingly, almost every individual of medical necessity develops a relationship with a pharmacy, the result of which is a growing dependency on pharmaceutical remedies and medications needed to resolve the complaints and medical issues one has. Thankfully, these necessary interventions restore a sense of well-being and function that otherwise may not be possible.

Prescription medications (as well as herbal remedies) are prescribed and dosed for the effect they can have on disease processes and basic physiology. The dosing considers age, body weight, type and severity of disease, side-effects, and drug interactions with other medications also being taken.

Improvements in overall health that can arise from improving disease states, improved lifestyle (exercise, diet, sleep, and stress management), dietary supplements, redox replenishment, and Nrf2 and EGR1 guided gene-expression activators, can have an effect on the use of and need for taking medicines. Accordingly, it is important to not change or alter their use without proper supervision from your prescribing physicians and health professionals.

Having said that, if and as health improvements are qualitatively and quantitatively realized, it may be prudent to discuss this with your supervising health professional(s) to determine if adjustments in required medications are appropriate.

It is important to realize that as cellular health improves it may lessen the need for medical interventions such as prescribed medications. There are many factors, variables and considerations at play including the degree of health compromise, genetic status, and lifestyle variables. These must be all considered together and discussed with a competent health professional in determining the wisdom and/or rate at which any adjustments – if any – are made in existing pharmacologic interventions.

Redox Detoxification

It is important to NOT reduce or delete medications without first consulting with the prescribing provider, who would then determine suitability and best method for doing so, if at all.

With this said, if you want to change the conversation you have with your prescribing health providers, begin a redox lifestyle!

About the Author

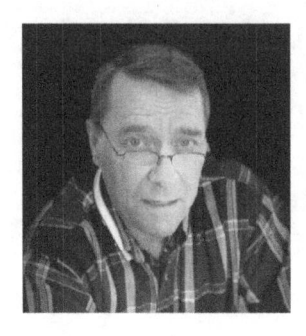

Dr. Lee Ostler graduated with a bachelor's degree in Biology/Zoology with emphasis in biochemistry and physiology from Brigham Young University and earned his Doctor of Dental Surgery degree from the University of Washington School of Dentistry. His general dental practice has an emphasis on advanced cosmetic dentistry, bite rehabilitation, periodontal and oral-systemic health management, dental sleep medicine, and TMJ and craniomandibular therapy.

He received advanced training at the Las Vegas Institute for Advanced Dental Studies, has been a clinical instructor with LVI in Las Vegas, and at the LVI Continuums held at Baylor University and the University of Kentucky dental schools. He is currently a clinical and didactic lecturer at Pacific Northwest University of Health Sciences College of Osteopathic Medicine.

He is a founding member, past president and board member, and advisory council member of the American Academy for Oral Systemic Health, an international organization focusing on co-management of oral-systemic healthcare for health professionals.

He founded and operated an education and consulting company teaching health professionals the science and practice of oral-systemic health principles. He has presented and lectured to health professionals on principles of cosmetic dentistry, TMJ and craniomandibular treatment, oral-systemic health, and redox biology health applications.

He is founder and program chair for the Eastern Washington Medical Dental Summit, an annual gathering of physicians, dentists, and allied health professionals. He is author of Redox Matters: Connecting the Dots Between Redox Biology and Health, along with several books that focus on the co-management of patients relative to varied specialty areas of oral health including, oral-systemic health, TMJ disorders, obstructive sleep apnea, and biologic dentistry. He maintains websites and participates in webcasts that relate to the science and utility of redox biology and its impact on oral and general health.

Most important of all, he adores his family – five children and 20 grandchildren.

Books by Dr. Lee Ostler:

Redox Matters

Redox Matters chronicles the discovery and stabilization of Redox Signaling. This is one of the most important medical breakthroughs of our lifetime. Redox signaling molecules are the deepest cell-signaling molecules ever discovered.

They are naturally produced in mitochondria and the cell. They control all cellular health functions. They live and work at the interface of energy and matter, where cellular communication activates biological programming and animates all cell processes - even the energy of life itself.

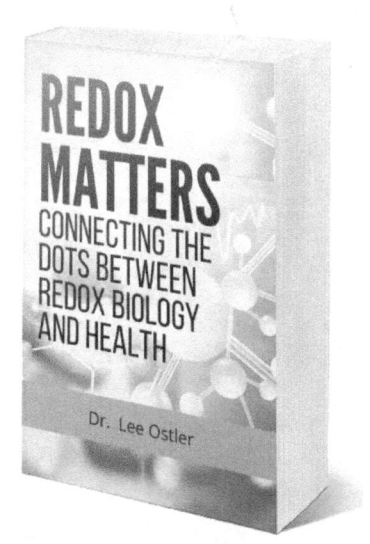

Redox "cell talk" is how cells know to respond to and prevent oxidation, inflammation, and disease. This is the innate *detect, repair, and replace* mechanism built into our cellular blueprints. And redox signaling activates it!

This is the "*Inner Doctor*." When it is awake and well, we are too! If not, we get more wrinkles, sagging skin, weight gain, gray air, lost memories, hurting joints, vascular problems, accelerated aging, immune disorders, hormone problems - and more medical intervention.

Visit www.RedoxMatters.com for more information about Redox Matters, and redox signaling.

End Notes

[1] https://www.who.int/news-room/fact-sheets/detail/noncommunicable-diseases.
[2] Centers for Disease Control; https://www.cdc.gov/chronicdisease/index.htm
[3] Raghupathi. An Empirical Study of Chronic Diseases in the United States: A Visual Analytics Approach to Public Health. Int J Environ Res Public Health. 2018 Mar; 15(3): 431.
[4] Martin. National Health Care Spending In 2019: Steady Growth For The Fourth Consecutive Year, Health Aff. 2020;40(1):1–11.
[5] Cumpstey. COVID-19: A Redox Disease—What a Stress Pandemic Can Teach Us About Resilience and What We May Learn from the Reactive Species Interactome About Its Treatment. Antioxidants & Redox Signaling. Nov 2021.1226-1268.
[6] Steele. Ultra-processed foods and added sugars in the US diet: evidence from a nationally representative cross-sectional study. BMJ Open 2016;6:e009892.
[7] Fast food consumption among adults in the United States, 2013-2016, CDC, National Center for Health Statistics.
[8] https://www.nytimes.com/2016/05/22/upshot/it-isnt-easy-to-figure-out-which-foods-contain-sugar.html#:~:text=A%20team%20of%20researchers%20at,some%20form%20of%20added%20sugar.
[9] https://sugarscience.ucsf.edu/hidden-in-plain-sight/#.YeM8ZP7MKUk
[10] Lichtman. Discrepancy between Self-Reported and Actual Caloric Intake and Exercise in Obese Subjects. N Engl J Med 1992; 327:1893-1898.
[11] Enstrom. "Health Practices and Cancer Mortality among Active California Mormons," in Latter-day Saint Social Life: Social Research on the LDS Church and its Members (Provo, UT: Religious Studies Center, Brigham Young University, 1998), 441–460.
[12] Orlich. Vegetarian Dietary Patterns and Mortality in Adventist Health Study 2. JAMA Intern Med. 2013 Jul 8; 173(13): 1230–1238.
[13] Mendeley. Proanthocyanidins in grape seeds: An updated review of their health benefits and potential uses in the food industry. Journal of Functional Foods, Volume 67, April 2020, 103861.
[14] Lieber. Relationships Between Nutrition, Alcohol Use, and Liver Disease. National Institute on Alcohol Abuse and Alcoholism. https://pubs.niaaa.nih.gov/publications/arh27-3/220-231.htm
[15] Cederbaum. Alcohol metabolism. Clin Liver Dis. 2012 Nov; 16(4): 667–685.
[16] Goldstein. Alcohol Consumption and Cancer of the Oral Cavity and Pharynx from 1988 to 2009: An Update. Eur J Cancer Prev. 2010 Nov; 19(6): 431–465.
[17] Alcohol use and burden for 195 countries and territories, 1990–2016: a systematic analysis for the Global Burden of Disease Study 2016. Aug 23, 2018. https://doi.org/10.1016/S0140-6736(18)31310-2

[18] Diaz-Vegas. Is Mitochondrial Dysfunction a Common Root of Noncommunicable Chronic Diseases? Endocr Rev. 2020 Jun 1;41(3):bnaa005.
[19] Fam. The liver, key in regulating appetite and body weight. Adipocyte, 2012, Oct 1; 1(4):259-264.
[20] Karastergiou. Sex differences in human adipose tissues – the biology of pear shape. Biol Sex Differ. 2012; 3: 13.
[21] Bellentani. Epidemiology of non-alcoholic fatty liver disease. Dig Dis. 2010;28(1):155-61.
[22] Maciejewska. Metabolites of arachidonic acid and linoleic acid in early stages of non-alcoholic fatty liver disease—A pilot study. Prostaglandins & Other Lipid Mediators, Volume 121, Part B, September 2015, Pages 184-189.
[23] Luukkonen. Effect of a ketogenic diet on hepatic steatosis and hepatic mitochondrial metabolism in nonalcoholic fatty liver disease. Proc Natl Acad Sci U S A. 2020 Mar 31; 117(13): 7347–7354.
[24] Johnson. Dietary sugars intake and cardiovascular health: a scientific statement from the American Heart Association. Circulation. 2009;120:1011-20.
[25] https://www.hsph.harvard.edu/nutritionsource/carbohydrates/added-sugar-in-the-diet/#ref27
[26] Sano. Sodium–glucose cotransporters: Functional properties and pharmaceutical potential. Journal of Diabetes Investigation, Vol 11, Issue 4, July 2020, P 770-782.
[27] Vos. Dietary Fructose Consumption Among US Children and Adults: The Third National Health and Nutrition Examination Survey. Medscape J Med. 2008; 10(7): 160.
[28] Douard. Regulation of the fructose transporter GLUT5 in health and disease. Am J Physiol Endocrinol Metab. 2008 Aug; 295(2): E227–E237.
[29] Gugliucci. Formation of Fructose-Mediated Advanced Glycation End Products and Their Roles in Metabolic and Inflammatory Diseases. Adv Nutr. 2017 Jan; 8(1): 54–62.
[30] Galvan. Real-time in vivo mitochondrial redox assessment confirms enhanced mitochondrial reactive oxygen species in diabetic nephropathy. Kidney Int. 92, 1282–1287 (2017).
[31] Fang. Fructose drives mitochondrial metabolic reprogramming in podocytes via Hmgcs2-stimulated fatty acid degradation. Signal Transduction and Targeted Therapy volume 6, Article number: 253 (2021).
[32] Williams. Fructose affects the growth of long bones in mice independent of ketohexokinase. https://doi.org/doi:10.7282/t3-gg6e-4682
[33] Campbell. Fructose-induced hypertriglyceridemia: A review, in Nutrition in the Prevention and Treatment of Abdominal Obesity, 2014
[34] https://www.ncbi.nlm.nih.gov/books/NBK22395/
[35] Jamnik J, et al. Fructose intake and risk of gout and hyperuricemia: a systematic review and meta-analysis of prospective cohort studies. BMJ Open. 2016;6(10)
[36] Added Sugars on the New Nutrition Facts Label | FDA

[37] https://thehealthsciencesacademy.org/wp-content/uploads/2014/08/The-Health-Sciences-Academy_65-Names-Of-Sugar.pdf

[38] Kawabata. A high-fructose diet induces epithelial barrier dysfunction and exacerbates the severity of dextran sulfate sodium-induced colitis. Int J Mol Med. 2019 Mar;43(3):1487-1496.

[39] Kim. Gut microbiota and metabolic health among overweight and obese individuals. Scientific Reports volume 10, Article number: 19417 (2020).

[40] Kovatcheva-Datchary. Nutrition, the gut microbiome and the metabolic syndrome. Best Pract. Res. Clin. Gastroenterol. 27, 59–72.

[41] Moreira. Gut microbiota and the development of obesity. Nutr. Hosp. 27, 1408–1414.

[42] Circu. Redox biology of the intestine. Free Radic Res. 2011.Nov:45(11-12): 1245-1266.

[43] Chen. TLR ligand decreases mesenteric ischemia and reperfusion injury0-induced gut damage through TNF-alpha signaling. Shock. 2008;30:563-570.

[44] Paray. Leaky Gut and Autoimmunity: An Intricate Balance in Individuals Health and the Diseased State. Int J Mol Sci. 2020 Dec; 21(24): 9770.

[45] Dumitrescu. Oxidative Stress and the Microbiota-Gut-Brain Axis. Oxidative Medicine and Cellular Longevity, 2018, article ID 2406594.

[46] Campbell. Control and dysregulation of redox signalling in the gastrointestinal tract. Nat Rev Gastroenterol Hepatol. 2019 Feb;16(2):106-120.

[47] Guzman. Microbiome, and the intestinal epithelium: An essential triumvirate? BioMed Research International, vol 2013, Article ID 425146.

[48] Jones. Redox signaling mediated by gut microbiota. Free Radical Res. 2013 Nov; 47(11): 950-957.

[49] Laura Dumitrescu. Oxidative Stress and the Microbiota-Gut-Brain Axis. Oxidative Medicine and Cellular Longevity, vol. 2018, Article ID 2406594, 2018.

[50] Neish. Redox signaling mediates symbiosis between the gut microbiota and the intestine. Gut Microbes. 2014 Mar 1; 5(2): 250-253.

[51] National Center for Health Statistics, 2013-2016, CDC

[52] Araujo. Prevalence of Optimal Metabolic Health in American Adults: National Health and Nutrition Examination Survey 2009–2016. Metabolic Syndrome and Related Disorders Vol. 17, No. 1.

[53] Srikanthan. Muscle mass index as a predictor of longevity in older adults. The American Journal of Medicine, February 20, 2014.

[54] Abdelaal. Morbidity and mortality associated with obesity. Ann Transl Med. 2017 Apr; 5(7): 161.

[55] Cnop. Mechanisms of pancreatic beta-cell death in type 1 and type 2 diabetes. Diabetes 2005 Dec; 54(suppl 2): S97-S107.

[56] Meier. The collateral circulation of the heart. BMC Med. 2013; 11: 143.

[57] https://www.nia.nih.gov/health/alzheimers-disease-fact-sheet

[58] https://www.heart.org/-/media/phd-files-2/science-news/2/2021-heart-and-stroke-stat-

update/2021_heart_disease_and_stroke_statistics_update_fact_sheet_at_a_glance.pdf

[59] Lustig. Metabolical. Metabolical: The Lure and the Lies of Processed Food, Nutrition, and Modern Medicine. 2021. Harper Collins.

[60] Perry. Leptin Mediates a Glucose-Fatty Acid Cycle to Maintain Glucose Homeostasis in Starvation. Cell. 2018 Jan 11;172(1-2):234-248.e17.

[61] Cnop. Mechanisms of pancreatic beta-cell death in type 1 and type 2 diabetes. Diabetes 2005 Dec;54 (suppl 2): S97-S107.

[62] Serrenho. The role of ghrelin in regulating synaptic function and plasticity of feeding-associated circuits. Front. Cell. Neurosci., 27 May 2019.

[63] Levonen. Redox regulation of antioxidants, autophagy, and the response to stress: implications for electrophile therapeutics. Free Radic Biol Med. 2014 Jun;71:196-207.

[64] Miller. Nutritional Ketosis and Mitohormesis: Potential Implications for Mitochondrial Function and Human Health. Journal of nutrition and Metabolism, vol 2018, Article ID 5157645.

[65] Goodpaster. Metabolic flexibility in health and disease. Cell Metab. 2017 May 2; 25(5): 1027–1036.

[66] Chen. A vicious circle between insulin resistance and inflammation in nonalcoholic fatty liver disease. Lipids in Health and Disease volume 16, Article number: 203 (2017).

[67] Cox. Nutritional ketosis alters fuel preference and thereby endurance performance in athletes. Cell Metabolism 24, 256-268, Aug 2016.

[68] https://www.webmd.com/diabetes/keto-diet-for-diabetes

[69] https://www.sciencedirect.com/topics/agricultural-and-biological-sciences/ketone-bodies.

[70] Jensen. Effects of ketone bodies on brain metabolism and function in neurodegenerative disease. International journal of molecular sciences, November 2020.

[71] Daines. The Therapeutic Potential and Limitations of Ketones in Traumatic Brain Injury. Front. Neurol., 22 October 2021.

[72] Takahashi. Roles and Regulation of Ketogenesis in Cultured Astroglia and Neurons Under Hypoxia and Hypoglycemia. ASN Neuro, September 2014.

[73] Guzman. Is there an astrocyte-neuron ketone body shuttle? Trends Endocrinol Metab. May-Jun 2001

[74] Achanta. β-Hydroxybutyrate in the Brain: One Molecule, Multiple Mechanisms. Neurochem Res. 2017 Jan;42(1):35-49.

[75] Takahashi. Metabolic compartmentalization between astroglia and neurons in physiological and pathophysiological conditions of the neurovascular unit. Neuropathology, Feb 2020.

[76] Newmanβ-Hydroxybutyrate: a signaling metabolite. Annu Rev Nutr 2017;37:51-76.

[77] Milder. Acute oxidative stress and systemic Nrf2 activation by the ketogenic diet. Neurobiol Dis. 2010 Oct;40(1):238-44.
[78] Miyauchi. Up-regulation of FOXO1 and reduced inflammation by β-hydroxybutyric acid are essential diet restriction benefits against liver injury. PNAS Vol 116, No 27. June 13, 2019.
[79] Puchowicz. Neuroprotection in diet-induced ketotic rat brain after focal ischemia. J Cereb Blood Flow Metab. 2008 Dec;28(12):1907-16.
[80] Liskiewicz. Upregulation of hepatic autophagy under nutritional ketosis. J Nutr Biochem. 2021 Jul;93:108620.
[81] Imai. It takes two to tango: NAD+ and sirtuins in aging/longevity control. NPJ Aging Mech Dis 2016;2:16017-16017.
[82] Mattson. Intermittent metabolic switching, neuroplasticity and brain health. Nat Rev Neurosci 2018;19:63-80.
[83] Paoli. Ketosis, ketogenic diet and food intake control: A complex relationship. February 2015 Frontiers in Psychology 6:27.
[84] Bornstein. Differential effects of mTOR inhibition and dietary ketosis in a mouse model of subacute necrotizing encephalomyelopathy. Neurobiology of Disease, Volume 163, February 2022, 105594.
[85] Rius-Perez. PGC-1α, Inflammation, and oxidative stress: An integrative view in metabolism. Oxidative Medicine and Cellular Longevity. Volume 2020, Article ID 1452696.
[86] Fisher. Understanding the physiology of FGF21. Annu Rev Physiol 2016;78:223-241.
[87] Lee. Physiological functions of cyclic ADP-ribose and NAADP as calcium messengers. Annu Rev Pharmacol Toxicol 2001;41:317-345.
[88] Elamin. Ketone-Based Metabolic Therapy: Is Increased NAD + a Primary Mechanism? Front Mol Neurosci. 2017 Nov 14;10:377.
[89] Elamin. Ketogenic Diet Modulates NAD+-Dependent Enzymes and Reduces DNA Damage in Hippocampus. Front. Cell. Neurosci., 30 August 2018.
[90] Kolb. Ketone bodies: from enemy to friend and guardian angel. BMC Medicine volume 19, Article number: 313 (2021).
[91] O'Hearn. The therapeutic properties of ketogenic diets, slow-wave sleep, and circadian synchrony. Current Opinion in Endocrinology & Diabetes and Obesity: October 2021 - Volume 28 - Issue 5 - p 503-508.
[92] Stubbs. A Ketone Ester Drink Lowers Human Ghrelin and Appetite. Obesity (Silver Spring). 2018 Feb;26(2):269-273.
[93] Albert-Garay. High glucose concentrations induce oxidative stress by inhibiting Nrf2 expression in rat Müller retinal cells in vitro. January 2022Scientific Reports 12(1).
[94] Buranasin. High glucose-induced oxidative stress impairs proliferation and migration of human gingival fibroblasts. PLoS ONE 13(8):e0201855; August 2018.
[95] Zhao. Neuroprotective effects of an Nrf2 agonist on high glucose-induced damage in HT22 cells. Biological Research volume 52, Article number: 53 (2019)

[96] De Toledo. Unravelling the health effects of fasting: a long road from obesity treatment to healthy life span increase and improved cognition. Annals of Medicine, Volume 52, 2020 - Issue 5.

[97] Takahashi. Roles and Regulation of Ketogenesis in Cultured Astroglia and Neurons Under Hypoxia and Hypoglycemia. ASN Neuro, Sept. 2014.

[98] Takahashi. Metabolic compartmentalization between astroglia and neurons in physiological and

[99] Calabrese. Hormesis: from mainstream to therapy. J Cell Commun Signal. 2014 Dec; 8(4): 289–291.

[100] Mattson. Hormesis defined. Ageing Res Rev. 2008 Jan; 7(1): 1–7.

[101] Barcena. Mitohormesis, an antiaging paradigm. International Review of Cell and Molecular Biology, Volume 340, 2018, Pages 35-77.

[102] Janssen. Mito-Nuclear Communication by Mitochondrial Metabolites and Its Regulation by B-Vitamins. Front. Physiol., 12 February 2019.

[103] Woo. Mitochondrial Stress Signals Revise an Old Aging Theory. Cell Volume 144, Issue 1, 7 January 2011, Pages 11-12

[104] Bell. Mild oxidative stress activates Nrf2 in astrocytes, which contributes to neuroprotective ischemic preconditioning. Proc Natl Acad Sci U S A. 2011 Jan 4;108(1):E1-2; author reply E3-4.

[105] Zimmerman. When less is more: hormesis against stress and disease. Microb Cell. 2014 May 5; 1(5): 150–153.

[106] Ristow. Mitohormesis: Promoting Health and Lifespan by Increased Levels of Reactive Oxygen Species (ROS). Dose Response. 2014 May; 12(2): 288–341.

[107] Naoi. Mitochondria in Neuroprotection by Phytochemicals: Bioactive Polyphenols Modulate Mitochondrial Apoptosis System, Function and Structure. Int J Mol Sci. 2019 May; 20(10): 2451.

[108] Mattson. Neurohormetic phytochemicals: Low-dose toxins that induce adaptive neuronal stress responses. Trends in Neurosciences 2006 Nov;29(11):632-9.

[109] Son. Hormetic dietary phytochemicals. Neuromolecular Med. 2008;10(4):236-46.

[110] https://openbiotechnologyjournal.com/VOLUME/13/PAGE/68/FULLTEXT/#r29

[111] Kao. Determination of flavonoids and saponins in Gynostemma pentaphyllum (Thunb.) Makino by liquid chromatography-mass spectrometry. Anal Chim Acta 2008; 626(2): 200-11.

[112] Wcislo. Colorectal cancer prevention by wheat consumption. Wheat and Rice in Disease Prevention and Health, 2014.

[113] Akiyama. Antibacterial action of several tannins against Staphylococcus aureus. J Antimicrob Chemother 2001; 48(4): 487-91.

[114] Chowanski. A review of bioinsecticidal activity of solanaceae alkaloids. Toxins (Basel). 2016 Mar; 8(3): 60.

[115] Eggler. Chemical and biological mechanisms of phytochemical activation of Nrf2 and importance in disease prevention. Recent Adv Phytochem. 2013; 43: 121–155.

[116] Mattson. Ibid. Neurohormetic phytochemicals.

[117] Mattson. Ibid. Dietary factors, hormesis and health.
[118] Martucci. Mediterranean diet and inflammaging within the hormesis paradigm. Nutrition Reviews, Volume 75, Issue 6, June 2017, Pages 442–455.
[119] Esposito. Prevention and control of type 2 diabetes by Mediterranean diet: a systematic review. Diabetes Res Clin Pract. 2010 Aug;89(2):97-102.
[120] Martucci. Mediterranean diet and inflammaging within the hormesis paradigm. Nutr Rev. 2017 Jun; 75(6): 442–455.
[121] Rahman. Potential therapeutic role of phytochemicals to mitigate mitochondrial dysfunction in Alzheimer's disease. Antioxidants, 2021, 10, 23.
[122] Nakamura. Electrophiles in Foods: The Current Status of Isothiocyanates and Their Chemical Biology. Biosci Biotechnol Biochem. 2010;74:242–255.
[123] Rahman. Ibid.
[124] Forman. Para-hormesis: An innovative mechanism for the health protection brought by antioxidants in wine. Nutrition and Aging, vol. 2, no. 2-3, pp. 117-124, 2014.
[125] Son. Ibid.
[126] Dinkova-Kostova. Direct and indirect antioxidant properties of inducers of cytoprotective proteins. Mol Nutr Food Res. 2008;52:S128–S138.
[127] Eggler. Chemical and biological mechanisms of phytochemical activation of Nrf2 and importance in disease prevention. Recent Adv Phytochem. 2013; 43: 121–155.
[128] Son. Hormetic Dietary Phytochemicals. Neuromolecular Med. 2008; 10(4): 236-246.
[129] https://www.sciencedirect.com/topics/medicine-and-dentistry/mitochondrial-respiration
[130] Sandoval-Acuna. Polyphenols and mitochondria: An update on their increasingly emerging ROS-scavenging independent actions. Archives of Biochemistry and Biophysics, Volume 559, 1 October 2014, Pages 75-90.
[131] Murakami. Hormesis-Mediated Mechanisms Underlying Bioactivities of Phytochemicals. Current Pharmacology Reports volume 6, pages325–334 (2020).
[132] Froman. How Do Nutritional Antioxidants Really Work: Nucleophilic Tone and Para-Hormesis Versus Free Radical Scavenging in vivo. Free Radic Biol Med. 2014 Jan 8.
[133] Ursini. Redox Homeostasis: The Golden Mean of Healthy Living. Redox Biology, January 2016.
[134] Juhasz. Hormetic response of resveratrol against cardioprotection. Exp Clin Cardiol. 2010 Winter; 15(4): e134–e138.
[135] Pal. Hormetic Potential of Sulforaphane (SFN) in Switching Cells' Fate Towards Survival or Death. Mini Rev Med Chem. 2016;16(12):980-95.
[136] Bao. Benefits and Risks of the Hormetic Effects of Dietary Isothiocyanates on Cancer Prevention. PLoS One. 2014; 9(12): e114764.
[137] Rattan. Curcumin's Biphasic Hormetic Response on Proteasome Activity and Heat-Shock Protein Synthesis in Human Keratinocytes. Annals of the NY Academy of Sciences. May 10, 2006. Published online.

[138] Fedullo. Hormetic Effects of Bioactive Compounds from Foods, Beverages, and Food Dressing: The Potential Role in Spinal Cord Injury. Oxidative Medicine and Cellular Longevity, Vol 2021, Article ID 6615752.

[139] Sanchez-Arreguin. Generation of BSA-capsaicin Nanoparticles and Their Hormesis Effect on the Rhodotorula mucilaginosa Yeast. Molecules. 2019 Aug 1;24(15):2800.

[140] Vargas. Hormesis and synergy: pathways and mechanisms of quercetin in cancer prevention and management. Nutrition Reviews, Volume 68, Issue 7, 1 July 2010, Pages 418–428.

[141] Calabrese. Does green tea induce hormesis? Dose Response. 2020 Jul-Sep; 18(3): 1559325820936170.

[142] Wang. Hormesis as a mechanistic approach to understanding herbal treatments in traditional Chinese medicine. Pharmacology & Therapeutics, Volume 184, April 2018, Pages 42-50.

[143] Dinkova-Kostova. Direct and indirect antioxidant properties of inducers of cytoprotective proteins, Mol. Nutr. Food Res., 52 (2008), pp. S128-S138.

[144] Calabrese. Cellular stress responses, hormetic phytochemicals and vitagenes in aging and longevity. Biochimicaet Biophysica Acta (BBA) - Molecular Basis of Disease, Volume 1822, Issue 5, May 2012, Pages 753-783.

[145] Son. Ibid. Hormetic dietary phytochemicals.

[146] Mattson. Dietary factors, hormesis and health. Ageing Res Rev. 2008 Jan; 7(1): 43–48.

[147] Radak. Exercise and hormesis: oxidative stress-related adaptation for successful aging. Biogerontology. 2005;6(1):71-5.

[148] Peake. Modulating exercise-induced hormesis: Does less equal more? Applied Physiology, Vol 119, Issue 3, Aug 2015, p 172-189.

[149] Gustavo. Translational Control: Implications for Skeletal Muscle Hypertrophy. Clinical Orthopaedics and Related Research: October 2002 - Volume 403 - Issue - p S178-S187.

[150] Peake. Ibid.

[151] Topf. Quantitative proteomics identifies redox switches for global translation modulation by mitochondrially produced reactive oxygen species. Nature Communications, Volume 9, Article number: 324 (2018).

[152] Dupuy. An Evidence-Based Approach for Choosing Post-exercise Recovery Techniques to Reduce Markers of Muscle Damage, Soreness, Fatigue, and Inflammation: A Systematic Review With Meta-Analysis. Front. Physiol., 26 April 2018.

[153] Nieman. Influence of a redox-signaling supplement on biomarkers of physiological stress in athletes: a metabolomics approach. FASEB Journal, Experimental Biology 2012 Meeting Abstracts, Vol 26, Issue S1, p lb713

[154] www.amazingmolecules.com

[155] Dodd. Ros-mediated activation of NF-κB and Foxo during muscle disuse. Muscle and Nerve. October 7, 2009, p 110-113.

[156] Chopard. Molecular events and signalling pathways involved in skeletal muscle disuse-induced atrophy and the impact of countermeasures. Journal of Cellular and Molecular Medicine. Vol 13, Issue 9b, Sept 2009, p 3032-3050.
[157] Cros. Upregulation of M-creatine kinase and glyceraldehyde3-phosphate dehydrogenase: two markers of muscle disuse. Am J Physiol. 1999; 276: R308–16.
[158] Buresh. A tutorial on oxidative stress and redox signaling with application to exercise and sedentariness. Sports Med Open. 2015 Dec; 1: 3.
[159] Parker. Exercise and Glycemic Control: Focus on Redox Homeostasis and Redox-Sensitive Protein Signaling. Frontiers in Endocrinology, 05 May 2017, 8:87.
[160] Williams. Walking Versus Running for Hypertension, Cholesterol, and Diabetes Mellitus Risk Reduction. Arteriosclerosis, Thrombosis, and Vascular Biology. 2013;33:1085–1091.
[161] Myers. Exercise and cardiovascular health. Circulation. 2003;107:e2–e5.
[162] Musci. Exercise-Induced Mitohormesis for the Maintenance of Skeletal Muscle and Healthspan Extension. Sports (Basel). 2019 Jul; 7(7): 170.
[163] Ristow. Antioxidants prevent health-promoting effects of physical exercise in humans. Proc. Natl. Acad. Sci. U. S. A., 106 (2009), pp. 8665-8670.
[164] Gomez-Cabrera. Decreasing xanthine oxidase-mediated oxidative stress prevents useful cellular adaptations to exercise in rats. J Physiol. 2005 Aug 15;567(Pt 1):113-20.
[165] Calabrese. Cellular stress responses, hormetic phytochemicals and vitagenes in aging and longevity. Biochimica et Biophysica Acta (BBA) - Molecular Basis of Disease, Volume 1822, Issue 5, May 2012, Pages 753-783.
[166] Ristow. How increased oxidative stress promotes longevity and metabolic health: the concept of mitochondrial hormesis (mitohormesis). Exp. Gerontol., 45 (2010), pp. 410-418.
[167] Hadacek. Hormesis and a Chemical Raison D'être for Secondary Plant Metabolites. Dose Response. 2011; 9(1): 79–116.
[168] Liu. Health-Promoting Components of Fruits and Vegetables in the Diet12. Adv. Nutr. 2013;4:384S–392S.
[169] Petroski. Is There Such a Thing as "Anti-Nutrients"? A Narrative Review of Perceived Problematic Plant Compounds. Nutrients. 2020 Oct; 12(10): 2929.
[170] Bora. Anti-nutritional factors in foods and their effects. Journal of Academia and Industrial Research (JAIR), Vol 3, Issue 6, Nov 2014.
[171] https://www.hsph.harvard.edu/nutritionsource/anti-nutrients/
[172] Shewry. Do we need to worry about eating wheat? Nutr Bull. 2016 Mar; 41(1): 6–13.
[173] Gasbarrini. Origin of celiac disease: How old are predisposing haplotypes? World J Gastroenterol. 2012 Oct 7; 18(37): 5300–5304.
[174] Samtiya. Plant food anti-nutritional factors and their reduction strategies: an overview. Food Production, Processing and Nutrition volume 2, Article number: 6 (2020).

[175] Preet. Antinutrients and digestibility (in vitro) of soaked, dehulled and germinated cowpeas. Nutr Health. 2000;14(2):109-17.
[176] Chen. Mitophagy: An emerging role in aging and age-associated diseases. Front. Cell Dev. Biol., 26 March 2020.
[177] Rabinowitz. Autophagy and metabolism. Science. 2010 Dec 3; 330(6009): 1344–1348.
[178] Gelino. Autophagy – an emerging anti-aging mechanism. J Clin Exp Pathol. 2012 Jul 12; Suppl 4: 006.
[179] Barbosa. Hallmarks of aging: An autophagic perspective. Front. Endocrinol., 09 January 2019.
[180] Cadwell. Crosstalk between autophagy and inflammatory signalling pathways: balancing defense and homeostasis. Nature Reviews Immunology volume 16, pages661–675 (2016).
[181] Lee. Autophagy, mitochondria and oxidative stress: cross-talk and redox signalling. Biochem J. 2012 Jan 15;441(2):523-40.
[182] Plaza-Zabala. Autophagy and Microglia: Novel Partners in Neurodegeneration and Aging. Int J Mol Sci. 2017 Mar; 18(3): 598.
[183] Glick. Autophagy: cellular and molecular mechanisms. J Pathol. 2010 May;221(1):3-12.
[184] Hamel. Insulin Inhibits Peroxisomal Fatty Acid Oxidation in Isolated Rat Hepatocytes. Endocrinology, Volume 142, Issue 6, 1 June 2001, Pages 2702–2706.
[185] ScienceDirect, High Carbohydrate Diet. https://tinyurl.com/4fxkvdyb
[186] Kanasaki. Relevance of Autophagy Induction by Gastrointestinal Hormones: Focus on the Incretin-Based Drug Target and Glucagon. Front. Pharmacol., 16 May 2019.
[187] Ding. The importance of autophagy regulation in obstructive sleep apnea. Sleep Breath. 2021 Sep;25(3):1211-1218.
[188] Cheng. Short-Term Sleep Fragmentation Dysregulates Autophagy in a Brain Region-Specific Manner. Life (Basel). 2021 Oct 16;11(10):1098.
[189] He. Circadian rhythm of autophagy proteins in hippocampus is blunted by sleep fragmentation. Chronobiology International 33(5):1-8. April 2016.
[190] Turcotte. Skeletal Muscle Insulin Resistance: Roles of Fatty Acid Metabolism and Exercise. Phys Ther. 2008 Nov; 88(11): 1279–1296.
[191] Thyfault. Metabolic inflexibility in skeletal muscle: a prelude to the cardiometabolic syndrome? J Cardiometab Syndr. Summer 2006;1(3):184-9.
[192] Sandri. Autophagy in skeletal muscle. FEBS Letters. Autophagy. Vol 584, Issue 7. April 2, 2010.
[193] Mizushima. In vivo analysis of autophagy in response to nutrient starvation using transgenic mice expressing a fluorescent autophagosome marker. Mol. Biol. Cell, 15, (2004), 1101– 1111.
[194] Kelley. Skeletal muscle fat oxidation: timing and flexibility are everything. J Clin Invest. 2005 Jul 1; 115(7): 1699–1702.

[195] Cox. Nutritional Ketosis Alters Fuel Preference and Thereby Endurance Performance in Athletes. Cell Metab. 2016 Aug 9;24(2):256-68.
[196] de Magalhaes. Meta-analysis of age-related gene expression profiles identifies common signatures of aging. Bioinformatics 2009: 25: 875–881.
[197] Aman. Autophagy in healthy aging and disease. Nature Aging volume 1, pages634–650 (2021)
[198] Ibid. Yan.
[199] Ibid. Plaza-Zabala.
[200] Sanada. Sources of Chronic Inflammation in Aging. Front Cardiovasc Med. 2018; 5: 12.
[201] https://www.sciencedirect.com/topics/nursing-and-health-professions/glycation
[202] Tessier. Health effects of dietary Maillard reaction products: the results of ICARE and other studies. Amino Acids. 2012 Apr;42(4):1119-31.
[203] Ansari. Amadori Glycated Proteins: Role in Production of Autoantibodies in Diabetes Mellitus and Effect of Inhibitors on Non-Enzymatic Glycation. Aging Dis. 2013 Feb; 4(1): 50–56.
[204] Yan. Autophagy as a regulator of cardiovascular redox homeostasis. Free Radic Biol Med. 2017 Aug; 109: 108–113.
[205] Ibid. Yan.
[206] Guo. Oxidative stress, mitochondrial damage and neurodegenerative diseases. Neural Regen Res. 2013 Jul 25; 8(21): 2003–2014.
[207] Gurusamy. Autophagy, redox signaling, and ventricular remodeling. Antioxid Redox Signal. 200 Aug; 11(8): 1975-1988.
[208] He. Regulation mechanisms and signaling pathways of autophagy. Annu Rev Genet. 2009; 43: 67–93.
[209] Navarro-Yepes. Oxidative Stress, Redox Signaling, and Autophagy: Cell Death Versus Survival. Antioxid Redox Signal. 2014 Jul 1; 21(1): 66–85.
[210] Liu. Hepatic Autophagy Is Suppressed in the Presence of Insulin Resistance and Hyperinsulinemia. J of Biological Chemistry. Vol 284, Issue 45, p 31484-31492, November 2009.
[211] Zhang. Redox signaling: Potential arbitrator of autophagy and apoptosis in therapeutic response. Free Radical Biology and Medicine, Volume 89, December 2015, Pages 452-465.
[212] Op Cit. Yan.
[213] Chen. Superoxide is the major reactive oxygen species regulating autophagy. Cell Death Differ. 2009 Jul; 16(7):1040-52.
[214] Wu. Physical Exercise and Selective Autophagy: Benefit and Risk on Cardiovascular Health. Cells. 2019 Nov; 8(11): 1436.
[215] Freese. The sedentary (r)evolution: Have we lost our metabolic flexibility? F1000Research vol. 6 1787. 2 Oct. 2017, doi:10.12688/f1000research.12724.2
[216] Lee. β-cell autophagy: Mechanism and role in β-cell dysfunction. Molecular Metabolism, Volume 27, Supplement, September 2019, Pages S92-S103.

[217] Bharath. Selective Autophagy in Hyperglycemia-Induced Microvascular and Macrovascular Diseases. Cells. 2021 Aug 17;10(8):2114.
[218] Wang. Resveratrol-enhanced autophagic flux ameliorates myocardial oxidative stress injury in diabetic mice. J Cell Mol Med. 2014 Aug; 18(8):1599-611.
[219] Bhattacharya. Is autophagy associated with diabetes mellitus and its complications? A review. EXCLI J. 2018; 17: 709–720.
[220] Kasacka. Autophagy in adipose tissue of patients with obesity and type 2 diabetes. Mol Cell Endocrinol. 2015 Jul 5; 409():21-32.
[221] Haung. KCa3.1 mediates dysfunction of tubular autophagy in diabetic kidneys via PI3k/Akt/mTOR signaling pathways. Sci Rep. 2016 Mar 31; 6():23884.
[222] Goncalves. Schwann cell interactions with axons and microvessels in diabetic neuropathy. Nat Rev Neurol. 2017 Mar; 13(3):135-147.
[223] Li. Autophagy impairment mediated by S-nitrosation of ATG4B leads to neurotoxicity in response to hyperglycemia. Autophagy. 2017 Jul 3; 13(7):1145-1160.
[224] Piano. Involvement of Autophagic Pathway in the Progression of Retinal Degeneration in a Mouse Model of Diabetes. Front Cell Neurosci. 2016; 10():42.
[225] Bhattacharya. Ibid.
[226] Liu. Targeting Autophagy for the Treatment of Alzheimer's Disease: Challenges and Opportunities. Front. Mol. Neurosci., 22 August 2019.
[227] Pomilio. Glial alterations from early to late stages in a model of Alzheimer's disease: evidence of autophagy involvement in Aβ internalization. Hippocampus 26, 194–210, 2016.
[228] She. Release the autophage brake on inflammation: the MAPK14/p38α-ULK1 pedal. Autophagy 14, 1097–1098, 2018.
[229] https://www.integrativenutrition.com/blog/what-is-functional-nutrition
[230] Valko. Free radicals and antioxidants in normal physiological functions and human disease. Int J Biochem Cell Biol. 2007; 39(1):44-84.
[231] Bouayed. Exogenous antioxidants—Double-edged swords in cellular redox state. Oxid Med Cell Longev. 2010 Jul-Aug; 3(4): 228–237.
[232] Bouayed. Ibid.
[233] Martin. Reactive oxygen species as double-edged swords in cellular processes: low-dose cell signaling versus high-dose toxicity. Hum Exp Toxicol. 2002 Feb; 21(2):71-5.
[234] Bouayed. Ibid.
[235] Pandey. Plant polyphenols as dietary antioxidants in human health and disease. Oxid Med Cell Longev. 2009 Nov-Dec; 2(5):270-8.
[236] Pettegrew. Acetyl-L-carnitine physical-chemical, metabolic, and therapeutic properties: relevance for its mode of action in Alzheimer's disease and geriatric depression. Mol Psychiatry 5, 616–632 (2000).
[237] Zanelli. Mechanisms of ischemic neuroprotection by acetyl-L-carnitine. Ann N Y Acad Sci. 2005 Aug;1053:153-61.

[238] Traina. The neurobiology of acetyl-L-carnitine. Frontiers in Bioscience-Landmark / Articles / Volume 21 / Issue 7 / 10.2741/4459.
[239] Choi. Carnitine induces autophagy and restores high-fat diet-induced mitochondrial dysfunction. Metabolism
Volume 78, January 2018, Pages 43-51.
[240] Piovesan. Acetyl-L-carnitine treatment increases choline acetyltransferase activity and NGF levels in the CNS of adult rats following total fimbria-fornix transection. Brain Res. 1994 Jan 7;633(1-2):77-82.
[241] Choline – Fact Sheet for Health Professionals. https://ods.od.nih.gov/factsheets/Choline-HealthProfessional/
[242] Nur. Revealing the Reversal Effect of Galangal (Alpinia galanga L.) Extract Against Oxidative Stress in Metastatic Breast Cancer Cells and Normal Fibroblast Cells Intended as a Co- Chemotherapeutic and Anti-Ageing Agent. Asian Pac J Cancer Prev. 2020; 21(1): 107–117.
[243] Kaushik. Protective effect of Alpinia galanga in STZ induced diabetic nephropathy. Pak J Biol Sci. 2013 Aug 15;16(16):804-11.
[244] Saha. Central nervous system stimulant actions of Alpinia galanga (L.) rhizome: a preliminary study. Indian J Exp Biol. 2013 Oct;51(10):828-32.
[245] Srivastava. Effect of Alpinia galanga on Mental Alertness and Sustained Attention With or Without Caffeine: A Randomized Placebo-Controlled Study. J Am Coll Nutr. Nov-Dec 2017;36(8):631-639.
[246] Singh. Neuroprotective effect of Alpinia galanga (L.) fractions on Aβ(25-35) induced amnesia in mice. J Ethnopharmacol, 2011 Oct 31;138(1):85-91.
[247] Singh. An Overview on Ashwagandha: A Rasayana (Rejuvenator) of Ayurveda. Afr J Tradit Complement Altern Med. 2011; 8(5 Suppl): 208–213.
[248] Singh. Ibid.
[249] Salve. Adaptogenic and Anxiolytic Effects of Ashwagandha Root Extract in Healthy Adults: A Double-blind, Randomized, Placebo-controlled Clinical Study. Cureus. 2019 Dec; 11(12): e6466.
[250] Tardy. Vitamins and Minerals for Energy, Fatigue and Cognition: A Narrative Review of the Biochemical and Clinical Evidence. Nutrients. 2020 Jan 16;12(1):228.
[251] Kennedy. B Vitamins and the Brain: Mechanisms, Dose and Efficacy—A Review. B Vitamins and the Brain: Mechanisms, Dose and Efficacy—A Review. 2016.
[252] Huskisson. The role of vitamins and minerals in energy metabolism and well-being. The Journal of International Medical Research. 2007; 35: 277-289.
[253] Laquale. B-complex vitamins' role in energy release. Bridgewater State University Virtual commons. https://vc.bridgew.edu/cgi/viewcontent.cgi?article=1029&context=mahpls_fac
[254] Mittleman. Branched-chain amino acids prolong exercise during heat stress in men and women. Med Sci Sports Exerc. 1998 Jan;30(1):83-91.
[255] Xiao. NAD(H) and NADP(H) Redox Couples and Cellular Energy Metabolism. Antioxid Redox Signal. 2018 Jan 20; 28(3): 251–272.

[256] Pirinen. Niacin Cures Systemic NAD + Deficiency and Improves Muscle Performance in Adult-Onset Mitochondrial Myopathy. Cell Metab. 2020 Jun 2;31(6):1078-1090.e5.

[257] Massudi. Age-associated changes in oxidative stress and NAD+ metabolism in human tissue. PLoS One. 2012;7(7):e42357.

[258] Ganji. Niacin inhibits vascular oxidative stress, redox-sensitive genes, and monocyte adhesion to human aortic endothelial cells. Atherosclerosis. 2009 Jan;202(1):68-75.

[259] Gong. Nicotinamide riboside restores cognition through an upregulation of proliferator-activated receptor-γ coactivator 1α regulated β-secretase 1 degradation and mitochondrial gene expression in Alzheimer's mouse models. Neurobiology of Aging, Volume 34, Issue 6, June 2013, Pages 1581-1588.

[260] Ilkhani. Niacin and Oxidative Stress: A Mini-Review. J Nutri Med Diet Care 2:014. 2016.

[261] Wu. Niacin Inhibits Vascular Inflammation via the Induction of Heme Oxygenase-1. Circulation, Vol. 125, No. 1, 2012;125:150-158.

[262] Ismail. Vitamin B5 (d-pantothenic acid) localizes in myelinated structures of the rat brain: Potential role for cerebral vitamin B5 stores in local myelin homeostasis. Biochemical and Biophysical Research Communications Volume 522, Issue 1, 29 January 2020, Pages 220-225.

[263] Selhub. Folate, vitamin B12 and vitamin B6 and one carbon metabolism. J Nutr Health Aging. 2002;6(1):39-42.

[264] Ettinger. Metals and metallothionein, in Nutritional Pathophysiology of Obesity and its Comorbidities. 2017.

[265] Baird. Metallothionein protects against oxidative stress-induced lysosomal destabilization. Biochem J. 2006 Feb 15;394(Pt 1):275-83.

[266] Dalto. Pyridoxine (Vitamin B6) and the Glutathione Peroxidase System; a Link between One-Carbon Metabolism and Antioxidation. Nutrients. 2017 Mar; 9(3): 189.

[267] Green. Vitamin B12 deficiency. Nat. Rev. Dis. Primers. 2017;3:17040.

[268] Camfield.

[269] Aytemir. Assessment of autonomic nervous system functions in patients with vitamin B12 deficiency by power spectral analysis of heart rate variability. Pacing Clin Electrophysiol. 2000 Jun;23(6):975-8.

[270] Beitzke. Autonomic dysfunction and hemodynamics in vitamin B12 deficiency. Auton Neurosci. 2002 Apr 18;97(1):45-54.

[271] Kennedy D.O. B Vitamins and the Brain: Mechanisms, Dose and Efficacy—A Review. Nutrients. 2016;8:68.

[272] Hooshmand. Homocysteine and holotranscobalamin and the risk of Alzheimer disease: a longitudinal study. Neurology. 2010 Oct 19;75(16):1408-14.

[273] Miller. Vitamin B12, demyelination, remyelination and repair in multiple sclerosis. J Neurol Sci. 2005 Jun 15;233(1-2):93-7.

[274] Tiemeier. Vitamin B12, folate, and homocysteine in depression: The Rotterdam Study. Am. J. Psychiatry. 2002;159:2099–2101.

[275] Doets. Vitamin B12 intake and status and cognitive function in elderly people. Epidemiol. Rev. 2013;35:2–21.

[276] Koury. New insights into erythropoiesis: the roles of folate, vitamin B12, and iron. Annu Rev Nutr. 2004;24:105-31.Camfield. The Effects of Multivitamin Supplementation on Diurnal Cortisol Secretion and Perceived Stress. Nutrients. 2013 Nov; 5(11): 4429–4450.

[277] Ankar. Vitamin B12 Deficiency. https://www.ncbi.nlm.nih.gov/books/NBK441923/

[278] Roberts. Biochemical-physiological correlations in studies of the γ-aminobutyric acid system. Brain Res. 8, 1–35.

[279] Zhu. In vivo NAD assay revels the intracellular NAD contents and redox state.

[280] Yamatsu. The Improvement of Sleep by Oral Intake of GABA and Apocynum venetum Leaf Extract. J Nutr Sci Vitaminol (Tokyo). 2015;61(2):182-7

[281] Ngo. An Updated Review on Pharmaceutical Properties of Gamma-Aminobutyric Acid. Molecules 2019, 24(15), 2678.

[282] Ngo. An Updated Review on Pharmaceutical Properties of Gamma-Aminobutyric Acid. Molecules 2019, 24(15), 2678. 93, 11–21.

[283] Calvo. Dynamic Regulation of the GABAA Receptor Function by Redox Mechanisms. Molecular Pharmacology September 2016, 90 (3) 326-333.

[284] Termsarasab. Medical treatment of dystonia. J Clin Mov Disord. 2016;3:19.

[285] Calvo, Ibid.

[286] Tildesley. Salvia lavandulaefolia (Spanish Sage) enhances memory in healthy young volunteers. Pharmacol Biochem Behav. 2003;75:669–74.

[287] Scholey. An extract of Salvia (sage) with anticholinesterase properties improves memory and attention in healthy older volunteers. Psychopharmacology (Berl). 2008;198:127–39.

[288] Lopresti. Salvia (Sage): A Review of its Potential Cognitive-Enhancing and Protective Effects. Drugs R D. 2017 Mar; 17(1): 53–64.

[289] Luchicchi. Illuminating the role of cholinergic signaling in circuits of attention and emotionally salient behaviors.
Front Synaptic Neurosci. 2014; 6():24.

[290] Savelev. Synergistic and antagonistic interactions of anticholinesterase terpenoids in Salvia lavandulaefolia essential oil. Pharmacol Biochem Behav. 2003;75:661–8.

[291] Huang. Neurotrophins: roles in neuronal development and function. Annu Rev Neurosci. 2001; 24():677-736

[292] Zacchigna. Neurovascular signaling defects in neurodegeneration. Nat Rev. 2008; 9: 169–181.

[293] Bowling. Deconstructing brain-derived neurotrophic factor actions in adult brain circuits to bridge an existing informational gap in neuro-cell biology. Neural Regen Res. 2016 Mar; 11(3):363-7.

[294] Bianca. EGR3 immediate early gene and the brain-derived neurotrophic factor in bipolar disorder. Frontiers in Behavioral Neuroscience, 12, Article 15.
[295] Siamilis. The effect of exercise and oxidant-antioxidant intervention on the levels of neurotrophins and free radicals in spinal cord of rats. Spinal Cord. 2009; 47: 453–457.
[296] Siamilis. Ibid.
[297] Lopresti. Ibid.
[298] Chang. Oxidative Stress and <i>Salvia miltiorrhiza</i> in Aging-Associated Cardiovascular Diseases. Oxid Med Cell Longev. 2016; 2016():4797102.
[299] Lopresti. Ibid.
[300] Seol. Antidepressant-like effect of Salvia sclarea is explained by modulation of dopamine activities in rats. J Ethnopharmacol. 2010 Jul 6; 130(1):187-90.
[301] Kavvadias. Constituents of sage (Salvia officinalis) with in vitro affinity to human brain benzodiazepine receptor. Planta Med. 2003 Feb; 69(2):113-7.
[302] Pereira. Neurobehavioral and genotoxic aspects of rosmarinic acid. Pharmacol Res. 2005 Sep; 52(3):199-203.
[303] Lopresti. Ibid.
[304] Iuvone. The spice sage and its active ingredient rosmarinic acid protect PC12 cells from amyloid-beta peptide-induced neurotoxicity. J Pharmacol Exp Ther. 2006 Jun;317(3):1143-9.
[305] Ververis. Greek Sage Exhibits Neuroprotective Activity against Amyloid Beta-Induced Toxicity. Evidence-Based Complementary and Alternative Medicine, Volume 2020, Article ID 2975284.
[306] Porres-Martinez. Major selected monoterpenes α-pinene and 1,8-cineole found in Salvia lavandulifolia (Spanish sage) essential oil as regulators of cellular redox balance. Pharm Biol. 2015 Jun;53(6):921-9.
[307] Smith. Guaraná's Journey from Regional Tonic to Aphrodisiac and Global Energy Drink. Evid Based Complement Alternat Med. 2010 Sep;7(3):279-82.
[308] Yonekura. Bioavailability of catechins from guaraná (Paullinia cupana) and its effect on antioxidant enzymes and other oxidative stress markers in healthy human subjects. Food Funct. 2016 Jul 13;7(7):2970-8.
[309] Bittencourt. The protective effects of guaraná extract (Paullinia cupana) on fibroblast NIH-3T3 cells exposed to sodium nitroprusside. Food and Chemical Toxicology, Volume 53, March 2013, Pages 119-125.
[310] Fukumasu. Paullinia cupana Mart var. sorbilis, guaraná, reduces cell proliferation and increases apoptosis of B16/F10 melanoma lung metastases in mice. Braz J Med Biol Res. 2008 Apr;41(4):305-10.
[311] Bittencourt. Ibid.
[312] Arantes. Mechanisms involved in anti-aging effects of guarana (Paullinia cupana) in Caenorhabditis elegans. Braz J Med Biol Res. 2018 Jul 2;51(9):e7552.
[313] Krewer. Habitual Intake of Guaraná and Metabolic Morbidities: An Epidemiological Study of an Elderly Amazonian Population, Phytotherapy Research (2011), 10.1002/ptr.3437.

[314] Babu. Green tea catechins and cardiovascular health: an update. Curr Med Chem. 2008;15:1840–1850.
[315] Bonadiman. Guarana (Paullinia cupana): Cytoprotective effects on age-related eye dysfunction. Journal of Functional Foods, Volume 36, September 2017, Pages 375-386.
[316] Haskell. A double-blind, placebo-controlled, multi-dose evaluation of the acute behavioral effects of guaraná in humans. J Psychopharmacol. 2007 Jan;21(1):65-70.
[317] Kennedy. Improved cognitive performance in human volunteers following administration of guarana (Paullinia cupana) extract: comparison and interaction with Panax ginseng. Pharmacol Biochem Behav. 2004 Nov;79(3):401-11.
[318] Basile. Antibacterial and antioxidant activities of ethanol extract from Paullinia cupana Mart. Journal of Ethnopharmacology, Volume 102, Issue 1, 31 October 2005, Pages 32-36.
[319] Portella. Guaraná (Paullinia cupana Kunth) effects on LDL oxidation in elderly people: an in vitro and in vivo study. Lipids Health Dis. 2013; 12: 12.
[320] Dias. L-Theanine promotes cultured human Sertoli cells proliferation and modulates glucose metabolism. Eur J Nutr. 2019 Oct;58(7):2961-2970.
[321] Zeng. L-Theanine Ameliorates D-Galactose-Induced Brain Damage in Rats via Inhibiting AGE Formation and Regulating Sirtuin1 and BDNF Signaling Pathways. Oxidative Medicine and Cellular Longevity, 2021, Article ID 8850112.
[322] Mi-Ran. Neuroprotective Effect of L-Theanine on Aβ-Induced Neurotoxicity through Anti-Oxidative Mechanisms in SK-N-SH and SK-N-MC Cells. Biomol Ther. 2011 May19(3):288-295.
[323] Kim. L-Theanine, an amino acid in green tea, attenuates beta-amyloid-induced cognitive dysfunction and neurotoxicity: Reduction in oxidative damage and inactivation of ERK/p38 kinase and NF-kappa B pathways. Free Radical Biology and Medicine 47(11):1601-10, 2009.
[324] Zeng. l-Theanine attenuates liver aging by inhibiting advanced glycation end products in d-galactose-induced rats and reversing an imbalance of oxidative stress and inflammation Experimental Gerontology, Volume 131, March 2020, 110823.
[325] Kim. l-Theanine, an amino acid in green tea, attenuates β-amyloid-induced cognitive dysfunction and neurotoxicity: Reduction in oxidative damage and inactivation of ERK/p38 kinase and NF-κB pathways.
Free Radical Biology and Medicine, Volume 47, Issue 11, 1 December 2009, Pages 1601-1610.
[326] Zeng. L-Theanine Ameliorates D-Galactose-Induced Brain Damage in Rats via Inhibiting AGE Formation and Regulating Sirtuin1 and BDNF Signaling Pathways. Oxidative Medicine and Cellular Longevity, 2021, Article ID 8850112.
[327] Tan. Evaluation on the alleviating physical fatigue function of theanine compound preparation, J Tea Sci, 32 (2012), pp. 530-534.
[328] Hidese. Effects of L-Theanine Administration on Stress-Related Symptoms and Cognitive Functions in Healthy Adults: A Randomized Controlled Trial. Nutrients. 2019 Oct; 11(10): 2362.

[329] Baba. Effects of l-Theanine on Cognitive Function in Middle-Aged and Older Subjects: A Randomized Placebo-Controlled Study. J Med Food. April 2021; 24(4): 333–341.

[330] Owen. The combined effects of L-theanine and caffeine on cognitive performance and mood. Nutr Neurosci. 2008 Aug;11(4):193-8.

[331] Raj. l-Theanine ameliorates motor deficit, mitochondrial dysfunction, and neurodegeneration against chronic tramadol induced rats model of Parkinson's disease. Drug Chem Toxicol. 2021 Jul 1;1-12.

[332] Kim. l-Theanine, an amino acid in green tea, attenuates β-amyloid-induced cognitive dysfunction and neurotoxicity: reduction in oxidative damage and inactivation of ERK/p38 kinase and NF-κB pathways. Free Radical Biology and Medicine. 2009;47(11):1601–1610.

[333] Takeshima. l-Theanine protects against excess dopamine-induced neurotoxicity in the presence of astrocytes. J Clin Biochem Nutr. 2016 Sep;59(2):93-99.

[334] Di. L-theanine protects the APP (Swedish mutation) transgenic SH-SY5Y cell against glutamate-induced excitotoxicity via inhibition of the NMDA receptor pathway. Neuroscience. 2010 Jul 14;168(3):778-86.

[335] Nobre. L-theanine, a natural constituent in tea, and its effect on mental state. Asia Pac J Clin Nutr. 2008;17 Suppl 1:167-8.

[336] Adhikary. l-theanine: A potential multifaceted natural bioactive amide as health supplement. Asian Pacific Journal of Tropical Biomedicine, Volume 7, Issue 9, September 2017, Pages 842-848.

[337] Dratman. The many faces of thyroxine. AIMS Neurosci. 2020; 7(1): 17–29.

[338] Wasinski. Tyrosine Hydroxylase Neurons Regulate Growth Hormone Secretion via Short-Loop Negative Feedback. Journal of Neuroscience 27 May 2020, 40 (22) 4309-4322.

[339] Young. L-tyrosine to alleviate the effects of stress? J Psychiatry Neurosci. 2007 May; 32(3): 224.

[340] Schultz. Why NAD+ Declines during Aging: It's Destroyed. Cell Metab. 2016. June 14; 23(6): 965–966.

[341] Kosciuk. Updates on the Epigenetic Roles of Sirtuins. Curr Opin Chem Biol. 2019 Aug; 51: 18–29.

[342] Zhu. In vivo NAD assay revels the intracellular NAD contents and redox state in healthy human brain and their age dependences. Proc. Natl. Acad. Sci. 2015; 112:2876–2881

[343] Sakellariou. Redox homeostasis and age-related deficits in neuromuscular integrity and function. J Cachexia Sarcopenia Muscle. 2017 Dec; 8(6): 881–906.

[344] Shade. The Science Behind NMN–A Stable, Reliable NAD+Activator and Anti-Aging Molecule. Integr Med (Encinitas). 2020 Feb; 19(1): 12–14.

[345] Xie. Nicotinamide mononucleotide ameliorates the depression-like behaviors and is associated with attenuating the disruption of mitochondrial bioenergetics in depressed mice. J Affect Disord. 2020 Feb 15;263:166-174.

[346] Allen. Mitochondria and Mood: Mitochondrial Dysfunction as a Key Player in the Manifestation of Depression. Front. Neurosci., 06 June 2018.
[347] Mahady. Ginsengs: a review of safety and efficacy. Nutr Clin Care. 2000;3:90–101.
[348] Kiefer. Panax ginseng. Am Fam Physician. 2003 Oct 15;68(8):1539-1542.
[349] Rattan, Hormesis-Based Anti-Aging Products: A Case Study of a Novel Cosmetic. Dose Response, Volume 11, Issue 1, January 12, 2012.
[350] Calabrese. Hormesis and Ginseng: Ginseng Mixtures and Individual Constituents Commonly Display Hormesis Dose Responses, Especially for Neuroprotective Effects. Molecules. 2020 Jun; 25(11): 2719.
[351] Podbielska. Myelin Recovery in Multiple Sclerosis: The Challenge of Remyelination. Brain Sci. 2013 Sep; 3(3): 1282–1324.
[352] Martinez. Phosphatidylserine and Signal Transduction: Who Needs Whom? Science Signaling. 17 Jan 2006, Vol 2006, Issue 318, p. pe3.
[353] Glade. Phosphatidylserine and the human brain. Nutrition. 2015 Jun;31(6):781-6.
[354] Glade. Ibid.
[355] Glade. Ibid.
[356] Neves. A new insight on elderberry anthocyanins bioactivity: Modulation of mitochondrial redox chain functionality and cell redox state. Journal of Functional Foods, Volume 56, May 2019, Pages 145-155.
[357] Alam. Hydroxycinnamic acid derivatives: a potential class of natural compounds for the management of lipid metabolism and obesity. Nutrition & Metabolism volume 13, Article number: 27 (2016).
[358] Szwajgier. The Neuroprotective Effects of Phenolic Acids: Molecular Mechanism of Action. Nutrients. 2017 May; 9(5): 477.
[359] Li. Health-promoting effects of the citrus flavanone hesperidin. Rev Food Sci Nutr. 2017 Feb 11;57(3):613-631.
[360] Rizza. Citrus Polyphenol Hesperidin Stimulates Production of Nitric Oxide in Endothelial Cells while Improving Endothelial Function and Reducing Inflammatory Markers in Patients with Metabolic Syndrome. The Journal of Clinical Endocrinology & Metabolism, Volume 96, Issue 5, 1 May 2011, Pages E782–E792,
[361] Matias. Flavonoid Hesperidin Induces Synapse Formation and Improves Memory Performance through the Astrocytic TGF-β1. Front. Aging Neurosci., 13 June 2017.
[362] https://www.sciencedirect.com/topics/pharmacology-toxicology-and-pharmaceutical-science/narirutin
[363] Chen. Protective effects of sweet orange (Citrus sinensis) peel and their bioactive compounds on oxidative stress. Food Chem. 2012;135:2119–2127.
[364] Pontifex. Citrus Polyphenols in Brain Health and Disease: Current Perspectives. Front. Neurosci., 19 February 2021.
[365] Zou. Antioxidant activity of citrus fruits. Food Chem. 2016 Apr 1;196:885-96.

[366] Oboh. Effect of citrus peels-supplemented diet on longevity, memory index, redox status, cholinergic and monoaminergic enzymes in Drosophila melanogaster model. J Food Biochem. 2021 Feb;45(2):e13616.

[367] Anjum. Memory boosting effect of citrus juices. World Journal of Pharmacy and Pharmaceutical Sciences, 7(9):211-219, Aug 2018.

[368] Panossian. The adaptogens rhodiola and schizandra modify the response to immobilization stress in rabbits by suppressing the increase of phosphorylated stress-activated protein kinase, nitric oxide and cortisol. Drug Target Insights. 2007; 2:39–54.

[369] Amsterdam. Rhodiola rosea L. as a putative botanical antidepressant. Phytomedicine. 2016 Jun 15;23(7):770-83.

[370] Anghelescu. Stress management and the role of Rhodiola rosea: a review. Int J Psychiatry Clin Pract. 2018 Nov;22(4):242-252.

[371] Tang. Salidroside protects against bleomycin-induced pulmonary fibrosis: activation of Nrf2-antioxidant signaling, and inhibition of NF-κB and TGF-β1/Smad-2/-3 pathways. Cell Stress Chaperones. 2016 Mar;21(2):239-49.

[372] Song. Inhibitory effects of salidroside on nitric oxide and prostaglandin E2 production in lipopolysaccharide-stimulated RAW 264.7 macrophages. J Med Food. 2013;16:997–1003. doi: 10.1089/jmf.2012.2473.

[373] Li. Rhodiola rosea L.: an herb with anti-stress, anti-aging, and immunostimulating properties for cancer chemoprevention. Curr Pharmacol Rep. 2017 Dec; 3(6): 384–395.

[374] Khazdair. The effects of Crocus sativus (saffron) and its constituents on nervous system: A review. Avicenna J Phytomed. Sep-Oct 2015;5(5):376-91.

[375] Hausenblas. Saffron (Crocus sativus L.) and major depressive disorder: a meta-analysis of randomized clinical trials. J Integr Med. 2013 Nov;11(6):377-83.

[376] Gout. Satiereal, a Crocus sativus L extract, reduces snacking and increases satiety in a randomized placebo-controlled study of mildly overweight, healthy women. Nutr Res. 2010 May;30(5):305-13.

[377] Abu-Izneid. Nutritional and health beneficial properties of saffron (Crocus sativus L): a comprehensive review. Crit Rev Food Sci Nutr. 2020 Dec 17;1-24.

[378] Mehdizadeh. Cardioprotective Effect of Saffron Extract and Safranal in Isoproterenol-Induced Myocardial Infarction in Wistar Rats. Iran J Basic Med Sci. 2013 Jan; 16(1): 56–63.

[379] Potnuri. Crocin attenuates cyclophosphamide induced testicular toxicity by preserving glutathione redox system. Biomedicine & Pharmacotherapy, Volume 101, May 2018, Pages 174-180

[380] Frederickson. Importance of Zinc in the Central Nervous System: The Zinc-Containing Neuron. The Journal of Nutrition, Volume 130, Issue 5, May 2000, Pages 1471S–1483S.

[381] Blakemore. Zinc as a Neuromodulator in the Central Nervous System with a Focus on the Olfactory Bulb. Front Cell Neurosci. 2017; 11: 297.

[382] Pfeiffer. Zinc, the brain and behavior. Biol Psychiatry. 1982 Apr;17(4):513-32.

[383] Mott. Unraveling the role of zinc in memory. PNAS February 22, 2011 108 (8) 3103-3104.
[384] Dabbagh-Bazarbachi. Zinc Ionophore Activity of Quercetin and Epigallocatechin-gallate: From Hepa 1-6 Cells to a Liposome Model. J. Agric. Food Chem. 2014, 62, 32, 8085–8093.
[385] Adlard. Cognitive loss in zinc transporter-3 knock-out mice: a phenocopy for the synaptic and memory deficits of Alzheimer's disease? J Neurosci. 2010 Feb 3; 30(5):1631-6.
[386] Adlard. Ibid.
[387] Grabrucker. Brain-Delivery of Zinc-Ions as Potential Treatment for Neurological Diseases: Mini Review. Drug Deliv Lett. 2011 Sep; 1(1): 13–23.
[388] Szewczyk. Zinc homeostasis and neurodegenerative disorders. Front Aging Neurosci. 2013 Jul 19;5:33.
[389] Read. The role of zinc in antiviral immunity. Adv Nutr. 2019 Jul; 10(4): 696–710.
[390] Urbano. The role of phytic acid in legumes: antinutrient or beneficial function? J Physiol Biochem. 2000 Sep;56(3):283-94.
[391] Petroski. Ibid.
[392] https://www.hsph.harvard.edu/nutritionsource/anti-nutrients/lectins/
[393] Petroski. Is There Such a Thing as "Anti-Nutrients"? A Narrative Review of Perceived Problematic Plant Compounds. Nutrients. 2020 Oct; 12(10): 2929.
[394] Yau. Lectins with Potential for Anti-Cancer Therapy. Molecules. 2015 Mar; 20(3): 3791–3810.
[395] Son. Hormetic dietary phytochemicals. Neuromolecular Med. 2008; 10(4): 236–246.
[396] Zhang. Hormetic effect of panaxatriol saponins confers neuroprotection in PC12 cells and zebrafish through PI3K/AKT/mTOR and AMPK/SIRT1/FOXO3 pathways. Scientific Reports 7(1):41082, January 2017.
[397] Martinez-Villaluenga. Alpha-galactosides: antinutritional factors or functional ingredients? Crit Rev Food Sci Nutr. 2008 Apr;48(4):301-16.
[398] Pusztai. Antinutritive effects of wheat-germ agglutinin and other N-acetylglucosamine-specific lectins. Br J Nutr. 1993 Jul;70(1):313-21.
[399] Kottgen. The lectin properties of gluten as the basis of the pathomechanism of gluten-sensitive enteropathy. Klin Wochenschr. 1983 Jan 17;61(2):111-2.
[400] Filer. Aspartame Metabolism in Normal Adults, Phenylketonuric Heterozygotes, and Diabetic Subjects. Diabetes Care 1989 Jan; 12(1): 67.
[401] Rycerz. Effects of aspartame metabolites on astrocytes and neurons. Folia Neuropathol. 2013;51(1):10-7.
[402] Aspartame: Decades of Science Point to Serious Health Risks. https://usrtk.org/sweeteners/aspartame_health_risks/
[403] Malik. Long-Term Consumption of Sugar-Sweetened and Artificially Sweetened Beverages and Risk of Mortality in US Adults. Circulation. 2019;139:2113–2125.
[404] Humphries. Direct and indirect cellular effects of aspartame on the brain. European Journal of Clinical Nutrition volume 62, pages451–462 (2008).

[405] Choudhary. Revisiting the safety of aspartame. Nutr Rev. 2017 Sep 1;75(9):718-730.
[406] Palumaa. Biological redox switches. Antioxid Redox Signal. 2009 May;11(5):981-3.
[407] Belanger. Brain energy metabolism: focus on astrocyte-neuron metabolic cooperation. Cell Metabolism, vol. 14. No 6, p 724-738, 2011.
[408] Coyle. Oxidative stress, glutamate, and neurodegenerative disorders. Science. Vol 262. No. 5134, pp 689-695, 1993.
[409] Wojsiat. Oxidant / antioxidant imbalance in Alzheimer's disease: Therapeutic and diagnostic prospects. Oxidative Medicine and Cellular Longevity. Vol 2018, Article ID 6435861.
[410] La Berge. How the Ideology of Low Fat Conquered America. Journal of the History of Medicine and Allied Sciences, Volume 63, Issue 2, April 2008, Pages 139–177. https://doi.org/10.1093/jhmas/jrn001.
[411] Harvard Health Publishing. New Thinking on Saturated Fat. Sept 1, 2010, Harvard Medical School.
[412] Harvard T.H. Chan School of Public Health. Fats and Cholesterol. https://www.hsph.harvard.edu/nutritionsource/what-should-you-eat/fats-and-cholesterol/
https://www.hsph.harvard.edu/news/hsph-in-the-news/low-fat-diets-failed-experiment/
[413] Hatanaka. Oleic, Linoleic and Linolenic Acids Increase ROS Production by Fibroblasts via NADPH Oxidase Activation. PLoS One. 2013; 8(4): e58626.
[414] Ramsden. Lowering dietary linoleic acid reduces bioactive oxidized linoleic acid metabolites in humans. Prostaglandins Leukot Essent Fatty Acids. 2012 Oct; 87(4-5): 135–141.
[415] Fuhrman. The hidden dangers of fast and processed food. Am J Lifestyle Med. 2018 Sep-Oct; 12(5): 375–381.
[416] Zhang. The changes in the volatile aldehydes formed during the deep-fat frying process. J Food Sci Technol. 2015 Dec; 52(12):7683-96.
[417] Lee. Cooking oil fumes and lung cancer: a review of the literature in the context of the U.S. population. J Immigr Minor Health. 2013 Jun; 15(3):646-52.
[418] Knobbe. The 'Displacing Foods of Modern Commerce' Are the Primary and Proximate Cause of Age-Related Macular Degeneration: A Unifying Singular Hypothesis. Medical Hypotheses Volume 109, November 2017, Pages 184-198.
[419] Nakar. AMPK and PPARdelta agonists are exercise mimetics. Cell. 2008 Aug 8; 134(3):405-15.
[420] Goodpaster. Metabolic flexibility in health and disease. Cell Metab. 2017 May 2; 25(5): 1027–1036.
[421] Luigi. Effects of Ketone Bodies on Endurance Exercise. Curr Sports Med Rep. 2018 Dec;17(12):444-453.
[422] Roessner. What is metabolomics all about? BioTechniques, Vol 46, No. 5, April 25, 2018.

[423] Gieger. Genetics meets metabolomics: A genome-wide association study of metabolite profiles in human serum. PLoS Genet. 4:e1000282.

[424] Thamsen. The Redoxome, Proteomic Analysis of Cellular Redox Networks. Curr Opin Chem Biol. 2011 Feb; 15(1): 113–119.

[425] Nieman. Metabolomics Results. Human Performance Laboratory, North Carolina Research Campus and Appalachian State University.

[426] Duke, DHMRI, UNC, NC State, UNC Charlotte, NC Central, NC A&T State, UNC Greensboro, and Appalachian State. www.ncresearchcampus.net

[427] https://ncrc.appstate.edu/people

[428] Martinez-Reyes. Mitochondrial TCA cycle metabolites control physiology and disease. Nat Commun 11, 102 (2020).

[429] Zechner. Fat signals – lipases and lipolysis in lipid metabolism and signaling. Cell Metab, 2012 Mar 7;15(3):279-91.

[430] Liu. Peroxisomal regulation of redox homeostasis and adipocyte metabolism. Redox Biol. 2019 Jun; 24: 101167.

[431] Lopaschuk. Myocardial fatty acid metabolism in health and disease. Physiological Reviews, Vol 90, Issue 1, January 2010, pgs 207-258.

[432] Tumova. Excess of free fatty acids as a cause of metabolic dysfunction in skeletal muscle. Physiol. Res. 65:193-207, 2016.

[433] Maccarrone. Redox regulation and metabolic syndrome. Cell Death and Differentiation, 13 May 2011, 18(7):1234-1236.

[434] Horton. The metabolic responses to stress and physical activity, Institute of Medicine (US) Committee on Military Nutrition Research; Marriott BM, editor, National Academies Press, 1994.

[435] Wolfe. Fat metabolism in exercise. Adv Exp Med Biol. . 1998;441:147-56.

[436] www. med.libretexts.org/Courses/Dominican_University/DU_Bio_1550%3A_ Nutrition_(LoPresto)/1%3A_Basic_ Concepts_in_Nutrition

[437] https://www.stonebridge.uk.com/blog/food-and-drink/5-principles-of-nutrition/

[438] https://www.freshcityfarms.com/blogs/three-principles-for-good-health

[439] http://www.crossfitdafonz.com/da-blog/2019/11/1/the-10-principles-of-nutrtion

[440] https://www.dietaryguidelines.gov/sites/default/files/2020-12/DGA_2020-2025_StartSimple_ withMyPlate_English_color.pdf

[441] https://www.nutrition.gov/expert-q-a

[442] https://www.fao.org/nutrition/education/food-dietary-guidelines/regions/countries/united-states-of-america/en/

[443] https://www.pcrm.org/good-nutrition/nutrition-programs-policies/2020-2025-dietary-guidelines

[444] Koning. Low-carbohydrate diet scores and risk of type 2 diabetes in men. American Journal of Clinical Nutrition. Feb 2011, 93(4):844-50.

[445] Banach. Low carbohydrate diets are unsafe and should be avoided. ESC Press Release: https://www.escardio.org/The-ESC/Press-Office/Press-releases/Low-carbohydrate-diets-are-unsafe-and-should-be-avoided

[446] Ibid. https://www.pcrm.org/good-nutrition/nutrition-programs-policies/2020-2025-dietary-guidelines

[447] https://tinyurl.com/etrj3z3n

[448] Ibid. European Society of Cardiology – Low carbohydrate diets are unsafe and should be avoided, August 28, 2018.

[449] Ibid, Koning, Low-carbohydrate diet scores and risk of type 2 diabetes in men.

[450] Niaz. Extensive use of monosodium glutamate: A threat to public health? EXCLI J. 2018; 17: 273–278.
Published online 2018 Mar 19.

[451] USA Today, Miriam Fauzia, June 25, 2021; Fact check: MSG doesn't cause neurological disorders, is safe overall for human consumption.

[452] Saxena. Food Color Induced Hepatotoxicity in Swiss Albino Rats, Rattus norvegicus. Toxicol Int. 2015 Jan-Apr; 22(1): 152–157. 10.4103/0971-6580.172286

[453] https://www.nhlbi.nih.gov/health-topics/education-and-awareness/heart-truth/about

[454] https://www.cbsnews.com/news/coke-fit-to-be-the-face-of-heart-health/

[455] https://www.health.harvard.edu/blog/is-there-a-link-between-diet-soda-and-heart-disease-201202214296

[456] Pastore. Analysis of glutathione: implication in redox and detoxification. Clinica Chimica Acta, Volume 333, Issue 1, 1 July 2003, Pages 19-39.

Made in United States
Cleveland, OH
09 September 2025